Healing Through the Arts for Non-Clinical Practitioners

Jenny Bopp
Westtown School, USA

Amy M. Grebe
Zinnia Consulting and Design, USA

Joanna Hope Denny
Pellisippi State Community College, USA

A volume in the Advances in Medical Technologies and Clinical Practice (AMTCP) Book Series

IGI Global
DISSEMINATOR OF KNOWLEDGE

Published in the United States of America by
IGI Global
Medical Information Science Reference (an imprint of IGI Global)
701 E. Chocolate Avenue
Hershey PA, USA 17033
Tel: 717-533-8845
Fax: 717-533-8661
E-mail: cust@igi-global.com
Web site: http://www.igi-global.com

Library of Congress Cataloging-in-Publication Data

Names: Bopp, Jenny, 1986- editor.
Title: Healing through the arts for non-clinical practitioners / Jenny Bopp, Amy M. Grebe, and Joanna Hope Denny, editors.
Description: Hershey, PA : Medical Information Science Reference, [2019]
Identifiers: LCCN 2018010749| ISBN 9781522559818 (hardcover) | ISBN 9781522559825 (ebook)
Subjects: LCSH: Arts--Therapeutic use. | Art therapy for youth. | Mind and body therapies. | Families. | Music therapy.
Classification: LCC RC489.A72 H43 2019 | DDC 616.89/1656--dc23 LC record available at https://lccn.loc.gov/2018010749

This book is published in the IGI Global book series Advances in Medical Technologies and Clinical Practice (AM
(ISSN: 2327-9354; eISSN: 2327-9370)

British Cataloguing in Publication Data
A Cataloguing in Publication record for this book is available from the British Library.

Advances in Medical Technologies and Clinical Practice (AMTCP) Book Series

Srikanta Patnaik
SOA University, India
Priti Das
S.C.B. Medical College, India

ISSN:2327-9354
EISSN:2327-9370

Mission

Medical technological innovation continues to provide avenues of research for faster and safer diagnosis and treatments for patients. Practitioners must stay up to date with these latest advancements to provide the best care for nursing and clinical practices.

The **Advances in Medical Technologies and Clinical Practice (AMTCP) Book Series** brings together the most recent research on the latest technology used in areas of nursing informatics, clinical technology, biomedicine, diagnostic technologies, and more. Researchers, students, and practitioners in this field will benefit from this fundamental coverage on the use of technology in clinical practices.

Coverage

- Clinical High-Performance Computing
- Biomechanics
- Medical Imaging
- Medical informatics
- Nutrition
- Telemedicine
- Clinical Nutrition
- Patient-Centered Care
- Diagnostic Technologies
- Nursing Informatics

IGI Global is currently accepting manuscripts for publication within this series. To submit a proposal for a volume in this series, please contact our Acquisition Editors at Acquisitions@igi-global.com or visit: http://www.igi-global.com/publish/.

The Advances in Medical Technologies and Clinical Practice (AMTCP) Book Series (ISSN 2327-9354) is published by IGI Global, 701 E. Chocolate Avenue, Hershey, PA 17033-1240, USA, www.igi-global.com. This series is composed of titles available for purchase individually; each title is edited to be contextually exclusive from any other title within the series. For pricing and ordering information please visit http://www.igi-global.com/book-series/advances-medical-technologies-clinical-practice/73682. Postmaster: Send all address changes to above address.

Titles in this Series

For a list of additional titles in this series, please visit: www.igi-global.com/book-series

Electrocardiogram Signal Classification and Machine Learning Emerging Research and Opportunities
Sara Moein (Mount Sinai School of Medicine, USA)
Medical Information Science Reference • copyright 2018 • 196pp • H/C (ISBN: 9781522555803) • US $160.00 (our price)

Research Advancements in Pharmaceutical, Nutritional, and Industrial Enzymology
Shashi Lata Bharati (North Eastern Regional Institute of Science and Technology, India) and Pankaj Kumar Chaurasia (Babasaheb Bhimrao Ambedkar Bihar University, India)
Medical Information Science Reference • copyright 2018 • 549pp • H/C (ISBN: 9781522552376) • US $255.00 (our price)

Microbial Cultures and Enzymes in Dairy Technology
Şebnem Öztürkoğlu Budak (Ankara University, Turkey) and H. Ceren Akal (Ankara University, Turkey)
Medical Information Science Reference • copyright 2018 • 413pp • H/C (ISBN: 9781522553632) • US $265.00 (our price)

Multifunctional Nanocarriers for Contemporary Healthcare Applications
Md. Abul Barkat (K.R. Mangalam University, India) Harshita A.B. (K.R. Mangalam University, India) Sarwar Beg (Jubilant Generics, India) and Farhan J. Ahmad (Jamia Hamdard, India)
Medical Information Science Reference • copyright 2018 • 602pp • H/C (ISBN: 9781522547815) • US $265.00 (our price)

Biomedical Signal and Image Processing in Patient Care
Maheshkumar H. Kolekar (Indian Institute of Technology Patna, India) and Vinod Kumar (Indian Institute of Technology Roorkee, India)
Medical Information Science Reference • copyright 2018 • 312pp • H/C (ISBN: 9781522528296) • US $265.00 (our price)

Next-Generation Mobile and Pervasive Healthcare Solutions
Jose Machado (University of Minho, Portugal) António Abelha (University of Minho, Portugal) Manuel Filipe Santos (University of Minho, Portugal) and Filipe Portela (University of Minho, Portugal)
Medical Information Science Reference • copyright 2018 • 286pp • H/C (ISBN: 9781522528517) • US $245.00 (our price)

IGI Global
DISSEMINATOR OF KNOWLEDGE

701 East Chocolate Avenue, Hershey, PA 17033, USA
Tel: 717-533-8845 x100 • Fax: 717-533-8661
E-Mail: cust@igi-global.com • www.igi-global.com

List of Reviewers

Sarah Joy Baker, *Eastern University, USA*
Sheetal B. Barde, *Symbiosis International University, India*
Jennifer Lynne Bird, *Oxbridge Academy, USA*
Peter Bowersox, *Coalition for Christian Outreach, USA*
Rebecca Bowersox, *Mosaic Norristown, USA*
Callie B. Dean, *Eastern University, USA*
Linda Ellington, *Southern New Hampshire University, USA*
Kara Fontes, *Tempo! Music Therapy Services, USA*
Danica Frazier, *Independent Researcher, USA*
Robert Frazier, *Immaculata University, USA*
Tessa L. Hitz, *Eastern University, USA*
Stephanie Land, *Thomas Jefferson University, USA*
Fran Lieberman, *Westtown School, USA*
Melissa Lucchesi, *Voices, Inc., USA*
Brianne Murphy, *Transformation Yoga Project, USA*
Suet Ferng Tan, *Eastern University, Singapore*
Leah Throckmorton, *Achievement House Cyber Charter School, USA*
Karin Tollefson-Hall, *James Madison University, USA*
Carlee Zajatz, *Zajatz Creative Arts Therapy, USA*

Table of Contents

Section 3
Learning Adaptive Responses

Section 4
Mastery and Self-Regulation

Section 5
Arts-Based Post-Traumatic Growth Assessments

Detailed Table of Contents

be simplistic yet are purposeful. However, developmental psychologists point out that stories are not innocent as they always have a message. These emotionalized messages have been told over centuries and yet the messages are often lost, unappreciated, and unheard in the clutter of assumptions, caveats, data, and the fear that the storyteller will not be taken seriously.

Societies rely on first responders to save lives. What happens when the wellbeing of these crisis workers is compromised by daily exposure to crisis and trauma? This chapter describes a developed and tested arts-based intervention aimed at mitigating the trauma response through positive resource reinforcement. Specifically designed to be used in a non-clinical setting, the intervention features the drawing of a mandala capturing images and symbols of safety and was tested to ascertain the efficacy of its ability to increase positive affect, decrease negative affect, and reinforce connections to positive resources in participants.

The prevalence of traumas such as sexual violence is difficult to measure. However, it is fairly widely accepted that 1 in 5 women and 1 in 33 men will be a victim of sexual violence in her or his lifetime. Because of complicating factors to this type of trauma, survivors may not readily identify themselves as that. Healing arts and yoga help survivors to process traumatic energy and thoughts without having to delve into those dark and painful caverns. This chapter shares first person experience of sexual violence and navigating healing, as well as professional experience with other survivors, to illustrate the importance of trauma-informed healing and expressive arts when healing from trauma.

This chapter describes a 17-year partnership between the James Madison University Art Education Center and the Virginia Mennonite Retirement Community. The collaboration centers on a service-learning experience for pre-service art educators to provide art instruction to the residents of the retirement community. In 2009, the author became the coordinator of this service-learning experience and instructor for its corresponding art education course. The art education students work with independent living and memory care residents of the retirement community. Being a part of a collaborative, long-term program with the retirement community has provided tremendous learning experiences for the author, her students, the residents, and the retirement community staff regarding the power of art making in an intergenerational setting. This chapter includes a literature review, examples of artwork made in the program, descriptive observations, and reflections on the author's experience working with students and residents in the retirement community.

Section 3
Learning Adaptive Responses

Our responses to the world around us are often informed by our past experiences. Past experiences, whether positive or negative, often hold great power in our present state of being. If left unresolved, past traumatic experiences can hinder present growth of body, mind and spirit, due to an inhibited ability to cope with the past. The following chapters provide tools for non-clinicians to utilize and teach to those they serve in order to help move away from maladaptive responses and adopt more positive, adaptive responses.

In this chapter, the author explores her personal experience with depression and the healing through applied community theater. The author discusses how her autobiographical performance is similar to aspects of drama therapy, mindfulness, and cognitive behavioral therapy. The author explores how four common treatment goals for depression can be addressed through the process of writing, rehearsing, and performing an autobiographical performance. Advice is given to non-clinical practitioners on how to address depression among their clients. Findings from this case study promote that applied community theater, in addition to traditional treatments, can serve as catalyst for furthering the healing of depression.

This chapter explores how embroidery as a visual mapping tool can address situations of historical trauma and increase community resilience through a process of conscientisation and grassroots organizing. The author will draw from her fieldwork with a group of indigenous Wayuu women in the Guajira Peninsula in northern Colombia, a region that has been significantly affected by climate change and decades of armed conflict. The women created embroidered maps of their daily lives, analyzed these maps for common themes and challenges, identified the root causes of the oppression they experience daily, and discussed action steps to address these power disparities. The author suggests that embroidery is a powerful healing tool for engaging indigenous women in a dignified manner by illuminating their narratives of resilience in order to address historical trauma.

Writing as an art form helps people heal physically, emotionally, and spiritually. This chapter uses the theory of narrative inquiry to present a first-person case study of the author's writing life dovetailed with research illustrating how writing helps people heal. Writing methods will help educators, patients, people experiencing struggles, and anyone who wants to transfer thoughts to the page. Writing helps people cope with adversity, reframe situations to show a more optimistic attitude, and feel safe because the written page will not judge its author. Journal prompts serve as resources for the reader to begin or continue a writing practice.

Everyone has a story to tell, but because of trauma, not everyone can use words to tell it. The purpose of this chapter is to demonstrate an arts-based, trauma-informed, hope-infused movement and storytelling curriculum for adults (ages 19+) who are in recovery from various addictions or traumatic experiences. The curriculum was implemented with a group of five people selected by the supervising agency (Kingdom Recovery) to assess whether or not it proved beneficial to the participants. Assessment methods included before/after class experiences, a movement assessment checklist, and an evaluation survey. The curriculum consisted of seven lessons lasting 90 minutes each, and the goal of the curriculum was to promote life-skill building, healing, and hope. At the end of the seven-week time period, subjects performed pieces they choreographed throughout the sessions as a celebration of their accomplishments and hard work. The goals of the curriculum were accomplished successfully and 100% of the participants noticed an increase in their confidence, empathy, and creativity.

Too often a traumatic experience can hinder a person's ability to self-regulate and gain mastery over their emotional responses. Unfortunately, the absence of mastery and self-regulation can result in the development of mental illness, feelings of hopelessness, depression, etc. These can be crippling and prevent people from leading full and healthy lives. The following chapters offer strategies for non-clinicians to help their constituents develop mastery of life skills and self-regulation in their everyday lives.

This chapter emphasizes several key concepts concerning mental illness in today's society. The author strongly believes that mental health recovery is possible and that it is an individualized journey. People struggling with mental health issues can find hope and healing through the use of artistic expression. This chapter is designed to encourage and inspire others to use everyday items and turn them into art. The author describes how collaboration can be a key ingredient to the success of the healing that takes place while doing art together.

The motivation of this chapter is to add to the literature about the practice of teaching dance with a critical and somatic approach and to contribute to illuminating the reality of negotiating power in the dance classroom and the complexity of the influence of cultural values on this dynamic. This chapter reflects on the process of teaching a dance curriculum that explores identity to three different cultural groups in order to gain knowledge of best practices for nurturing somatic authority and providing meaningful choice opportunities while developing dance skills.

This study supports the value of collaborative visual artmaking in the pursuit of strong relationships, healthy bonding, and the development of the whole child. Based on educational, artistic, and child development theory, this mixed-methods study utilized arts-based collaborative experiences to measure potential growth in the areas of bonding, attachment, and relationship development between child and caregiver pairs (dyads). Through informal art-making sessions, caregivers and their child experienced collaborative artmaking and rated their own personal view of their relationship and bond with their dyad partner in pre and post-assessment surveys, through interviews and storytelling, and through observation using a bonding assessment chart. It was found that collaborative artmaking does indeed have a positive effect on the deepening of relationships and supports an increase in positive family behaviors and dynamics.

This chapter discusses the collaboration of community musicians and community music therapists working to create a community orchestral dialogues experience for youth patterned after a Middle Eastern model. The author explores the definitions of community musicians, music therapy and community music therapy, and how these definitions diverge and converge. The author explains and discusses Orchestral Dialogues: Accepting Self, Accepting Others and the learning that took place for the youth involved, as well as for the staff, both community musicians and community music therapists. The final section of the chapter provides lessons learned and implications for future collaborations for community musicians and community music therapists.

As tools and strategies are gained to assist in our care for others, it is important to assess the effects of our work. Arts-based Post-traumatic Growth Assessments help us to understand how our work benefits others and can help us better guide our groups toward healing. These assessments also aid in the continued improvement of our programming, and help us build concrete data that we may later find useful. There are many methods for measuring success and growth in arts based work, several of which can be found in these next chapters.

This chapter explores the suitability of an arts-based approach to the spiritual assessment of adolescents. Spirituality is a notoriously difficult concept to define, much less to measure. However, many practitioners in both religious and secular settings are increasingly concerned about promoting spiritual development

Foreword

It lay on my shoulder heavy. I turned my head and momentarily froze as I saw the muzzle of an automatic rifle pointed directly at my neck. I grabbed the pot of fear boiling up from my gut. I decided it would be in my self-survival interest to hold that pot of fear and not spill my emotions in the direction of a voice that was now becoming stronger.

"Sir, Sir, SIR! Where are you going?"

I want to go home. That was my first thought, like a small child running to his mother. But I could neither fly home nor fight the situation. The fear was now turning to anger. The boiling pot was beginning to burn as my physical space was threatened. I was at a border crossing in a war zone where tensions were high and violence hovered waiting to swoop down with falcon speed. I would not be prey; I bolstered myself and held on.

I looked at the border officer with all the respect I could muster and became very confused. Here was a woman holding a weapon of death—and carrying new life. She was pregnant, her belly pushing the uniform beyond its limits.

"SIR! Where are you going?" She repeated sharply.

My mind was sorting for a response, one that might appeal to her nurturing side and encourage her to pull the gun from my shoulder. My mother's voice was now in my head, "Nathan, a soft answer turneth away wrath."

"I'm going to the Kampala to judge a youth choir festival." I managed a smile as I responded.

"Hmph." She grunted with unconcern and pulled the gun to her side as she waved me on.

I did judge the choir festival. In the middle of devastating poverty and what I now know as the trauma of war, I watched children and youth dance and sing with cathartic vigor that released their fear and anger and helped to bind their scattered emotions within a safe space. Then, the destination and purpose seemed so insignificant. What reasonable good could a music educator, or any creative artist, do in a place filled with so much hatred and violence? So much poverty--so many problems. That was nearly thirty-five years ago. It was in a nascent time of creative arts therapy, ethnomusicology, and creative education, of which I would begin to study and apply in similar contexts.

Since that time, I have continued to witness firsthand the injustices of war—death, human trafficking, and forced human migration, among a long list of rights withheld and needs denied by aggression at the point of a gun, or spear, or fist. My anger was sparked by that single incident and has been continually ignited by similar ones. My hope, witnessed in the play of those children, led me to encourage and engage creative people in responding to injustice with love, compassion, empathy and the healing power of art-making wherever they find themselves.

This encouragement and engagement became expressed through the co-founding of BuildaBridge International with my colleague Dr. Vivian Nix-Early, a psychologist and music therapist. For the next twenty years we developed and implemented a conceptual and practical model for trauma-informed art making for children and families living in the contexts of poverty and crisis. Our work and training focused on creating safe spaces for hope, healing and resilience.

Over the course of nearly twenty years through my teaching and non-profit work, I have met and worked with well over 1,000 remarkable creative artists who understand the therapeutic nature of art-making in the non-clinical context. They serve their communities as artists, ministers, social workers, educators, and therapists. At times these creative people are prophets who stand on the edge of society providing a window to the reality of our world. Their art serves as a mirror where we are forced to see ourselves at our best, and our worst. They bring a critical awareness to a world many of us do not know exists, even in our own neighborhoods, and they call us to action. At other times these creative people are healers who painstakingly work with survivors of abuse, torture, and trafficking-- invisible people in the shadows--where a quiet presence of compassionate, empathic, and collaborative souls with shared life experience work out hopeful futures.

Two of these collaborative souls, of whom I am proud to call former students, are Amy Grebe and Jenny Bopp. Along with their co-editor, J. Hope Denny, they are exemplary in their non-clinical service to marginalized communities through art making. They have also seen the need to collaboratively share practical research and models of arts-based trauma-informed interventions in this excellent collection that will add to a growing body of practical models to inform the work of creative artists serving children, families and communities.

There are at least four basic questions that provide a guide for engaging art making in transformation:

- How do we increase access to the therapeutic role of the arts ?
- How do we meet the holistic growth of children and family who have limited access to education, social capital, wealth and health (holistic well-being)?
- What method or model provides a preventive structure for building resilience, hope and healing?
- What naturally re-occurring resources already exist in a community?

The chapters of *Healing Through the Arts for Non-Clinical Practitioners* answer these questions. The narratives of practitioners clearly convey models that work and that can be replicated. Grebe, Bopp, and Denny were also careful to include a section most needed in this work that answers a fifth question: Are you making a difference and doing what you say you do? The section on *Assessment Measures* provides models based on arts-based research and assessment.

For me this book is a celebration. Several chapters written by former students are based on their graduate research. I am proud. At the same time, I celebrate with all the authors on their service to communities around the world through a variety of art forms. It gives me hope for the future. It is exactly the kind of book I could have used in 1982 when I began my journey.

J. Nathan Corbitt
BuildaBridge International, USA & Eastern University, USA

Preface

INTRODUCTION

The 1969 book *The Other 23 Hours* provided a framework for child care workers to integrate elements of healing into their regular interactions with the children in their care. It supported the timeless premise that healing is not solely regulated to a one-hour therapy session, but is likely more quickly achieved when being addressed around the clock (Trieschman, Whittaker, & Brendtro, 1969). While the book was specifically written for non-clinically trained child care workers, the premise is universal and timeless. Emotional and mental healing can take place outside of the clinical realm.

The use of art in healing is equally universal and timeless. For example, Aboriginal philosophy subscribes to the belief that healing is not a separate art (Dufrene, 1991). Likewise, healing is not limited to only the physical illness, but encompasses psychological, social, and spiritual ills as well (Dufrene, 1991). For nearly all of history, healers and shamans have called on drumming, dance, song, and visual arts to bring healing and balance. Despite ever growing technological advances, the healing practices rooted in our ancestors remain powerful today.

This book is built on those two premises; using the universal benefits of the arts to provide healing outside the clinical realm. The compiled chapters examine and describe arts-based interventions and experiences that support the healing process. The interventions and activities described in this book are by no means a replacement for traditional therapy. Rather, this book and its authors seeks to fill those other 23 hours.

IMPACT OF TRAUMA

Post-traumatic stress disorder (PTSD) was introduced as a psychiatric disorder in 1980 with its inclusion in the third edition of the American Psychiatric Association's (APA) Diagnostic and Statistical Manual of Mental Disorders (DSM-III). At the time, it was understood that "a traumatic event was conceptualized as a catastrophic stressor that was outside the range of usual human experience" (Freidman, 2016). This then established the criterion for diagnosis of PTSD. The understanding and definition of trauma and PTSD was developed in response to the horrors of the first 60 years of the 20th century such as the Holocaust, the nuclear bombings of Hiroshima and Nagasaki, and the two world wars. The experience of trauma, however, has existed as long as humans have.

A World Health Organization survey found that 70.4% of respondents had experienced a traumatic event (Kessler et al., 2017). In the United States, up to 20% of those who experience trauma develop PTSD (Nebraska Department of Veterans Affairs, 2016). Recent epigenetic studies are finding that trauma can even become woven into DNA and passed down through generations. The likelihood of developing behavior or psychological disorders is increased with exposure to traumatic events, but the risk of developing these disorders increases if one's ancestors experienced trauma – regardless of your personal experience (Gapp et al., 2016).

More anecdotally, teachers in both grade school and higher education are noting a steep increase in the number of students who struggle cognitively and behaviorally. In schools, PTSD symptoms are often misdiagnosed as Attention Deficit and Hyperactivity Disorder (ADHD), depression, anxiety, or learning disabilities. Unfortunately, trauma symptoms that are left undiagnosed or are misdiagnosed can later manifest into further mental illnesses.

Over the nearly 40 years since the APA's recognition of PTSD, the understanding of trauma and stressor-related disorders have grown considerably and with it, vast amounts of trauma treatment models for therapists. And yet, as Howard Bath (2015) points out, little is written or shared regarding the great post traumatic growth that can occur in the other 23 hours.

While the editors approach healing through a trauma-informed lens, it is simultaneously recognized that not all healing is a response to trauma and its subsequent symptoms. However, there is a universality to trauma interventions that provides healing and respite from numerous behavioral and psychological disorders and so justifies disseminating information on healing through this trauma-informed lens.

POST-TRAUMATIC GROWTH AND HEALING

Arts-based trauma interventions use sensory experiences that are predictable, integrate both sides of the brain, and support emotional skills. Through this approach, participants can experience positive brain changes and work towards resiliency and post-traumatic growth (Behrens, 2014). Wentling and Behrens (2018) outline five steps of a treatment protocol which is based on the neurobiology of trauma. These steps, of which three are discussed below, helps a trauma victim to properly process the traumatic experience without re-traumatization. Applying all five steps within this neurobiological framework requires the training possessed by clinical practitioners. However, three of these steps can be used in everyday environments without risking re-traumatization and are likely already inadvertently facilitated. These three steps include:

Providing Safety and Trust

In addition to creating a physically safe environment in which to work, Bath (2015) suggests creating "social safety in peer and adult relationships; emotional safety through acceptance, empathy, and compassion; and cultural safety in a world where diversity can be marked by discrimination" (p. 6).

Unlearning Maladaptive Responses and Learn Adaptive Responses

Often in an attempt to either mask psychological symptoms or numb emotional pain, maladaptive coping mechanisms are adopted. Unfortunately, these coping mechanisms lead further away from healing.

Instead, interventions should be designed to help "facilitate perceptual changes of self, others, and person's inner world" and "undo reactive responses" (Berhens, 2014, p. 4).

Developing Coping and Self-Mastery

Interventions should aim to explore how to respond appropriately to external circumstances or events while managing strong emotions and impulses (Bath, 2015).

Although not all chapters specifically address trauma or are designed around a neurobiological method to post-traumatic growth and healing, all authors have described methods in which to incorporate one or more of these healing steps into art making. It is likely that many who facilitate art making in community settings are already implementing these steps almost instinctually. With greater understanding, non-clinical practitioners can deepen the impact for those they serve by increasing the intentionality with which they incorporate these healing steps.

HEALING THROUGH THE ARTS

The arts are used to build skill (mastery), yield products in which the artists and their community can take pride, build sense of self, build social networks, and present no risk of failure. Effective arts programs are designed ... to provide access to connection with friends, family, and extended community and access to ways of giving meaning to experiences, feelings, and observations. (Basting, 2006, p. 17)

Just as the shaman recognized the need for a balanced, holistic approach to healing, the arts provide the necessary tools to achieve balanced, holistic healing. Holistic arts-based experiences are body centered, provide a container for expressed thoughts and feelings, foster meaning through the use of metaphor, build relationships, and aid in the re-establishment of creativity.

Body Centered

Art therapist Mindy Jacobson-Levy coined the phrase "Art Before Words." Experiencing a traumatic event shuts down the part of the brain responsible for language while the fear center records the trauma as visual and sensory memories (Rausch et al., 1996). This leaves many people unable to verbalize their experience or reactions. The arts access both visual and sensory memories and provide the ability for a non-verbal telling. As narrative and context are put to the created art, memories can be properly integrated, shifting away from the fear center and releasing the body from its fight/flight/freeze response.

Container

Processing thoughts and feelings through the creative process allows the creator to pour into the container of art. This pouring provides distance from the issues and provides a new perspective to deepen discernment or acceptance. The distance allows one to see more clearly what is in front of them that cannot be seen while inside. The container also provides respite from the emotions attached to the hurt or anger.

Metaphor

Similar to the distance created by using art as a container, drawing upon metaphors during the creative process helps to create distance or detachment from painful memories. Much of art is expressed or communicated through metaphor. Creating a metaphor to represent the experience removes the emotional connection, allowing the creator to figuratively work out a path forward or a resolution to a problem. Once understood or resolved externally, it can be more easily internalized.

Relational

Building and growing relationships naturally occur in the creative process. Actors, dancers, and musicians are in constant communication both verbally and non-verbally throughout the rehearsal and performance process. Visual artists build intimate relationships with their materials, trusting in their tools to bring their message to life. Simultaneously, the creator is relying on the relationship and communication between their own body, mind, and spirit to carry out their vision - a relationship that is often shattered during the traumatic experience.

Creation

For a person experiencing trauma, accessing their creative side can aid in the regulation of affect as well as help them make meaning out of the traumatic experience (Phillips, 2012). Tantamount to post traumatic growth is the ability to create a new path forward, a new mindset, or a new way of coping. The process of art making builds agency and efficacy not only in the ability to create, but in problem solving, higher level reasoning, and self-regulation. These skills developed in the safety of an art making session can be transferred to other areas of life.

NON-CLINICAL PRACTITIONERS

Rapidly changing political and environmental climates are contributing to the rising instances of trauma and the subsequent symptoms are likely to continue to manifest in more people, particularly those in vulnerable populations. Educators, social workers, and community leaders are often undereducated about the impact and implications of trauma in classrooms, with congregations, and other community settings. In response, it becomes critically important for those working with these populations to have access to methods that support trauma treatments and post traumatic growth. Too often, well-meaning leaders cause more harm in their attempt to help by unknowingly working beyond appropriate healing boundaries.

Carving out those treatment steps that are available to non-clinical practitioners may result in the examination of other activities that similarly offer brain-based sensory experiences that can be used as either a standalone activity or integrated into educational or community activities. In providing educators, clergy, social workers, and other community leaders with tools that build upon their own knowledge and expertise, individuals will be empowered to reclaim their lives after traumatic experiences, and potentially mitigate intergenerational trauma and the trauma cycle.

ORGANIZATION OF THE BOOK

This compilation of chapters offers strategies and experiential ideas for those who do not possess clinical licenses to implement into their daily work practices. The opening chapter shares three healing stories that while based on real lives, are nearly generic because they are so universal and timeless - they are undoubtedly similar to stories any reader of this book has encountered in their own lives. These stories help to ground later academically heavy chapters in reality.

The book is further organized into three sections corresponding with the steps of post-traumatic growth and finishes with two assessment strategies for evaluating post-traumatic growth and healing. Each section offers replicable arts-based research and interventions. Straying slightly from the norm of academic writing, many chapters are written from the first-person perspective. The evolution from trauma victim to survivor and further on to thriver is a testament to the potent healing power of the arts and a process critical of understanding.

Chapter 1 demonstrates the ability to create opportunities to use the arts to heal. The author has included three narratives, both his personal story as a professional artist, but non-clinical practitioner, and those of his students. These narratives illustrate the effect of the arts on individuals dealing with trauma and poverty.

Chapter 2 reviews the literature on storytelling as an art form and discusses the benefits of how this artform can be used with people who have experienced traumatic events. The author provides some sample techniques that can be modified for community use.

Chapter 3 explores the concept of vicarious trauma as experienced by crisis workers. It examines the use of a mandala art making experience as an intervention to increase positive affect and decrease in negative affect. The author further explores the use of art as a connection to participants' positive resources surrounding the theme of safety.

Chapter 4 utilizes a first-person account to describe the effects of trauma on the body, mind, and spirit. The author discusses initiatives aimed at helping those who have experienced trauma, one centered in the arts and another that specifically focuses on yoga as an avenue of healing.

Chapter 5 presents the experiences of pre-service teachers engaged in the teaching of art classes for intergenerational students. The author outlines student engagement in this embedded service learning activity, and explores the benefits for both the student and elderly members of a retirement community.

Chapter 6 explores depression from a first-person perspective, both as a clinician and as one who struggles with depression. The author describes her personal experiences with autobiographical community theater performance, an alternative treatment grounded in expressive arts therapy, and compares this experience to a branch of drama therapy: Self-Revelatory Performance. Relationships between the author's theatrical experience and five of the typical psychotherapeutic goals for someone seeking clinical treatment for depression is discussed.

Chapter 7 addresses the issue of historical trauma in the context of an indigenous group of women in Columbia. The chapter explores the use of embroidery as an art form and healing process to help women express their individual and collective stories. The author includes a follow-up with the Wayuu women who participated in this study.

Chapter 8 explores the use of narrative writing in the healing process. This chapter provides processes of how to incorporate narrative writing to assist in teaching, to aid in the healing of emotional pain, to understand physical pain, to address spirituality, and as an art form itself.

Chapter 9 provides a movement and storytelling-based framework for working for adults who are in recovery from various addictions or traumatic experiences. The author utilizes this framework to build a seven-week healing curriculum of dance and movement. The experiences of sample participants and their reflections on the process are discussed.

Chapter 10 presents the process of collaborative art making as a means of healing for persons with diagnosed mental illness. This chapter discusses the benefits and considerations of group art making in the context of a psychiatric rehabilitation program.

Chapter 11 utilizes the lens of social justice to approach the field of dance as an avenue of healing. This chapter explores the pedagogy of dance instruction, the role of the teacher, and the teacher-student relationship. The author argues that redefining classroom culture promotes dancers' meaningful choices, which can foster healing and wholeness.

Chapter 12 examines how the visual arts may support and enhance family relationships through collaborative creativity and art making experiences. The author outlines an arts-focused intervention to promote bonding, social-emotional connection, and relational ability. This intervention, used in a study of families with children between the ages of 2 to 10 years old, demonstrated positive growth in the parent-child relationship.

Chapter 13 considers the divide between community musicians and music therapists. The author presents one approach to bridge this divide by focusing on deep listening and transformative dialogue. Implications and lessons learned from the program are discussed.

Chapter 14 introduces an arts-based approach to spiritual assessment, which can be applied to community-based youth development programs. The chapter provides an overview of the role of spirituality in youth development, and describes the benefits of adopting an arts-based approach to assessment. Two assessment activities which demonstrate this approach are included.

Chapter 15 concludes with the concept of utilizing arts-based assessment as a means to evaluating post-traumatic growth. The author outlines how to develop an art-based assessment by demonstrating the process in a study of teenage pregnancy rooted in the context of Asian culture. Approaches of questionnaires, observations, and interviews are explored.

Jenny Bopp
Westtown School, USA

Amy M. Grebe
Zinnia Consulting and Design, USA

J. Hope Denny
Pellissippi State Community College, USA

REFERENCES

Basting, A. (2006). Arts in dementia care: This is not the end…it's the end of this chapter. *Generations (San Francisco, Calif.)*, *30*(1), 16–20.

Bath, H. (2015). The three pillars of traumawise care: Healing in the other 23 hours. *Reclaiming Children and Youth*, *23*(4), 5–11.

Behrens, G. A. (2014, May 26). *Art in healing panel: Neurobiology of trauma and the arts* [PowerPoint Slides].

Bromet, E., Karam, E., Koenen, K. C., & Steine, D. J. (2018). *Trauma and posttraumatic stress disorder: Global perspectives from the WHO world mental health surveys*. Academic Press.

Dufrene, P. (1991). Utilizing the arts for healing from a Native American perspective: Implications for creative Arts therapies. *Canadian Journal of Native Studies*.

Freidman, M. J. (2016). *PTSD history and overview*. Retrieved from https://www.ptsd.va.gov/professional/ptsd-overview/ptsd-overview.asp

Gapp, K., Bohacek, J., Grossmann, J., Brunner, A. M., Manuella, F., Nanni, P., & Mansuy, I. M. (2016). Potential of environmental enrichment to prevent transgenerational effects of paternal trauma. *Neuropsychopharmacology*, *41*(11), 2749–2758. doi:10.1038/npp.2016.87 PMID:27277118

Nebraska Department of Veterans Affairs. (2016). *Post traumatic stress disorder*. Retrieved from http://www.ptsd.ne.gov/what-is-ptsd.html

Phillips, A. (2012, March 7). *Art and trauma: Creativity as a resiliency factor*. Retrieved from https://www.goodtherapy.org/blog/art-and-trauma-creativity-as-a-resiliency-factor-0307124

PTSD United. (2013). *PTSD statistics*. Retrieved from http://www.ptsdunited.org/ptsd-statistics-2/

Rausch, S. L., van der Kolk, B. A., Fisler, R. E., & Alpert, N. M. (1996). A symptom provocation study of posttraumatic stress disorder using positron emission tomography and script-driven imagery. *Archives of General Psychiatry*, *53*(5), 380–387. doi:10.1001/archpsyc.1996.01830050014003 PMID:8624181

Trauma and PTSD in the WHO World Mental Health Surveys. (2017). Retrieved from https://www.tandfonline.com/doi/full/10.1080/20008198.2017.1353383

Trieschman, A., Whittaker, J., & Brendtro, L. (1969). *The other 23 hours: Child-care work with emotionally disturbed children in a therapeutic milieu*. Piscataway, NJ: Transaction.

Wentling, B., & Behrens, G. A. (2018). Case study of early childhood trauma using a neurobiological approach to music therapy. *Music Therapy Perspectives*, *36*(1), 131. doi:10.1093/mtp/miy003

Section 1

Introduction

Chapter 1
Music, the Arts, and Healing

Rodney Luther Whittenberg
Melodyvision, USA

ABSTRACT

The goal of this chapter is to demonstrate the ability to create opportunities to use the arts to heal. The author has included three narratives, both his personal story as a professional artist, a non-clinical practitioner, and those of his students. These narratives illustrate the effect of the arts on individuals dealing with trauma and poverty. Time and time again, as indicated in these narratives, the arts can be called on to provide respite and relief from fear, anxiety, and hurting. The arts are a touchstone that can be revisited throughout a lifespan regardless of age or stage or even circumstance.

INTRODUCTION

The bow lands on a string, the reed vibrates with a push of air, the stick hits the drum and the snares rattle against the bottom head, the needle lands on the record, the mp3 player translates digital bits of zeros and ones to an analogue signal and the space is filled with these sounds...

These sounds. How can sounds created over fifty years ago have the power to transform me? These sounds created in another part of the world. I can now sit in my car or living room or on a train and play back these sounds. These sounds go to the very core of the very essence, the soul. I am transported and transformed, and my body moves uncontrollably. I begin to cry or laugh or both at the same time and I have no power over it. It is as if I am under a spell. In these sounds and in these moments, everything about this experience is as real as anything I have ever experienced or ever will experience.

When these sounds end, I am not the same. I am forever changed. I have communed with something more powerful, more connected, more alive, and more whole. And that is not even the most salient, most true, or most amazing part of the experience of these sounds. What must the act of creating and performing these sounds do to the creator of this work? What must they be going through to create this work? To what depth did they go to find some kind of truth? What layers did they peel away? What did they heal?

DOI: 10.4018/978-1-5225-5981-8.ch001

Did Pete Townsend transform the alienation and devastation of his childhood growing up in post WW2 England by composing the rock opera *Tommy*? I believe he did for millions of his fans. Did Roger Waters transform his isolation by composing *The Wall*? I believe he did for his fans. Did Chuck D transform his anger at oppression and racism with “It Takes a Nation of Millions to Hold Us Back?” I believe he did for his fans. This is real power. Music has power. Art has power; the power to move, the power to transform, and the power to heal.

MY STORY

My mom told me that as a young baby I would crawl into the kitchen and pull the pots and pans out of the cupboard. I would sit in the middle of the floor and bang on the pots and pans and make up songs. I could sit there for hours. I also had an imaginary friend named Gutty. Gutty and I had many adventures together: safaris in Africa, climbing to the top of Mt Everest, and high tea with the Queen of England to name a few. It was my dad who introduced me to the creativity that already existed within me. He was always making up stories and trying to get us to laugh. He was always trying to improve what already existed.

It was dad who opened me up to music and movies. My dad’s business was in retail sales. He was the first African American to sell refrigerators and air conditioners at Sears and Roebucks in West Philadelphia in the late 1950’s, early 1960’s. He grew up very poor, living in the developmental period of his life during the great depression. He found solace in movies and salvation in music, but knew he had to get himself out of poverty. The arts and entertainment would be something he could enjoy and use as an escape while he focused on working hard at a good job and achieving the American dream. He never stopped going to the movies and listening to music. What was a significant part of his single life merged right into his family life.

By the time I came along he not only worked for Sears, but he would purchase run down houses. On his days off, Dad would say to me, “Hey Rod, you want to go play build-a-house?” I was quick to respond, “Yea!” Upon arrival, however, I quickly realized that this was not play time. The houses were always run down with holes in the floors, no refrigerator, sink or stove, and crawling with bugs and rodents.

It was great, though. I learned how to wire outlets and weld pipes, put up paneling and install drop ceilings. The big takeaway was the lesson that if you imagined something, if you saw something in your mind, and then worked really, really hard, the vision could become real. Within a year my dad had rented the house out to a family. That run down, broken down house had become a home. Dad had taught me about the power of creativity.

When I was about seven, my dad came home from work and let my mom, sister, and I know that he had written a song. Of course, my mom was like, “Here we go”, and I thought, “Wow! My dad wrote a song, yea!” My dad, had no musical training, but he was determined to send the song to legendary country singer Charley Pride. Since he needed someone to create the sheet music for his song, he looked in the phone book and found a composer and arranger, and he made an appointment.

I remember that it was a beautiful Sunday afternoon when my dad and I piled into the car for the drive into Center City. When we got to the house of the arranger, I had no idea my whole life was going to change. The door opened and I could not believe my eyes. There were musical instruments everywhere. We went up a spiral staircase to find a room with a big tape machine and long mixing board. The arranger asked my dad to sing his song into the microphone. Once my dad had sung his song, the guy asked me if I wanted to say something on the microphone. After I heard my own voice back, I was hooked. That day, that moment, has stuck with me through my entire life.

If you were to walk into the front door of my house now, you might be transported back to that house we visited with my dad. There are musical instruments everywhere and a similar giant tape machine.

Creativity played such a big part of my early life; from Legos to erector sets, discovering electronics and building electronic music synthesizers, to writing short stories and of course, music. I was about 13 the first time that music saved my life.

At age 13 I started breaking out in hives. None of the doctors could figure out why. At the end of fifth grade, I also had horrible stomach problems. After many tests and many doctors, it was concluded that it was nerves. Family therapy was prescribed. To give my parents credit, they tried, but therapy for a black family in the late sixties, early seventies was not to be. After a few sessions we stopped. My dad just refused to go.

My stomach eventually began to calm down by the beginning of sixth grade, but not the hives. My parents and doctors believed like my earlier stomach problems, the hives were caused by nerves. I was prescribed Atarax, an antihistamine, and it was horrible. I would be falling asleep all the time and had trouble focusing but the hives just would not end.

Around this same time in my life, I had discovered the music of Kitaro and Tangerine Dream. After falling asleep in the middle of a conversation with one of my best friends, I decided I had to try something different. So every day after school I would put on a recording of Kitaro or Tangerine Dream, turn the lights out and I would sit in the lotus position and breath. The music soothed me; it calmed me. I was practicing my own version of mindfulness before I even knew what being mindful was. I was doing a rudimentary form of meditation and the music supported my breathing and helped me clear my mind. The music saved me. The hives stopped. For the first time, I experienced a glimpse of peace.

I received my first guitar on my 15th birthday. My grandmother bought it for me from *8th Street Music* in Philadelphia. It was certainly not a great guitar, but it would do the job. I had been studying piano and dance and had also been playing keyboards in various garage bands since I was twelve. Receiving this guitar was a big step. For the next few years practicing, learning, and writing songs became my religion, and I prayed everyday. This was the second time music saved my life. Having something to put all of my fears, anxiety and frustration into changed my fears, anxiety and frustration into confidence and self-esteem.

At the time, I was a bit of a weirdo at school, and I did not fit in. To be honest, I was not trying to fit in. I was a weirdo and I liked it. I was a young black kid in the suburbs of Philadelphia. I would wear tie-dye shirts or punk rock t-shirts and I had a big wild afro. I carried a slide rule in my pocket, always had books about electronics or poetry, and I lived for rock and roll. I was pretty weird and the other kids let me know it. They would pick on me, make fun of my musical obsession and the way I dressed. Music, though, gave me solace, and the more I played, the more I felt settled into who I was. The better I got as a guitarist and songwriter, the more self-confident I became.

After high school graduation, I figured music would be my hobby and electronics would be my vocation. I got a job working for the Southeastern Pennsylvania Transportation Authority (SEPTA). I was told at the time I was hired that I would be a working electronics technician

as I had studied electronics in high school. Instead, I was put in the maintenance gang. It was my introduction to the real world. I could tell within a short time that working a 9-to-5 job was not for me. If you wanted to know whether I quit or was fired on my 18th birthday, it all depends on who you ask. The way I tell the story is that I quit because I had decided to pursue music as a career. By the time I was

19, I had sold my first jingle and was accepted to the University of the Arts where I planned to study jazz guitar and music composition. By the time I was 20, I had a manager and financial investor. I was on my way to stardom, or so I thought.

I continued learning everything I could about not only music, but about all of the arts. The arts not only saved my life, but they gave me a family and a community. My friends were all in the arts. We were an eclectic group that have since gone on to be a casting agent who discovered Leonardo DiCaprio, a sound man for major Hollywood films like the Matrix, an Academy Award nominated writer, a photographer film editor turned therapist and actor, a drummer and set designer for SNL, a celebrated graphics designer, an arts educator, and me.

But back in 1983, we were a just group of kids in Philadelphia trying to figure it all out. I was drinking it all in. At college, I met anti-feminist feminist and scholar Camille Paglia, and she opened my mind to new ways of thinking about art. She turned me on to films and books and painters. I was experimenting with music, film, poetry and dance while working with my friends' projects. It was an amazing time. Camille also told me that I was disconnected from myself and if I wanted to write better lyrics I needed to find someway of going deeper. This led me to work with a therapist and leadership coach, Elizabeth Hechtman. Her art is supporting growth and development in others and it was through our work that I began to understand how arts had the power to heal. With her lifelong guidance, I began to understand that there was something otherworldly about art making. One of my professors, composer Joe Costaldo, turned me on to two quotes that speak to the mystical, magical, spiritual power of the arts.

Great art communicates before it is understood (TS Eliot)

All art constantly aspires to the condition of music (Walter H Pater)

The ideas expressed in these quotes speak to the mystical, magical, spiritual power of the arts.

I was 25 and my band was happening. I was getting airplay on the major Philadelphia rock stations. My band was voted best band at the WMMR Street Beat awards. The band had an Anheuser Busch sponsorship, and we got paid well for gigs with lines of fans out the door and around the block. I had a road crew and a road manager. We had started playing festivals. Everything was going well. Admittedly, I still had to work some kind of day job. A friend introduced me to Pecki Witonski, the founder of the Banner Project, an anti-violence/anti-drug arts program. The program used the arts as a way of building self-esteem, and to give young people a constructive outlet for the emotional impact of the trauma, poverty and lack of support. This is where I truly learned and witnessed the healing power of the arts.

In the beginning, I was the "music person" as Pecki would call me. There were a handful of pre-written, pre-recorded songs we used in the program. It was not long before I started writing original songs for the program and then getting the kids to write their own songs. I saw how the kids blossomed through the process of collectively writing, performing, and recording songs. It did not solve all of their problems. In fact, I do not think it solved any of their problems, but what I did see was the beginning of a process of healing.

P'S STORY

By the summer of 1994, my rock star days were behind me. I had become executive director of the Banner Project. I was back in school continuing to study composition while starting up Melodyvision. At the time, Melodyvision was a music and audio production company. That summer, Banner Project was hired to run a program with the Woodrock Community Center in the Kensington neighborhood of Philadelphia. Our charge was to work with the youth to create a mural and write an original song and poem to be performed at the mural revealing program.

I had a powerful staff. Indigo was a teaching artist. Ashack was a poet and a painter while Bet was a singer and songwriter. We also worked with Mbali, a poet and art therapist. Most of the staff that summer had been doing community-based art education since the early 1970s. I might have been in charge, but I definitely learned quite a bit from my staff that summer. The most important thing that I learned was to just make space for creation. As a teaching artist, it was my responsibility to create a safe space and facilitate and support opportunities for others to make art.

We served somewhere between 100 and 150 kids, aged nine to sixteen, over our two week residency at Woodrock. By this time, the staff was a well-oiled machine as we had been working together for two years. We could anticipate the challenges of getting kids to open up in order to create and the emotional fallout that could follow a session of art making. We were a multi-cultural group and we drew from many cultures to teach our lessons.

To start each day, we drew on the Native American tradition of the talking stick. With each new group, we would encourage the kids to make the talking stick their own. We would start with a stick that one of the staff may have found in their backyard or in the park on their way to the program. The kids would bring in things to attach to the stick in some way and then the stick would be left with the school or center.

We would start the day by passing the talking stick and sharing challenging news and good news. One of the things I loved best about this ritual was seeing two kids who did not get along sitting across from each other. Maybe one of them was bullying the other, but talking with each other led to the discovery of shared experiences. These kids often faced divorcing parents, sick family members, or even someone from their family in jail. In a split second, those relationships could transform and friendships might be born. It might have been helpful if one particular student would have shared her background story during this ritual.

That particular summer we had a tough one; a young girl we will call P. P was disruptive, disrespectful, and just in general, challenging. She had been in some trouble and there was concern that she may be adjudicated. Each of the staff members spent time working with her one on one while painting the mural. She was angry, acting out and difficult, but we kept at it.

P was part of the program both summers we were there. The staff spent a lot of time talking about P and trying to figure what could be done to create space where she could constructively deal with whatever was going on. During the second summer, we hired her to be a student facilitator, hoping that might drive a shift in her attitude. That summer was not necessarily any better with P, just different. We still did not give up. After the program ended, we tried to stay in touch with P, but over the years we lost contact.

Five or six years later, a friend had asked me to play guitar at her performance in an annual, regional arts festival. After the performance, I was packing my guitar and amp into my car while a burglar alarm was going off in the building next to my car. False alarms are pretty common place in Philadelphia, so I did not think anything of it until a police van pulled around the corner. The officer on the passenger side shouts out, "Don't move!" The van pulls down the street a little further and parks. Both officers get out and begin walking toward me, I see that both are women, one black and one white.

The black officer begins to run toward me faster and faster. Unexpectedly, she jumps on me, begins crying and is somewhat hysterical. Through her tears she is mumbling, "Mr. Rodney, Mr. Rodney, I'm…" My girlfriend standing next to me was as confused as I was and quite curious. As the officer calmed down, I began to understand what she was saying. It was P, the young girl from Woodrock. She began to tell me how her life had turned around during her time with the program and time spent creating music, painting murals, and performing. My staff had helped her to see possibilities for herself and how she had to power to change her life.

Now she was a police officer and she was buying her first home. The emotional reunion left us all in tears. We talked for a bit on the corner and exchanged numbers before P had to go back to work. I have worked with so many kids over the years. For most, I might not ever know if I had any effect on them. Did I reach them? Did they get any of what we were trying to do? How grateful I am for an experience like this. It is experiences like that these that help me persevere with those rough kids, and affirms the healing power of the arts.

THE BROTHERS' STORY

Pecki had shut down the Banner Project in 1997. By 1999, I transferred the program to work under the fiscal sponsorship of another nonprofit organization, and renamed the program, Project RESPECT (Realizing Everyone's Special Potential, Everyone Working Together). The fiscal sponsorship did not last long and soon the community education component was rolled into Melodyvision along with music and video production. Our team had grown to include a videographer/editor and a composer.

Personally, my vision for myself was finally beginning to be realized. I had composed the score for my first film along with composing music for a few episodes of A&E's Biography show. The community education program now encompassed animation, filmmaking, music videos, production and appreciation, as well as intergenerational programming. HBO had hired me as a freelance segment producer for their show 30 by 30: Kids Flicks. Through that relationship that I had built with HBO Family, they licensed the videos that we created with the kids in the program.

Around this same time, the city of Philadelphia had created a Youth Opportunity Center (YOC) located in one of the empowerment zones in the city. An empowerment zone was an economically distressed area of the city that received grant funding and tax incentives to support economic rejuvenation and job creation. We were hired by the YOC to create a video program for adjudicated kids.

On our first day of class, two brothers sat at the back of the room, both just a few steps away from going to juvenile detention centers. That whole first class, the two brothers snickered and made fun of how I spoke and were generally disruptive. Slowly, as we began to show them how to tell stories using a camera, making special effects and dolly shots, they began to come around. We were able to take them on a tour of our local PBS affiliate.

Most of these kids, including the two brothers, had never ventured out of the 15 block radius of their neighborhood of North Philadelphia. Now they were seeing the city in new ways. We did video shoots all over the city and ended up premiering their films in a big theater in town. Friends and family were invited to the premier. Later all of the films created by the kids were sent to film festivals. All of the kids were excited to see their films being viewed, appreciated, and celebrated by others, but I could tell that the process held deeper meaning for the two brothers.

After a year, our contract with the YOC ended, but we had taught the teachers at YOC how to use the equipment and they continued making films. Anytime I was invited to participate in anything film related, whether it was to enter a film festival or judge a festival, or even if I heard about a student film festival, I would reach out to the kids we had worked with at YOC. The two brothers would always show up.

In the mid 2000s, we were asked to put together a video education program for 100 kids in Barbados. We hired the two brothers to be student teachers. This time they were going far beyond their 15 block radius and leaving the country. It could have been disastrous, but they were amazing as teacher mentors. Today the two brothers live in L.A. and work as professional filmmakers and DJs. They are raising families and are no longer in danger of going to jail. In fact, this past year one of the brothers was the editor on a major film released in theaters.

Mastering skills is an important part of the healing process. When teaching artists do for their students, the students lose the opportunity to figure things out on their own. What happens during the creative process is often mirrored in life. For these two brothers, the act of learning and mastering the video creation process was mirrored in their ability to overcome the emotional and behavioral challenges they faced in their teens. Finding healing through the arts allowed them to break the cycle they had been raised in, and transform their lives to provide a more stable, supportive environment for their own children.

THE NEXT LOOP IN THE CYCLE OF THESE STORIES

Even though we write stories with a beginning, middle, and an end, in reality, each story is just a loop in a cycle. Sometimes, we can break out of one cycle, but we will always find ourselves in another, forever starting a new beginning or moving to the end in the current loop of the cycle. For P and the two brothers, the arts played a critical role in the healing cycle of their teen years. For me, the arts have played a critical role in healing cycles throughout my entire life. I am committed to live a healthy, connected life that challenges me to grow. In addition to my work with a therapist, I have found music and other art forms to have a profound effect in my healing journey. My journey of creativity and love of the arts was sparked at birth. Now at 54, I have seen and experienced the healing power of the arts. They have saved me time and time again.

Many years ago, my friends and I tried to pin down the purpose of art in one of our weekly artist support group meetings. At the time, we felt that art's purpose was to comment on the human condition. My journey with art, however, has shown me that it is so much more. Art gives us the opportunity to create connection, connection with our deeper selves and connection with others. Art requires ego and humility. Art requires discipline and free thinking. It requires determination and patience. It demands honesty and truth and then tells us there is no such thing. It requires us to be present and to dream. It demands we learn the rules and then inspires us to break them. Despite the irony that the greatest art is often created by the least healthy - consider Wagner or Picasso - art's greatest purpose is in its innate ability to heal body, mind, and spirit.

Section 2
Creating Safe Spaces

Establishing a safe space for the people we serve is the first key to a non-clinical practitioner's success. When the atmosphere and people in a place are felt to be safe, the doors to uninhibited self-expression, discovery, and healing relationships are opened wide. The following chapters provide ideas and recommendations for developing places of safety and trust.

Chapter 2
Healing:
Use the Power of Your Voice Through Your Stories

Linda Marie Ellington
Southern New Hampshire University, USA

ABSTRACT

This chapter, per the author, is to convey the significance in facilitating healing through storytelling empowering individuals to reclaim and build sustainable lives for themselves. People will feel the force of passion and commitment in their stories as they reflect and become inspired to act. When we help identify a way to transfer hurt to healing, we move people to consider what they might become if they are "more" than the hurt—more determined, more prepared, more confident, and more empowered. The purpose of this chapter is to advocate the use of storytelling as an effective medium to embrace in the positive power, benefit, and effect that stories have in the healing cycle. Stories may appear to be simplistic yet are purposeful. However, developmental psychologists point out that stories are not innocent as they always have a message. These emotionalized messages have been told over centuries and yet the messages are often lost, unappreciated, and unheard in the clutter of assumptions, caveats, data, and the fear that the storyteller will not be taken seriously.

INTRODUCTION

Human beings are by nature storytellers. We tell stories to bring coherence to our lives. To make sense of the layers of events that occur in our lives and our interactions with others, we draw everything that happens to us together in a coherent story (Wielenga, 2013). Our stories are formed in constant dialogue with those events and people, and tell us how we perceive the events, the people around us, and ourselves in relationship to the experiences (Cobely, 2001).

The methodology used in writing this chapter was a literature review in which to advocate the use of storytelling as an effective medium to embrace the positive power, benefit, and effect that stories have in the healing cycle. However, this chapter is not to be prescriptive nor a case study of specific types of hurt, because the use of storytelling changes depending on the context. Rather this is a review of what

DOI: 10.4018/978-1-5225-5981-8.ch002

scholars have stated about storytelling approaches that can be a positive way to respond to different needs, depending on the specific hurt or trauma that affects individuals physically, emotionally, mentally, and spiritually. Stories are both art and solace, but they are not prescriptive nor can the telling or listening be forced (Good, 2003). This chapter identifies three storytelling opportunities for facilitators to utilize.

What this chapter does do is to portray a collective exploration, through a literature search, to find ways in which facilitators may have the adeptness to acknowledge and combat the darkness and bring sufferers to paths of action and healing. Thus, the purpose of this chapter is to retell the unending appetite for stories, use storytelling to build compassionate communities, and learn to give the gift of a story.

WHAT IS STORYTELLING?

Once upon a time there was an ancient form of communication called storytelling. It was a basic endeavor. One person talked and one or more people listened. Then it fell in disfavor. There are several theories why, but most likely it had something to do with the fact that storytelling did not involve remote controls, fast-forward buttons or joysticks (Strickler, 1990). Storytelling was not flashy. The sound was limited to what came out of a person's mouth; there were no special effects. Worst of all, you could not brag to your friends about having just spent a month's wages for a state-of-the-art-high-tech storytelling unit (1990).

However, storytelling has enjoyed a resurgence in recent years as it appears that people are desperate for human contact, or something as basic as looking for the warmth that storytelling provides. Scholars and storytellers such as Howard (1991) reiterate to their audience that storytelling is more personal than story reading. Through stories we are taken immediately to another world and put into an adventure that engages the psyche as we attempt to gain an understanding of the emotional conflict in the story. Fisher (1989) defined storytelling as a communication process by which humans break down complex information into narratives that are shared between individuals and amongst groups. Many scholars have denoted that storytelling is how we make sense of our lives, as it defines cultures, establishes values, standards, and helps us cope with the ever-changing environment.

Stories may appear to be simplistic yet are purposeful. However, developmental psychologists point out that stories are not innocent as they always have a message. These emotionalized messages have been told over centuries and yet the messages are often lost, unappreciated, and unheard in the clutter of assumptions, caveats, data, and the fear that the storyteller will not be taken seriously.

Relational Role of Storytelling

Tutu (2000) argued that we are all wounded victims as well as perpetrators, and all need to be healed. Healing occurs through, among other things, the rebuilding of relationships (as cited in Wielenga, 2013). Lederach (1997) contended that if we intentionally engage each other as humans-in-relationships then there is a road to recovery of the dignity and humanity of both the victim and perpetrator. Thus, healing begins (Hay, 1999 as cited in Wielenga, 2013).

Storytelling integrates relationships. The teller of the story can simply reinterpret the story or even create a new story. It is as though stories are made of clay which can be molded and then reworked and fashioned into a different mold (Sager, 2012). The story should not be a mere tool or a mere means to provide information or teach a skill. A story has an integrity; a life of its own. And, of course, the story can be the stimulus for a discussion that engages the listener, as well as the teller of the story (Sager, 2012).

Miller (1976) sits among the first to propose that the way to achieving trust and connectedness, and indeed psychological wellbeing, is through mutually empowering relationships (as cited in Wielenga, 2013). Developing this theme, Uhl-Bien (2006) argued that human beings are by their very nature gregarious creatures for whom relationships are defining elements of their identities and creativity. The study of such relationships is, therefore, the study of human nature itself (as cited in Wielenga, 2013). Considering the relational dynamics of facilitators, it is held that embracing the inter-relatedness of those we want to help will prove necessary if we are to be successful in navigating through guiding and supporting others in a healing process. The resulting bonds can create the opportunity for establishing deep connections and trusting relationships. According to Siegel:

The capacity of an individual to reflect upon the experiences of another person may be an essential ingredient in many forms of close, emotionally engaging relationships. This reflection is more than a conceptual ability; it permits the two individuals' minds to enter a form of resonance in which each is able to "feel felt" by the other. This intense and intimate form of connection is manifested in the non-verbal aspects of communication: facial expressions, eye contact, tone of voice, bodily movement, and timing of response. (1999, p. 89 as cited in McLean, 2014)

Experiences, anecdotes, and case studies (McLean & Troung-White, 2015) provided preliminary evidence of a relational construct that is characterized by one's ability to establish and nurture deep interconnectedness, respect, and trust with each relational encounter. Moreover, observations from the field of positive psychology over the last decade reveal that the creation of the type of high quality connections described by this construct can engender trust (Dutton & Heaphy, 2003) and the storyteller's sense of self (Roberts, 2007). McLean and Troung-White (2015) found in their study that such evidence is contained in the social fabric of inter-dependencies that make up a community and is revealed in the interactions of storytellers and listeners. These interactions are the myths, legends, and stories that are archived in the hearts and minds of their characters. To honor these stories, their authors, and the significant contribution of the stories, is wisdom to society.

Dutton and Heaphy (2003) proposed that such connectedness permits the exchange of "vital, life-giving nutrients that strengthen the bond making it healthy, flexible and resilient" (p. 263). Further, Roberts (2007) asserted that such bonds exude positive emotions that "can inspire individuals to enact their reflected best-self" (p. 33). The trail of evidence supporting such benefits of relational development as strong connectedness, a positive sense of self and an enduring source of social capacity serves as ample justification to better understand the importance storytelling.

Fundamental to relational theory is an understanding that growth and development are optimized in a context of connection (Fletcher, 1998, 1999). Empathy, vulnerability, emotional expression, the development of others, and an expectation that the relationship will provide growth opportunities for all involved were found within the research to be key to developing relationally (Fletcher, 1998, 1999). Non-clinical practice in this context is fluid and founded on a relationship between those who aspire to help others share their stories and those who want to tell their stories but are unsure as to how they will be perceived by the listener. Success is wholly dependent upon the capacity to build and sustain those human relationships (Kouzes & Posner, 2003a). Such relational elements within storytelling need a more evolved system than that of mere storyteller and story listener. It must be a fluid symbiosis of interaction that holds at its center a healthy respect for the interdependencies which serve as the lifeblood of the relationship.

The Role of Storytelling in Healing

Sharing stories has been described as a way to foster healing following conflict. Wielenga (2013) argued that the story is in itself not necessarily helpful, but sharing the story fosters the beginning of meaningful change (2013). In order for reconciliation to become reality, Lederach (1997) suggested that healing is most significantly validated through storytelling. He describes storytelling as a living, interactive process through which new ways of engaging and being with one another are born (as cited in Wielenga, 2013). Balcomb takes this further, saying that sharing stories has the biggest impact when we allow the story to be shattered and transformed by that of another. This includes the shattering of stereotypes, assumptions, and ideas that sustain the division between us (as cited in Wielenga, 2013).

Storytelling can be a powerful instrument when it evokes imagery, heightens emotions, challenges perceptions, and inspires. The benefit of storytelling is that it comprises a tale of a character caught in a situation unfolding from start to climax to resolution (Boje, 1991); e.g., describing the ideal, defining reality, then recognizing the problem, discovering solutions, and detecting the next steps. It is not just about telling the story, but about finding the strength and using their voice to tell the story on their own terms. Those voices have the right to record their experiences, as they understand them, including the triumphs and disappointments (Jaffer, 2015). A point to ponder is that telling the story can further a message when it is anchored to something emotional – thus the power of stories.

Being able to perceive reality in new and more varied ways and being able to better understand the complex dynamic between self and others and between one's own reality and the effect of external conditions are critical to any process of personal healing and possible reconciliation with others. In engaging our stories critically, we shift from the limitations of a narrow story towards the possibilities of change (Wielenga, 2013).

Stories give us a common ground for understanding one another and acting in ways that are more inclusive and less destructive. According to Staub, Pearlman and Miller (2003):

As with stories, healing is not an isolated activity undertaken by an individual. It is a process which inevitably involves the one who caused the wound as well as the people with whom we are in a relationship and the broader society around us. (p. 2 as cited in Wielenga, 2013)

If facilitators encourage healing through storytelling, there is then hope that these practitioners can help shape the context of joy and sorrow. This is achieved by providing a framework for the storytellers to fulfill their role with dignity and on their own terms; knowing this may be a painful process piecing together their story. Storytelling is an effective way of helping people understand and acquire conceptual information about the hurt and to engage them emotionally (Mistry, 2017). They are the pioneers of their story and it is extremely important to create the space in which they may be able to understand the historical context in which the dramas unfolded for them. The foundation of whatever means used to create this haven for their stories to be told, must be enveloped in having a way for them to express themselves, feel comfortable in affirming their experiences, and to be able to draw on the knowledge of their existence.

Denning (2011) proposed that stories increase understanding of life changes that nurture the consciousness and communicate a new reality that will flourish without adversarial debate. Thus, one of the fundamental intents behind storytelling as a healing process is that it has the possibility of helping to move from despair to hope. Harris and Barnes (2006) posited that storytelling is significant by the power of such stories as they illustrate the important message during a healing progression.

Story narratives help people make sense and meaning of their changing environment and is a fundamental way we all think and communicate. A story should, per Aristotle's model, contain the three forms of influence – logic, emotion, and character. Logic is the data that is used to support decisions. Emotion is what connects the message with the past experiences and feelings of the storyteller. Character is the amount of trustworthiness given to the storyteller as others listen. (Dolan & Naidu, 2013)

Give the Gift of a Story

The power of one voice giving a gift of a story is a way to promote learning; whether one is the storyteller or the listener (Militello & Guajardo, 2013). It nurtures the inner spirit, touches the heart, and can be as simple as using props such as paper, a handkerchief, shadow puppets, or props from anywhere, even from a saltshaker, all to enhance the story; bringing the ordinary into the extraordinary (McLaren, 2004). Through his lived experiences and research Dr. Houston stated, "Telling and listening to stories has the potential to alter behavior and improve health" (as cited in Parker-Pope, 2011, p. 1). Their stories transform their specific hurt into knowing they have earned the right to be the griot of their own tale, the hero or heroine of their own quest, and a member of their own remembering (Trent, 2017). They just need to be reminded of their enormous talents and abilities to render a world complete with their vision of their place in that world.

It is through their voices that storytellers share their intimate journey, hopefully in a safe place that facilitators have created. One way to create such a place is in a loose structure that frames the storytelling; asks them to tell where they have been or let them know they may retell to others what they choose to tell. Storytelling is about their experiences of relationships and they have their own permission to pay close attention to their inner life – to experience again through their story – because it is the site for growth. There is lovely symmetry between voice and context. Stories told from this view, the inner life, represent redefining and revising while asserting their place in their world. A story that remains in us continues to be painful.

Giving them the gift of storytelling fosters individuals to embrace courage in which they will want to share their deepest thoughts and thus proclaim their worth and dignity, healing their body, mind and spirit. As stories have the capacity to warm hearts, there is a momentary forgetfulness of the pain and struggles; stories enshrine in a circle of healing. Telling stories does not end pain, but is the beginning of nurturing positive traits: resilience, courage, empathy, compassion, loyalty, conscientiousness and openness. This in turn allows people to feel comfortable wearing the face of their true, authentic selves. It is the beginning of celebrating who they are and bringing healing to the hurting.

How do facilitators facilitate a new conversation that helps identify a path through numbness, fear, and painful cycles of hurt? By becoming engaged in their own learning of the significance of storytelling, and then becoming authentic helpers for others to tell their story. One way is to engage in experiential activities. For example, based on the research and the experiential workshops (*Daring Acts)* of Dr. Brown, she discusses how to promote being courageous, accepting vulnerability, and creating the safe place for storytellers to want to tell their story (National Storytelling Network, 2018). Rupi Kaur's poetry states, "If you were born with the weakness to fall, you were born with the strength to rise" (2015, p. 156). In her storytelling poetry she realized that her voice is stronger through the telling of a poem which expresses her hurt and healing. According to Kaur, poetry is a simple yet purposeful example of the physiognomies of a story.

Physiognomies of a Story

Erdrich's novel, *Tales of Burning Love*, awakens the consciousness of the need for storytelling and identifies effective storytelling forms that can be used effectively to heal fractures in the psyche, or to put it metaphorically, to at least soothe our collective toothache (Rosenberg, 2002). There needs to be a creative blending, which is often overlooked as critics seek originality and difference instead of continuity and wholeness. A rich storytelling experience may create a transformative magic, mystical as well as intellectual; making the whole cloth of narrative threads (Rosenberg, 2002).

Healing Ceremonies

Storytelling means "something that comes out of an experience and an understanding of that original view". It is an appreciative knowing that all views are centripetal toward the sacred center, an imaginative construct evoked in the inward-spiraling form of a ceremonial sand painting (Rosenberg, 2002, p. 117). Thus, storytelling "does not accept the brokenness of the present world as an immutable condition of things but invokes deeper patterns of order and meaning . . . as a means of restoring wholeness" (p. 117). For facilitators, this means we gain an understanding of storytelling as a poetic process of creating, transforming, and restoring. This vision is shared, not by the storyteller working alone or a single narrator spinning an isolated web. From the images in the mind of the storyteller, the healing ceremony builds momentum. Thus, language then takes on power. If the words are used properly in the context, whether in a singular or communal voice, oral form or as art, stories return us to ourselves and inspire us to partake in the ceremony of healing. Such a ceremony is described through the words written by Momaday in his essay, *The Way to Rainy Mountain:*

Once in a life, a man ought to concentrate his mind upon the remembered earth . . . to look at it from as many angles as he can, to wonder about it, to dwell upon it. This reintegrative process is particularly important for people who have become disoriented, who have suffered a kind of psychic dislocation of themselves in time and space. The act of storytelling, therefore, is a mystical recombination of past and present, a balancing of multiple perspectives in order to create harmony and psychic healing. (Rosenberg, 2002, p. 118)

A new sense of presence comes from stories of survivance; stories create a new consciousness, reject a notion of domination and oppression, celebrate courage, self-determination and liberation (Rodriguez, 2015). It is an art form or all-embracing expression that produces a story that has a spirit regarded as an element of life. When we share stories, they come to life. We have a responsibility to share stories: "Stories themselves have the power to protect us and even has the power to heal us because the stories are alive" (Rodriguez, 2015).

Language and power are inextricably linked. The spoken word pushes thoughts out of someone's head and into the open. This is often difficult, as it is a battle. However, it can be won through storytelling. Experiences, when packed in a story framework, become that catalyst to uncover the unsaid words which, if they remain inside us, allow the pain to remain. Even though the storyteller may not know the contour of the story and the story may have many disparate pieces of information to convey, it can be a game-changing moment in their healing.

As facilitators it is important to remember we are not the hero who will save the hurting, those hurting are the heroes. The practitioner's stance should be humble, a place of humility, and simply a compassionate voice helping the storytellers to get unstuck in their journey. The main role is to give guidance, confidence, or quiet space so that they can overcome their initial fears and enter into their storytelling conversation knowing there is no judgment.

Storytelling Into Practice

The aforementioned narrative from a small literature review is the launch of sharing with the reader thoughts and ideas of how to tap into the life force of storytelling, which has always been present in the universe. Much of the practice being shared is not so much about the trauma and victimization, but about the soul healing. Stories connect us to place, space, and each one is unique and has a purpose. Stories are not mere artifacts or products but have meaning and can bring healing to the storytellers who make them and those people who listen to them (Rodriquez, 2015).

Following are scenarios as they are shared across the landscape of not only education, but personal and professional venues as well. As this author traveled through the literature, the courage of the storytellers to tell their stories, inspired this writer to continue to travel on her chapter journey. Significant to her journey was hearing many voices as they collaborated in the research and writing of how stories have the panorama to impact healing.

To begin such a journey, a facilitator's mantra could be:

All life forms carry great intelligence. But trees do especially because they spend their entire lives, day and night, in rain, sleet, snow and sun, in deep meditation. So, they have much to impart. The key to communicating and gathering energy from a tree is to recognize the equality in the worth of all life, of the tree's life and your own. (Xochiquetzal & Garcia, 2005, p. 136 as cited in Rodriguez, 2015)

Storytelling has been the glue connecting people. An elegantly simple concept, storytelling as a tool can seem simplistic. However, successfully used it can achieve the objective (Clark, 2004). The objective in this section of the chapter is to unfold three simple scenarios, not complex, that facilitators may want to explore and use in the format in which they are described below, or a version that fits the environment in which the practitioner is working, or with what victim or perpetrator they are working with.

Scenario One: Totem Pole Art

A simplistic yet purposeful approach is to 'tell' their story using a totem pole or *mutupo* (Trent, 2017). To facilitate this approach, the facilitator should first learn the history and meaning of such a storytelling artifact. Then encourage and foster the creation of the storyteller's totem pole, as a mechanism for the story to be less frightening than words.

Totem poles serve many purposes beyond their beauty. Their meanings are as varied as the storytellers that make them. Can you imagine someone who feels they are fearful if asked to use words to tell their story, but with encouragement tell their stories in a visual, hands-on experience? Often using narrative is not understood by the people we are trying to help, because we as helpers may be using words that are not recognized or grasped by those we are trying to help.

By constructing a totem pole, two learning styles come into practice, that of hands-on and visual learning. Telling the story benefits both the narrator and the listener. Telling the story helps the narrator process the possibly traumatizing feelings and opens the door for restoration. The reasons for carving a totem pole remain the same as it did for the Aboriginal people. The story is told through symbols. The story symbols could be a myth or may be a story from life experiences of a person or family.

Here's a story to get you started. It is represented on a totem pole:

One day a woman was picking berries. By accident, she slipped on some bear droppings and spilled the berries. The woman became angry and blamed the bears for her bad luck. The bears heard the woman call them names and became very angry with her. They captured her and took her away to their village. At first the woman felt very sad. She missed her family and her own village. But Bear Father was kind to her. She married Bear Father and they had twin bear cubs. Many years later the woman went back to her village. She taught the people to always respect the bears and all living creatures.

On the pole is a carving of Bear Father who can be seen holding the two cubs. The people of the village are proud to honor the Bear Mother story and to have their respect for nature represented on their village pole. (Trent, 2017)

When using this approach, the facilitator may want to use metaphors when introducing the totem pole experience. Using metaphors conjures up visual images and a significant awareness to ensure the storytellers, who will be designing their own totem pole, know the context in which the metaphor is being used for. For example, if the practitioner says, "*You are a peach*", do the storytellers understand the meaning of that metaphor? If their real-life experiences have never been introduced to that metaphor, there may be a missed opportunity for the storyteller to meet the objective of this approach: to convey her message through the building of a totem pole (The New Indian Express, 2015).

Dr. Noonan, teacher of art therapy at Marylhurst University wrote in the magazine, *Words on the Wing* in 2002, about how metaphors of folktales can help patients in cancer therapy. He wrote, "living with cancer is hardly a fairy tale existence, yet the life portrayed in fairy tales metaphorically describes the inner journey traveled from illness to healing (as cited in National Storytelling Network, 2015).

Scenario Two: Sitting Around the Campfire

Another simple yet purposeful approach is to create a fun and safe place such as a pseudo campfire. Although a campfire scenario may seem insignificant initially, it provides an experience of being a member of a "tribe", and sitting in a circle sharing stories can touch the hearts and minds of everyone engaged in a virtual campfire (or real if possible). When moderating a campfire scenario, focus on therapeutic methods of healing. It is not a performance by the moderator (The New Indian Express, 2015). Performers cannot tell stories. A performer puts himself between the story and the listener (Yashinsky, 2004, p. 150). The facilitator or moderator allows the story to flow from the storyteller directly.

One story that could be shared to begin engaging the campfire folks to feel comfortable and safe is for the practitioner to tell the story of Osun. She is the Elegant Goddess of Love, who is connected to destiny and wisdom. Wouldn't this be a wonderful connection to those hurting who feel their destiny is to never break the cycle of pain? Sharing the message of Osun in a story format builds a relationship and thus an opportunity to build trust.

Osun is the African Goddess of Love and Sweet Waters. She is said to be the protector of the poor and the mother of all orphans. It is Osun who brings to them their needs in this life. Additionally, Osun is regarded as the healer of the sick, the bringer of song, music and dance, as well as depicted as a teacher. In art she is commonly shown as a charming young woman. In some cultures, she is depicted as a mermaid with a fish tale, perhaps as an allusion to her status as the goddess of sweet waters. She is associated with life's bright colors: gold, deep yellow, pink. (Trent, 2017)

Scenario Three: Digital Storytelling

Working in the health fields and attending many health conferences, Rodriquez stated, "There is a predominance of negative stories instead of positive stories about how people have survived adverse health conditions like diabetes, cancer, suicide, physical and emotional abuse, or alcoholism; the positive aspects have been left out of the stories" (2015, p. 109). Ongoing research collaborates Rodriquez's finding through the exploration into digital storytelling as one approach that provides a venue for people to be the storyteller, be it through poetry or prose, dancing or singing, or whatever method the storyteller chooses.

Digital storytelling not only addresses art education, computer technology, and interdisciplinary pedagogy, but it also allows storytellers to cultivate and apply their multiple literacy, artistic, and critical skills to give voice to issues affecting them (Chung, 2007). Advances in computer technology transform society into an environment where digital devices are indispensable. For example, the application of digital storytelling to art education offers tremendous potential for teaching contemporary visual art history to the digital generation. Digital stories derive their power through weaving images, music, narrative and voice together, thereby giving deep dimension to story's characters, situations and insights (Digital Storytelling Association, 2002 as cited in Chung, 2007).

Using this approach is characterized as "a possibility of recovering a centered sense of personal identity and significance" (Rosenberg, 2002, p. 120). Storytelling possesses some of the ceremonial magic and healing power which when transmitted fills the need for love and salvation. However, if using multiple narratives in the process of digitizing stories, be aware that the storytellers may tell their tales in a storytelling cycle; believing that there does not need to be one approved final version or one view of reality which dominates the rest (Rosenberg, 2002). Thus, the peril in beginning this type of storytelling is that storytellers will be discouraged to use the "storytelling cycle" as it may be seen as just "talk". What happens, then, is a perception by the storytellers that there are "no stories in this place"; meaning the facilitator structured the production, process, and even the vibration of the digital experience to be surrounded by a non-encouraging voice, but rather a "stick to the script" type protocol (Rodriguez, 2015).

Thus, as practitioners it is an important step to ensure everyone involved in the digital storytelling process has an understanding about the representation of digital storytelling, and all that it encompasses. The storytellers need to be given the oxygen within a digital environment as they may need to define, refine, and constantly tell their story. Repeatedly telling their story reignites the spark that fueled their courage to use the power of their voice.

A bricolage method is an approach facilitators may use by creating a makeshift studio. An example of how this can occur is:

The bricolage method favors the life world of storytellers working with visual art within a holistic and circular process. Holistic healing includes creative arts and is inclusive of digital storytelling. It captures the interrelatedness of creative arts, culture, and traditional healing and is consistent with holistic worldviews that stress balance, harmony and connectedness. (Archibald & Dewer, 2010, p. 6 as cited in Rodriguez, 2015, p. 83)

To begin such a journey within the makeshift studio, the steps to follow may enhance the experience:

- Introducing the idea that digital stories have a spirit and are living beings, not mere objective artifacts or products as mentioned in digital storytelling literature.
- Perhaps perform a ceremony before beginning to work on the digital process.
- Share with participants that the film creation needs a collaborative approach for "meaning-making".
- Express an appreciation for their resiliency through their strength, courage and bravery; not just surviving but thriving.

Then, before beginning the technical aspect of the filmmaking, share with them this story about the theory of "soul-wind":

As I am building a sacred fire, it starts with that small ember; you blow on it a little bit, and it begins to smoke. You keep feeding it and blowing on it a little more, until that flame comes to life. That is how it feels to build your digital stories. (Rodriguez, 2015, p. 251)

Healing does not end with this one approach, digital storytelling. It needs to be nurtured so the storytellers can continue to heal and create strength-based relationships. This is a deep and personal way of sharing a significant part of their lives. It is similar to producing a documentary in which the practitioner is in the role of cameraperson, and the storytellers are given the safe place to share their journey of being allowed to make meaning about their own life experiences through their own eyes, using their own voice.

CONCLUSION

Howe (2008) argued that stories are a foundational principle of autonomy, "no matter what form they take—history, drama, memoir, poem, painting, dance – seem to pull all the elements together" (p. x as cited in Rodriguez, 2015).

Research in various fields – neural biology, cognitive science, developmental psychology, clinical psychology, neural linguistics, education, information theory, knowledge management, organizational theory, anthropology, narratology, medical science, narrative therapy and, of course storytelling - agree that the human mind receives, processes, and responds to stories (Haven, 2007). This extraordinary truth is that storytelling is a method used to teach, to inspire, to inform and to educate.

One of the tasks of the facilitator is to make certain that the voices of those now silent, of those often forgotten, are heard if they voluntarily want to be heard (Welton, n.d.). Using their voices is a transformational experience in self-understanding and identity. Thus, their storytelling is with emancipatory intention to bring their feelings of isolation and loneliness into conversations with the facilitator or even with the group.

There is a transformative power of storytelling which shows a path, shines a light on the way, teaches us how to see, and reminds us of the greatest human possibilities (Feldman & Kormfield, 2018). Knowing stories are intangible, they have something solid that helps maintain a sense of purpose during times of healing. Storytelling to heal is nothing new. Aristotle told us this in "Poetics" that the art of storytelling is what gives us a shareable world. Health, disease, illness, death – we have been telling each other stories of these since the beginning of time.

What people are really looking for is some kind of human connection; a heart print. They do not want to stay camouflaged but are unsure how to stop blending into the environment. This is where facilitators can make a positive difference in other's lives – an ideal opportunity for connecting which when done well, the results can be outstanding. Human beings are, at times, lonesome animals. Yet, we spend all our life trying to be less lonesome. You are not alone as you thought (John Steinbeck as cited in Parker-Pope 2011).

Neuroscientist Anthony Damasio said, "Storytelling is something brains automatically do, naturally and implicitly. It should be no surprise that stories pervade the entire fabric of human connectedness" (2010, p. 293 as cited by Haven, 2014). In a keynote presentation, Syd Liberman quoted an elder in his community who stated, "If, at the end of our lives, we do not have stories, what have we got?" (Clark, 2004, p. 200).

REFERENCES

Boje, D. M. (1991). Learning story telling: Storytelling to learn management skills. *Journal of Management Education*, *49*(2), 279–294. doi:10.1177/105256299101500302

Chung, S. K. (2007). Art education technology: Digital storytelling. *Art Education*, *60*(2), 17–22.

Clark, E. (2004). *Around the Corporate Campfire*. Sammamish, WA: C&C Publishing.

Cobley, P. (2001). *Narrative*. London: Routledge.

Denning, S. (2011). *The leader's guide to storytelling: Mastering the art and discipline of business narrative*. San Francisco, CA: Jossey-Bass.

Dolan, G., & Naidu, Y. (2013). *Hooked: How leaders connect, engage and inspire with storytelling*. John Wiley & Sons. [Kindle Edition]. Retrieved from http://www.amazon.com/dp/

Duarte, N. (2010). *Resonate*. Hoboken, NJ: John Wiley & Sons.

Dutton, J., & Heaphy, E. (2003). The power of high quality connections. In K. Cameron, J. Dutton, & R. Quinn (Eds.), *Positive organizational scholarship* (pp. 263–278). San Francisco, CA: Berrett-Koehler.

Feldman, C., & Kornfield, J. (2015, April). Symposium conducted at the National Storytelling Network, Kansas City, MO.

Fisher, W. R. (1989). Clarifying the narrative paradigm. *Communication Monographs*, *56*(1), 55–58. doi:10.1080/03637758909390249

Fletcher, J. (1998). Relational practice: A feminist reconstruction of work. *Journal of Management Inquiry*, *7*(2), 163–186. doi:10.1177/105649269872012

Fletcher, J. (1999). *Disappearing acts: Gender, power, and relational practice at work*. Cambridge, MA: The MIT Press.

Good, J. (2003). Storytelling builds compassionate communities. *Edmonton Journal*. Retrieved from https://search.proquest.com/docview/252999613

Harris, J., & Kim Barnes, B. (2006). Leadership storytelling. *Industrial and Commercial Training*, *38*(7), 350–353. doi:10.1108/00197850610704534

Haven, K. (2007). *Story proof: The Science behind the startling power of story*. Westport, CT: Greenwood Publishing Group.

Healing through storytelling. (2015). *The New Indian Express*. Retrieved from http://proxy.stu.edu:2048

Howard, J. (1991). Entertainment spiritual warmth of storytelling art attracts listeners. *Las Vegas Review Journal*. Retrieved from https://search.proquest.com/docview/259857659

Jaffer, Z. (2015). *Healing our wounds through storytelling*. Retrieved from http://proxy.stu.edu:2048

Kaur, R. (2015). *Milk and honey*. Kansas City, MO: Andrews McMeel Publishing.

Kouzes, J., & Posner, B. (2003a). The five practices of exemplary leadership. In J. Gallos (Ed.), *Business leadership* (pp. 72–84). San Francisco, CA: John Wiley and Sons.

Lederach, J. P. (1997). *Building peace*. Washington, DC: United Institute of Peace.

McLaren, B. (2004). Learn to give the gift of a story. *The News*. Retrieved from https://search.proquest.com/docview/374985926

McLean, D. (2011). *Relationship agility and its impact on leader success – a case study*. Unpublished manuscript, Leadership and Change Program, Antioch University, Yellow Springs, OH.

McLean, D. (2014). *Understanding relational agility exploring constructs of relational leadership through story* (Doctoral Dissertation). Culver City, CA: Antioch University.

McLean, L., & Truong-White, H. (2015). Digital storytelling for transformative global citizenship education. *Canadian Journal of Education*, *38*(2).

Militello, M., & Guarjardo, F. (2013). Virtually speaking: How digital storytelling can facilitate organizational learning. *Journal of Community Positive Practice.*, *13*(2), 80–91.

Mistry, A. (2017). The art of storytelling: Cognition and action through stories. *The International Journal of the Arts in Society*, *09*(04), 301–324.

National Storytelling Network. (2018, Spring). *Healing Story Alliance Member's Newsletter*.

New Indian Express. (2015). *Healing through storytelling*. Retrieved from https://search.proquest.com/docview/1655891942

Parker-Pope, T. (2011. February). Healing through storytelling. *New York Times.*

Roberts, L. M. (2007). From proving to becoming: How positive relationships create a context for self-discovery and self-actualization. In J. Dutton & B. Rose (Eds.), *Exploring positive relationships at work: Building a theoretical and research foundation* (pp. 29–45). New York, NY: Psychology Press.

Rodriguez, C. (2015). *The Journey of a digital story: A Healing performance of mino-bimaadiziwin: The Good life* (Doctoral Dissertation). Retrieved from https://search.proquest.com/3731363

Rosenberg, R. (2002). Ceremonial healing and the multiple narrative tradition in Louise Erdrich's Tales of Burning Love. *Melus, 27*(3), 113. doi:10.2307/3250658

Sager, G. (2012, May). The art of storytelling. *Natural Life Magazine*, 21-23. Retrieved from https://search.proquest.com/2048

Saxberg, L. (1996). Storytelling comes alive as an art form. *The Ottawa Citizen.* Retrieved from https://search.proquest.com/docview/239974028

Strickler, J. (1990). Tell me a story: Storytellers hope ancient art can survive in modern society. *Star Tribune*. Retrieved from https://search.proquest.com/docview/418103779

Trent, T. (2017). *The Awakened Woman: Remembering and reigniting our sacred dreams.* New York: Simon & Schuster.

Welton, M. R. (n.d.). *Echoes of those now silent: Canadian women's associations as learning sites.* Retrieved from www.populareducation.co.za/sites/default/files

Wielenga, C. (2013). Shattered stories: Healing and reconciliation in the south African context. *Verbum Et Ecclesia, 34*(1), 1-8. Retrieved from https://search.proquest.com/docview/1635231523

Yashinsky, D. (2004). *Suddenly they heard footsteps.* Jackson, MS: University Press of Mississippi.

Chapter 3
Healing Our Heroes:
Creating an Arts-Based Intervention

Amy M. Grebe
Zinnia Consulting and Design, USA

ABSTRACT

Societies rely on first responders to save lives. What happens when the wellbeing of these crisis workers is compromised by daily exposure to crisis and trauma? This chapter describes a developed and tested arts-based intervention aimed at mitigating the trauma response through positive resource reinforcement. Specifically designed to be used in a non-clinical setting, the intervention features the drawing of a mandala capturing images and symbols of safety and was tested to ascertain the efficacy of its ability to increase positive affect, decrease negative affect, and reinforce connections to positive resources in participants.

INTRODUCTION

Emergency and crisis workers are our everyday heroes. They pull out us out of our darkest, scariest moments. We owe them depths of gratitude. Yet what happens when pieces of that dark and scary moment stay with these heroes? Not a day goes by that professional and volunteer crisis workers do not respond to a traumatizing event. While crisis workers are trained and prepared for the highly charged environment of emergency response, exposure to the events has significant impact on emotional and psychological well-being. Many suggestions of self-care activities are offered, but rarely do these provide immediate relief from the burgeoning emotions experienced during the event. Cumulative exposure and layering of empathetic response to traumatic events lead crisis workers to form maladaptive coping mechanisms, advancing the natural stress response to deepen into a disrupted belief system and vicarious trauma. Symptoms of vicarious trauma echo those of post-traumatic stress disorder (PTSD), having the potential to render crisis workers ineffective in their duties and creating one more victim of the disaster. By developing an arts based method for preventing vicarious trauma, this study seeks to add to the existing body of literature and best practices related to trauma disorder prevention.

DOI: 10.4018/978-1-5225-5981-8.ch003

Common to all groups of first responders is that, following a traumatic event, they will be among the first present at trauma sites and often the very first to attend to the victims. A look at the literature, however, shows that the first responder group as a whole is much less studied than victims of the same events that they attend. (Kleim & Westphal, 2011, p. 17)

Statistics specifically related to vicarious trauma in crisis workers are not readily available. Instead, the literature provides statistics on PTSD symptoms in crisis workers. It is unclear though, whether these symptoms are the result of direct exposure to the trauma experience or interaction with the trauma victims and aftermath of the crisis. As the symptoms of vicarious trauma and PTSD present similarly, statistics on PTSD in crisis workers may still provide insight into the depth of the problem and validation for further research.

Research examining symptoms of posttraumatic stress disorder (PTSD) in Chinese crisis workers found significantly higher rates of burnout and PTSD symptoms in the crisis workers than in nonclinical professions. Among these crisis workers exposed to traumatic events, 26% of the research participants demonstrated symptoms of PTSD. (Shakespeare-Finch, 2011) A specific study on Australian firefighters found 7% with severe levels of PTSD and an overwhelming 68% with moderate levels. Twenty-one percent (21%) of Japanese crisis workers reported with symptoms of PTSD due to their work following earthquakes, typhoons, and volcano eruptions (Kleim & Westphal, 2011). New Zealand studies found that 30% of paramedics and 46% of police officers exhibited moderate to high levels of PTSD symptoms (Regehr, 2001). The most recent study in the United States (US) indicates that of the 84% who have experienced a traumatic event, 34% go on to be diagnosed with a mental health disorder. Ten percent (10%) of US crisis workers are diagnosed with PTSD. While significantly lower than other countries, many cite negative repercussions in the workplace as a reason to avoid diagnosis and treatment (University of Phoenix, 2017).

Despite these alarming statistics, a larger volume of literature about emotional and psychological responses to trauma is written about the primary victim. Emotional and psychological impairments in crisis workers correlate to high personal and public costs. Maladaptive coping mechanisms adversely affect the ability to serve trauma victims. Considering the pervasiveness of emotional and psychological impairments in crisis workers, it is of critical importance to develop interventions based on an understanding of the risks that contribute to stress reactions and traumatic disorders (Kleim & Westphal, 2011, p. 21).

Art making serves as a vessel or container in which to hold cathartic emotional venting or facilitate the cognitive integration of the traumatic experience. Art making can offer a refuge from intense feelings of stress, anxiety, and terror; providing a container to capture the felt response to the trauma experience. Where verbal expression of the trauma experience may serve to retraumatize the participants, art making better moves the traumatized towards psychological and physical well-being. When the trauma occurs at such a depth to alter or disrupt belief systems and world view, creativity is the necessary tool for rebuilding schemas and reconnecting to self and reality.

BACKGROUND

Understanding previous studies and research on the emotional, cognitive, and psychological impact of traumatic experiences on crisis workers is critical to the successful building of a conceptual framework of the risk and protective factors associated with vicarious trauma. It is important to explore the work of the crisis responders and their exposure to traumatic experiences that provoke symptoms of secondary traumatic stress and vicarious trauma. Reviewing various literature provides definitions and parameters in which the developed intervention fits into the framework of the constructivist self-development theory (CSDT). The efficacy of previously tested interventions as well as recent research in the field of art therapy help to lay the groundwork on which the arts based, vicarious trauma intervention described in this chapter is built.

Exposure to Traumatic Experiences

"Crisis workers are front-line first responders for whom potential exposure to occupational trauma is a fact of daily life" (Beaton & Murphy, 1995, p. 51). These responders include medical personnel at accident and emergency sites, rescue disaster workers, firefighters, and police, among others, who have great probability of experiencing "traumatic events such as extreme violence, mass disasters, and infectious disease exposure" (Shakespeare-Finch, 2011, p. 1). While willingly entering into situations that threaten their own lives, first responders and disaster workers may work with traumatized survivors or may have the difficult task of recovering the dead (Kleim & Westphal, 2011). They may be exposed to the 'other side of the world' and face scenes of extreme poverty, abuse and neglect, patients harboring intense fear or mental illness, and terrible injustices (Young, 2005). When faced with these traumatic incidents, crisis workers are "frequently afflicted with mental health outcomes" (Kleim & Westphal, 2011, p. 18).

Mental Health Outcomes

Crisis workers will be affected by trauma in some way, whether through their contact with trauma victims, through graphic images of trauma and disaster, or through concern for their own safety and well-being (Nelson, 1996; Bell, Kulkarni, & Dalton, 2003). Repeated exposure to highly traumatized clients or traumatic events may lead crisis workers to experience secondary trauma stress (STS) or vicarious trauma (VT) (Bell, Kulkarni, & Dalton, 2003; Helm, 2011). "While not every practitioner who works with traumatized clients will develop vicarious traumatization, all are potentially at risk" (Helm, 1996, p. 18).

The terms secondary trauma stress (STS) and vicarious trauma (VT) are often used interchangeably in research literature. It is important to discern the difference between STS and VT as well as the terms compassion fatigue and burnout. While compassion fatigue and burnout are terms that commonly accompany and are defined similarly to STS and VT, neither present symptoms with the intense severity of STS and VT.

Secondary trauma stress is the result of those who work with trauma survivors and witness their stories and visual evidence. STS is an occupational hazard for crisis workers providing direct services to trauma victims. It is the stress "resulting from helping or wanting to help a traumatized or suffering person" (Figley, 1995, p. 7). Beaton and Murphy define the three operational components of STS as: "(1) Having witnessed or been confronted by actual or threatened death or injury, or by a threat to the physical integrity of oneself or others; (2) provocation by the stressor of responses of fear, horror, or helplessness; and (3) direct or indirect exposure to an exceptional mental or physical stressor, either brief or prolonged" (1995, p. 52). Secondary traumatic stress is unpreventable as stress is a natural and universal response to violent or disaster situations. The cumulative effects of this negative response, however, can be prevented from developing into a disorder (Yassen, 1995).

Immediately following a crisis, responders may experience symptoms of posttraumatic stress. Over time, this stress can build and begin to alter belief systems (Bober & Regehr, 2006). Crisis workers who experience a "change in their worldview or psychological frame of reference" (Pryce, Shackelford, & Price, 2007, p. 52) suffer from vicarious trauma. Vicarious trauma is defined as "the transformation that occurs in the inner experience of [crisis worker] that comes about as a result of empathic engagement with clients' trauma material" (Bell, Kulkarni, & Dalton, 2003, p. 464; Killian, 2008; Saakvitne & Pearlman, 1996).

Without early intervention, secondary trauma stress may develop into vicarious trauma which may present a manifestation of symptoms of post-traumatic stress disorder (PTSD) (Bourassa, 2011; Helm, 2011; Killian, 2008; Bell, Kulkarni, & Dalton, 2003). VT symptoms have the ability to "disrupt, dissolve, and destroy careers, families, and even lives" (Showalter, 2010). These symptoms may include fear and anxiety, sleep disturbance, hypervigilance, difficulty concentrating, and problems controlling anger. A distortion in the perception of safety and the ability to trust others may also be experienced (Killian, 2008; Setti & Argentero, 2014). Amidst the senselessness of disaster and crises, crisis workers may question their right to survive and thrive and develop survivor guilt and self-loathing (Helm, 1996). "Longer term reactions can include emotional and physical depletion, a sense of hopelessness, and a changed world view in which others are viewed with suspicion and cynicism" (Bober & Regehr, 2006, p. 2). Crisis workers rely on their mental and emotional well-being to effectively complete necessary tasks and support victims. "The deleterious effects of vicarious trauma can severely influence the work they do with clients" (Helm, 1996).

Constructivist Self-Development Theory

Repeated exposure to trauma challenges an individual's perception of reality. To cope, crisis workers may adapt an irrational or distorted belief system to protect themselves from the harm caused by trauma (Helm, 2011). McCann and Pearlman (1990) suggest the theory of constructivist self-development as a framework for understanding vicarious trauma. Constructivist self-development theory (CSDT) asserts that individuals develop their cognitive schemas based on their interactions and perceptions of the world. These schemas create mental templates of self and others (Regehr, 2001; Pearlman & Saakvitne, 1995). "CSDT understands the individual's adaptation to trauma as an interaction between his personality, personal history, the traumatic event and its context, within the social and cultural contexts for the event and its aftermath" (McCann & Pearlman, 1990b, p. 60). Helm (2011) posits that symptoms of vicarious trauma appear as adaptations to the traumatic event in order for the crisis worker to manage feelings and thoughts.

CDST also asserts that the changes in cognitive schemas have the potential to affect all aspects of a crisis worker's life and can accumulate layers as new trauma reinforces beliefs and schemas (Helm, 2011). According to this theory, exposure to trauma and crisis may affect five components of self or cognitive schemas. The five components that drive behavior and frame relationships are safety, trust, intimacy, control, and esteem. These affected components begin to alter an individual's frame of reference or his or her worldview, identity, and spirituality (Pearlman & Saakvitne, 1995).

Worldview incorporates an individual's general beliefs about the world, attitudes towards others, and beliefs surrounding justice and good versus evil. Identity refers to an individual's life story and their real and perceived relationship to others. Spirituality is described as an individual sense of connection to something greater than self (Pearlman & Saakvitne, 1995). Crisis workers who experience vicarious trauma have felt their sense of self threatened or compromised and adjust their frame of reference accordingly.

Though it is unclear, a crisis worker's trauma history may make him or her vulnerable to vicarious trauma. "Pearlman and McCann (1995) reported significantly more vicarious trauma symptoms in 60% of the therapists they surveyed who reported a personal history of trauma" (Bell, Kulkarni, & Dalton, 2003, p. 465). Other studies found that response to traumatic events is precipitated by biological determinants, cumulative life stressors, previous mental health problems, and a history of mental illness (Regher, 2001). Although there appears to be a high level of resilience to the work-related stress among those who regularly respond to trauma and disasters, there remains a significant potential for all crisis workers to succumb to the contagious effects of trauma and therefore, a heightened potential for vicarious trauma.

Regardless of susceptibility towards vicarious trauma, preventable measures should be taken to mitigate VT for the well-being of the crisis worker and those under his or her care.

Carefully designed prevention programs "based on research and applied to the specifics of the context, may be effective tools in promoting mental health" (Shakespeare-Finch, 2011, p. 2). Additionally, early intervention strategies should be designed specifically to lessen post-traumatic stress reactions and provide crisis workers with opportunities to heal and recover (Regehr, 2001; US Department of Health and Human Services, 2005). Developing these interventions through CSDT framework requires addressing both the individual's frame of reference and cognitive schemas. "This process of rebuilding a sense of self requires holistic transformation, as well developing a sense of purpose within meaningful social roles and relationships" (Van Lith, 2014, p. 20).

EFFICACY OF CURRENT VICARIOUS TRAUMA INTERVENTIONS

Self-Care

A culture of self-care has become the model for vicarious trauma intervention. Self-care can be defined as any measure taken to ensure well-being and support good health. Research indicates that self-care promotes resilience, decreases work related stress, and protects against VT (Lee & Miller, 2013; Bourassa, 2011). Self-care can help crisis workers enhance their care of others while balancing their life and work and ultimately, preventing or reducing symptoms of vicarious trauma (Showalter, 2010). Currently, the majority of organizations provide crisis workers with the following suggestions to prevent vicarious trauma:

- Adhere to established safety policies and procedures.
- Encourage and support coworkers.
- Recognize that "not having enough to do" or "waiting" are expected parts of disaster mental health response.
- Take regular breaks whenever you experience troubling incidents and after each work shift. Use time off to "decompress."
- Practice relaxation techniques such as deep breathing, meditation, and gentle stretching.
- Eat regular, nutritious meals and get enough sleep.
- Avoid alcohol, tobacco, drugs, and excessive caffeine.
- Stay in contact with your family and friends.

- Pace self between low and high-stress activities. (US Department of Health and Human Services, 2005)

Additional suggestions may include setting personal boundaries, accepting duties within the scope of experience and training, and engaging in pre-incident training and preparation.

Mental health professionals have long advocated that trauma victims be neither blamed for their victimization nor their trauma response. "When addressing the distress of colleagues, we have focused on the use of individual coping strategies, implying that those who feel traumatized may not be balancing life and work adequately and may not be making effective use of leisure, self-care, or supervision" (Bober & Regehr, 2006, p. 8). Yet, research by Bober and Regehr found no evidence that engaging in the above described recommended prevention methods successfully reduces stress or has an impact on vicarious trauma symptoms. Not only did these prescribed coping methods fail to reduce stress, crisis workers with disrupted belief systems are significantly less likely to engage in self-care in the first place (Bober & Regehr, 2006).

Crisis Debriefing Model

One such response to the need for early intervention methods to mitigate post-traumatic stress responses in crisis workers is the crisis debriefing model. The crisis debriefing model is "based on the premise that emergency service professionals possess the internal resources to deal with most work-related events but can benefit from limited extra assistance in extreme circumstances" (Regehr, 2001, p. 88). This intervention modality provides a group setting in which to vent experienced feelings. During a session, an event will be reviewed and discussed with particular attention placed on emotional and behavioral responses to the event. The facilitator is charged with helping the group to "normalize" their reactions and reinforce coping skills (Regehr, 2001). Therapists and counselors have raised concerns that the debriefing session may inadvertently re-traumatize some participants. As the group is sharing their memories of the event, graphic descriptions may set off the same neurobiological response felt during the initial trauma and may further imbed the perceived threat to self (Devilly, Gist, & Cotton, 2006; Regehr, 2001). "It is at this point that premature verbal psychological interpretation can do tremendous damage by cutting off expression altogether" (Kivnick & Erikson, 2010, p. 613). This is particularly true in those who are prone to stress or arousal (Devilly, Gist, & Cotton, 2006). Instead of preventing or mitigating the trauma response, the debriefing session has the potential to move the crisis worker closer towards vicarious trauma and PTSD.

Written Expression

Significant research has been conducted into the efficacy of promoting physical and psychological well-being through the written accounting of the traumatic experience (Henderson, Rosen, & Mascaro, 2007). Forming a narrative that merges the traumatic event with the emotional and mental process of the experience can create a cognitive integration. This cognitive restructuring serves to resolve the traumatic experience, as well as bring a sense of meaning to the event as insights are gained through the process of writing. Once a meaningful and integrated narrative is formed, it is hypothesized that the traumatic event can then be summarized, stored, and allowed to become a nonthreatening memory rather than a ghost that chronically haunts consciousness, subsequently leading to a decrease in psychological distress (Henderson, Rosen, & Mascaro, 2007).

Research suggests that using writing as an emotional catharsis for just a few moments over the course of three to four days brings about significant improvements in emotional well-being (Henderson, Rosen, & Mascaro, 2007). "Perhaps expressive writing improves both physical and psychological health because it allows individuals to form coherent narratives of their experiences, and the formation of coherent narrative may assist individuals in regulating and understanding their emotions" (Drake & Winner, 2012, p. 255).

Though this cognitive restructuring is of critical importance, like the crisis debriefing model, a written catharsis or venting may not provide relief for all crisis workers. "The written disclosure paradigm has been found to be ineffective among individuals with disordered cognitive processes or relatively severe depression" while some individuals process more successfully engaging in "visual-spatial exercises and experiences to verbal ones" (Henderson, Rosen, & Mascaro, 2007, p. 148). Additionally, studies indicate that art making offers more immediate affective benefits than writing activities that tend to produce results more long term (Drake & Winner, 2012).

Art Making as Vicarious Trauma Intervention

Crisis responders who experience a shift in their frame of reference as a result of exposure to traumatic events may be responsive to and greatly benefit from "short-term cognitive-behavioral interventions that help to modify maladaptive trauma-related appraisals" (Kleim & Westphal, 2011, p. 20). "Creativity is necessary in the process of rebuilding a new schema after the shattering of one's own belief system, of reconnecting with a changed reality, and of rediscovery of the mind-body connection" (Sutton, 2002, p. 76). Every person possesses creativity and therefore has the capacity to self-heal through the therapeutic process of art making (Camilleri, 2007). Art making allows those engaging in the activity the ability to communicate and make meaning while regulating emotion and discharging negative feelings through the creative process of self-expression (Drake & Winner, 2012). "Through emotional release and through reframing which arise through the art process or the visual content of art, new perceptions of the self and relationships are made possible" (Irving & The Union Institute, 1995).

Crisis workers finding difficulty or anxiety in articulating emotions or reactions through verbal means may have greater success releasing these feelings through artistic expression (Curry & Kasser, 2005; Irving & The Union Institute, 1995). Several studies have examined the efficacy of art making in comparison to written forms of release or reframing. Pizzaro's 2004 study examines the efficacy of art and writing in increasing positive mental health outcomes as well as participant retention in the therapies following a traumatic experience. While writing activities increased their mental health, art making participants found more enjoyment and were more likely to return to the art making activity than those in the writing group. Consistent with Pizarro, further studies found that art making provided them relief and increased their mood more effectively than writing (Drake, Coleman, & Winner, 2015; Van Lith, 2014). Participants understood that written or verbal forms of communicating their experiences would not have provided the same level of relief. "Instead, it was the symbolic and metaphorical meanings formed during the art making process that assisted in providing a sense of harmony, inner peace, social inclusiveness, and mental balance" (Van Lith, 2014, 28). Art making and the creative process allow the maker to fully experience and express emotions without distorting or inhibiting them as may happen with the interactive audience of a debriefing session. During the process of creating art, a trusting relationship builds between the art maker and the material. Emotions and memories that were previously inexpressible, now becomes expressible through the "external, impersonal, nonverbal nature of materials" (Kivnick & Erikson, 2010, p. 606 & 613).

While both art making and verbal expression may allow for an emotional release and a shift towards a more positive affect, art making moves beyond cognitive aspects to release and reframe the somatic experience. Emotions created by trauma and stress impact the physical body and may have lingering effects as these emotions settle and store themselves in the body. According to psychoanalytic theory, repressing feelings and emotions can lead to psychiatric symptomatology or psychosomatic symptoms (Kivnick & Erikson, 2010). Psychosomatic symptoms are decreased and released from the body through the art making experience of the visual expression coupled with the "tactile experience and kinaesthetic movement." The process of art making has far greater success than verbal expression in the interpretation of anxiety, stress, and somatic response (Irving & The Union Institute, 1995). Additionally, art making provides opportunities for "maintaining optimistic perseverance, seeking inner peace, and instituting contingency control" (Yassan, 2001, p. 188).

Venting, Distraction, and Positive Emotion

It is understood that art making brings about many positive results such as decreasing stress and anxiety, releasing somatic sensations, and increasing positive affect. In fact, using art making to let go of negative feelings is the underlying principle of art therapy (Drake & Winner, 2012). Several studies have gone on to examine what allows art making to be such a successful intervention; specifically, examining whether it is due to a cathartic release (venting) or a distraction from the stressor. In 2005, De Petrillo and Winner tested the key assumption that art making could repair mood, leaving the art makers feeling more positive and calm even in those participants who reportedly possessed no interest or ability in art. Their study built upon Pizarro's study and contained two drawing groups, one with a prompt that allowed participants to vent while the other prompted to draw something happy, and a control distraction group. All participants demonstrated an increase in positive mood though positive mood increased the most in the positive emotion group. Dalebroux et al.'s 2008 replication study supports these findings. "Art making is most beneficial for mood repair when the artist creates art with content associated with positive emotions" (Dalebroux, Goldstein, & Winner, 2008, p. 289). This study also determined that mood improved in the distraction condition group at a greater rate than in the venting or control condition groups.

When attention is given to a negative mood, it may lead to an attempt to repair the mood. Alternatively, giving energy to the negative mood may prolong and intensify the mood, making it more difficult to reach a more positive mood or affect. Venting the negative emotion may lead to rumination which only serves to deepen the emotion (Dalebroux et al., 2008; Drake et al, 2015). Distraction, or the prevention of focusing on only one thing, is more effective for self-regulating mood and moving away from negative affect (Thayer, Newman, & McClain, 1994). Drake and Winner further test the efficacy of distraction and venting in their 2012 study. Differing from the Dalebroux et al. study, this study provides the distraction condition with a neutral prompt rather than positive content. Regardless of the prompt, the research demonstrates again that art making as distraction is a more effective form of mood regulation than venting. Most recent research once again confirms that art making is more effective at short term mood repair than writing, while distraction is more effective at increasing positive affect than venting (Drake, Coleman, & Winner, 2015).

Mandalas

Art making can also serve as a vessel or container in which to hold cathartic emotional venting or facilitate the cognitive integration of the traumatic experience. Art making can offer a refuge from the intense emotions surrounding grief; providing a container to capture the felt response to the trauma experience. The imagination finds an unlimited way in which to express feelings and responses and the art work serves to archive the experience (Rappaport, 1998; Stuckey & Nobel, 2010). Rappaport states that "the first thing that comes to mind, is that art is a great container for difficult feelings, especially difficult feelings, volatile feeling like anger and rage. With trauma the rage is really big" (1998, p. 6). Art making provides a container to hold and facilitate forward movement or movement away from PTSD response (Rappaport, 1998).

Mandala drawing has been recognized as an art making activity "that lends itself particularly well to the symbolic expression and disclosure of a traumatic event" (DeLue, 1999; Henderson, Rosen, & Mascaro, 2007). In the field of art therapy, a mandala is generally considered any art form that is created in a circular fashion; a shape that can easily be viewed as a metaphoric container. Research indicates that those who drew within a circle experienced a more positive affect than those who drew within other shapes (Henderson, Rosen, & Mascaro, 2007).

The mandala functions as a symbolic representation of emotionally laden and conflicting material, yet at the same time provides a sense of order and integration to this material. In this manner, drawing a mandala is similar to a written disclosure in that it provides cognitive organization to complex emotional experiences (Henderson, Rosen, & Mascaro, 2007, p. 149).

The origins of the mandala can be traced back to Tibetan Buddhists who used mandalas to communicate complex philosophical ponderings. Mandalas were also used in meditative practices to induce altered states of consciousness (Fincher, 2014). Carl Jung was the first Westerner to recognize the healing properties of mandalas. He "suggested that the act of drawing mandalas had a calming and healing effect on its creator while at the same time facilitating psychic integration and personal meaning in life" (as cited in Henderson, Rosen, & Mascaro, 2007, p. 149). Jung understood the mandala to represent the inner journey of his patients to wholeness and wellness as they resolve inner conflicts (Fincher, 2014).

Creating mandalas is suggested in art therapy as a successful activity for centering, meditation, emotional expression, and self-soothing. Drawing and filling a mandala is found to be calming. The structure of the circle serves both to provide a sense of containment and to decrease anxiety. Csikszentmihalyi uses the word flow to describe the action of engaging in the creative process to provide distance from stressors (Metzl & Morrell, 2008). "The concept of flow thus offers a form of well-being for the creator, supporting creativity as a protective or promotive factor during adversity" (Metzl & Morrell, 2008, p. 309).

When presented with a blank, rectangular sheet of paper, many clients experience anxiety and the expectation of creating a "good picture." A starting point provided by the circle offers comfort (Mehlomakulu, 2012). Art psychotherapists rely on the comfort offered by the circle to help their clients discover self-awareness, self-expression, conflict resolution, and healing (Fincher, 1991; Henderson, Rosen, & Mascaro, 2007). What is created within, and sometimes outside, of the mandala provide insight for the therapist and help to map a treatment plan (Farrelly-Hansen, 2001).

Curry and Kasser (2005) designed a study to test the effectiveness of using mandalas to reduce anxiety. This study was based on earlier research by Belchamber in 1997 on the use of "coloring therapy". "When individuals color complex geometric forms, they are provided an opportunity to suspend their 'inner dialogue' (distraction) and to deeply engage in an activity that removes them from the flow of negative thoughts and emotion that can sometimes dominate their lives" (p. 81). A near meditative state can be achieved by coloring in the symmetrical shapes and patterns of a mandala. In replicating Curry and Kasser's study, van der Vennet (2012) found that greater decrease in anxiety occurred in study participants who colored a mandala in comparison to those who colored a plaid design or blank sheet of paper.

Henderson, Rosen, and Mascaro (2007) hypothesized that mandala drawing would greatly increase psychological and physical health not only immediately, but also at a one month follow session. Participants in the mandala drawing condition were asked to fill their circle with images related to their trauma experience while the control group was tasked with a still life drawing. Though their hypothesis for overall psychological well-being was not realized, the greatest outcome of the study was a significant decrease in PTSD symptoms (Henderson, Rosen, & Macaro, 2007). A replication study demonstrated opposite findings when the mandala drawing condition was not prompted to focus on the trauma experience. In this study, the control group showed greater signs of decreasing PTSD symptoms at the one month follow up (Henderson, 2007). Henderson further pursued the efficacy of mandalas in her 2012 study.

Positive affect has been shown to have a strengthening, uplifting effect on well-being and the ability to cope with stressors (Frederickson & Joiner, 2002), and interventions that increase people's experience of positive emotion can help to build their social, physical, and psychological resources (Fredrickson, 2008; Fredrickson et al., 2008; Lyubomirsky, King, & Diener, 2005; Russell & Fosha, 2008) (as cited in Henderson, 2012).

Negative emotions and affect formed as an adaptation to a trauma experience may threaten survival while positive affect broadens thinking and focus (Henderson, 2012). This study examined the ability to improve well-being by using the mandala to engage the whole self while exploring positive emotions rather than the trauma experience. Though the researcher was unable achieve the desired increase in psychological and physical well-being, study participants consistently demonstrated increased positive emotion and affect following each drawing session. Creating mandalas that express positive emotions "should prove be an effective intervention to produce sustained positive affect once the 'dose' is discovered (Henderson, 2012).

Background Summary

Vicarious trauma is unlikely to occur in one incident of trauma exposure, but rather through repeated exposure creating cumulative layering of stress. Vicarious trauma then occurs in that moment when the stress to body, mind, and spirit cause a break in perception of self and world. Crisis workers may find little relief from the very real and constant threat to safety and health of themselves and those with whom they work. Without relief, this external threat shifts to the internal threat of vicarious trauma and post-traumatic stress disorder with potentially devastating effects to self and others.

Interventions developed through the theoretical framework of the constructivist self-development theory would act in such a way as to slow or prevent cognitive restructuring towards a more negative frame of reference. In order to do so, it is suggested that crisis workers maintain a positive affect. This would allow them to remain open to positive resources for themselves, better cope with stressors, and remain better equipped to deal with the trauma experience.

Art making provides such an intervention. The very act of engaging in the process of art making is proven to lift spirits and maintain positive affect. Working within the mandala allows for holistic integration of mind, body, and spirit. Mandalas created specifically to express positive emotions or feelings allow the art maker the opportunity to externalize his or her positive resources, potentially solidifying his or her frame of reference before it can begin to unravel. At the least, art making will provide a concrete distraction from the many stressors facing crisis workers, disallowing rumination on negative thoughts and feelings. At best, art making may prove to be an effective intervention in the prevention or mitigation of vicarious trauma.

DEVELOPING AN INTERVENTION

What seems to be missing in the literature is arts based interventions as preventative measures for trauma related symptomatology. Similarly non-existent is literature on the effects of secondary trauma stress and vicarious trauma on crisis workers. Is it possible to prevent negative schema shifts; particularly within those populations most vulnerable to trauma experiences? And while these previous interventions may prove successful when led by the trained therapist, they are not practical for the non-clinical practitioner nor are they necessarily accessible to the trauma survivor or successful without a facilitator. As established through the review of literature, art making activities provide protection against the emotional and psychological risks associated with the trauma experience. While this intervention was not designed as a creative arts therapy method, it did build on the therapeutic properties of art making to bolster its success in achieving vicarious trauma intervention.

Considering these limitations, the author designed a trauma intervention and studied its effects on first responders in 2015. The available research at that time supported the findings of several previous studies on the use of mandalas as a healing tool (Curry & Kasser, 2005; Henderson et al., 2007; Henderson, 2012; van der Vennet & Serice, 2012); the use of art making as distraction to increase positive mood (Dalebroux et al., 2008; Drake et al., 2011; Drake & Winner, 2012); and the creation of art expressing positive emotions to increase mood (Dalebroux et al., 2008; Henderson, 2012). In addition to these three elements, the author was interested in exploring ways in which reinforce connections to positive resources possessed by the art maker. In the case of working with first responders or crisis workers, exploring positive resources around the theme of safety seemed most apropos. Therefore, the intervention designed included the drawing of a mandala capturing images and symbols of safety and was tested to ascertain the efficacy of its ability to increase positive affect, decrease negative affect, and reinforce connections to positive resources in participants.

Testing the Intervention

The study sought to prove two hypotheses. The first was that study participants would demonstrate an increase in positive affect and a decrease in negative affect immediately following the art making intervention. Changes in affect were measured by self-reported levels of emotions or feelings using the Positive and Negative Affect Survey (PANAS) (Watson, Clark, & Tellegen, 1988). The second hypothesis was that study participants would demonstrate a reinforced connection to their positive resources surrounding the theme of safety. This hypothesis was evaluated qualitatively by analyzing common themes found both in the mandala drawings as well as in the interview answers provided by the participants.

The demographics of the participants were collected through a pre-screening form. Demographic information collected included age, gender, ethnicity, and current employment or volunteer position as well as the use of any psychotropic drug use. The use of these drugs were a disqualifier and control aspect.

The research study consisted of a small sampling with 10 participants ranging in age from 25 to 44 years. The participants were 70% female and 30% male. The participants' race/ethnicity were African American/Black (20%), Caucasian/White (60%), Hispanic/Latino (10%), and Bi-Racial (10%). Current employment or volunteer positions were Firefighter (20%), Police Officers (20%), Emergency Medical Technician (30%), Emergency Room Nurse (10%), and Emergency Room Doctor (10%). All participants resided in the Greater Philadelphia area in urban communities.

The study used a pretest-posttest control group design with qualitative features. The intervention group and control group were assigned through random sampling. The PANAS was administered to the control group for three consecutive days followed by a debriefing meeting and short interview. The intervention group completed the pre-test PANAS on the first day of the study. On the second day of the study for the participant, the researcher met with the participant to administer the mandala drawing intervention. Each intervention participant was provided with oil pastels and a 12"x12" sheet of white paper containing a pre-drawn 10" mandala.

Following a brief introduction to the use of oil pastels, participants were given the following directions: *This circle represents your safe space. Within the circle, draw any objects or people that you would bring with you into this safe space. You might also draw a picture of a place that you already recognize to be safe. Please do not use any letters or words in your drawing.*

A posttest PANAS was administered again immediately following the art making activity. During the final session with the participants on the third day, a post-test PANAS was again administered after which the researcher met with the participants to conduct an interview in which to collect qualitative data and concluded with a debriefing which explained the full nature of the study and the purpose for withholding information about the expectations of the study.

Study Results

When the intervention group was asked to describe the experience of drawing in the mandala while focusing on the theme of safety, several common themes appeared as well as on their perceived change in mood between the start and end of the drawing activity.

Figure 1. Participant mandala: "This is my favorite spot along our usual run. My husband is always with me and we know just how far home it is from this point."

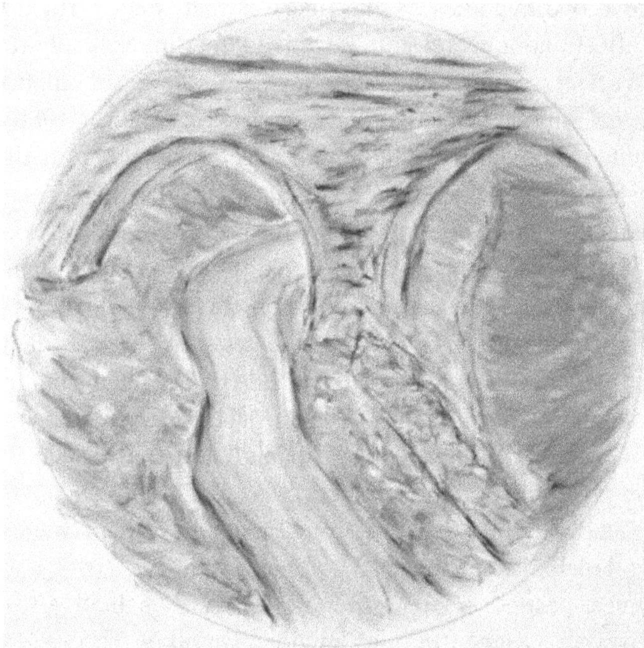

Table 1. Common themes among participants when asked to describe the mandala drawing experience

Common Themes	Participant Responses
The art making was distracting.	I was too involved in trying to remember what scene looked like that I was not thinking about anything else.
	This has been a good distraction from the news I received this morning.
	I enjoyed just thinking about myself for a while - I could block everything else out.
This was comforting.	If I were to look at this picture again, it would comfort me when I am down.
	It was comforting to think about safety.
	The churning motion (drawn in mandala) is comforting, I can rely on it.
I felt calm and focused.	I felt relaxed and at peace while I drew.
	I felt more focused because I had to really think about what made me feel safe.
	I was anxious to get started because I don't draw well, but after I started I began to feel calm.
This reminded me of what keeps me safe.	This made me think about what is important to me.
	I know that I am safe when I am with my husband.
	I have a lot of people protecting me.
	I need to remember this, it is part of my identity.

Regular Engagement in Art Making

Of the 5 participants in the intervention group, 60% felt that regularly engaging in art making in a manner similar to the safety-themed mandalas would be beneficial to their ability to stay focused and engaged in their work. Their additional comments are listed below.

- I don't have to be physically well to engage in this. I don't have to be physically active.
- This is very childish. I am very critical of what I do. This is childlike and I don't care to see myself doing this.
- Drawing is a different way of expressing myself and my emotions.
- This is something I don't normally do so it was a good thing to try today. If I did it every day, it would lose its effect over time. I would just be going through the motions.
- I feel like technology makes you absorb. It is constantly stimulating you so that you can't ever relax even when you trying to, this art making lets you release.

Figure 2. Participant mandala: "The giant tree next to my house makes me feel safe. It has stood for years through hurricanes, lightning, and snowstorms."

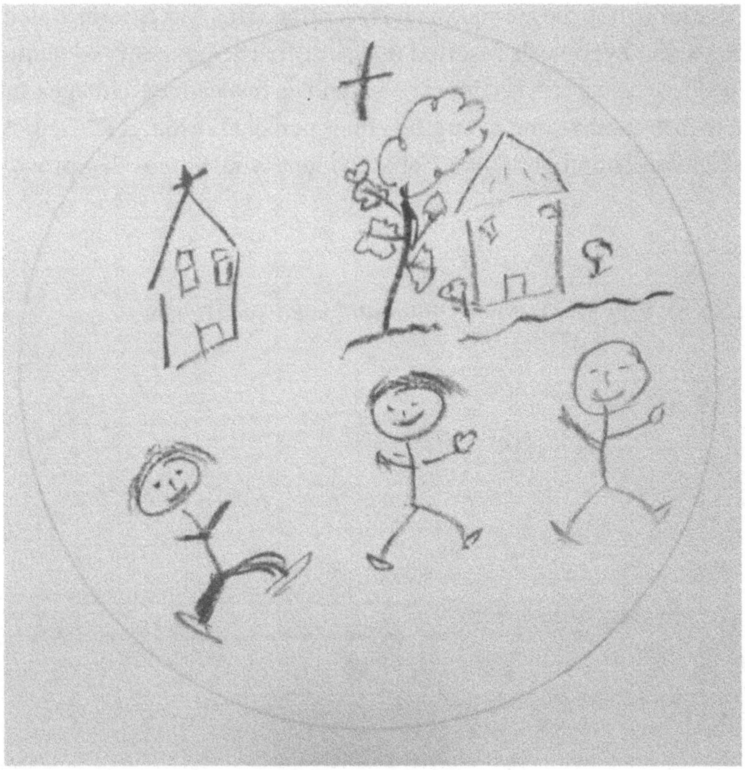

Perceived Change in Mood

Each participant in the intervention group was able to identify the emotion they brought into the mandala drawing activity. Most could attach it to an event or information learned earlier in the day. Each perceived a shift in their mood as they engaged in the art making, aware that the feeling was more positive than at the start. Two of the participants attributed the shift in mood to the act of drawing their mandala, while the other 3 felt the shift was due to reflecting on the theme of safety. One participant admitted that he felt better once the art making had concluded as some of his anxiety at the start was directly attached to having to engage in art making.

Findings from the self-reported PANAS scores support these narratives. Participants in the intervention group demonstrated an increase in positive affect that remained elevated above the pretest scores during the second posttest. Negative affect scores decreased following the intervention and similarly remained lower than pretest scores during the second posttest. The control group did not demonstrate these same results.

Study Discussion

The study results supported both hypotheses. The first hypothesis asserted that study participants who created safety-themed mandalas would demonstrate an increase in positive affect and a decrease in negative affect immediately following the art making intervention. This was demonstrated in the self-reported PANAS results. The second hypothesis asserted that study participants would demonstrate a reinforced connection to their positive resources. By drawing a mandala that captured images and symbols of safety, participants were able to "mobilize and strengthen their personal resources" (Setti & Argentero, 2014). All participants in the intervention group were able to identify resources that provide physical safety or

Figure 3. Mean PANAS Scores of the Intervention and Control Groups

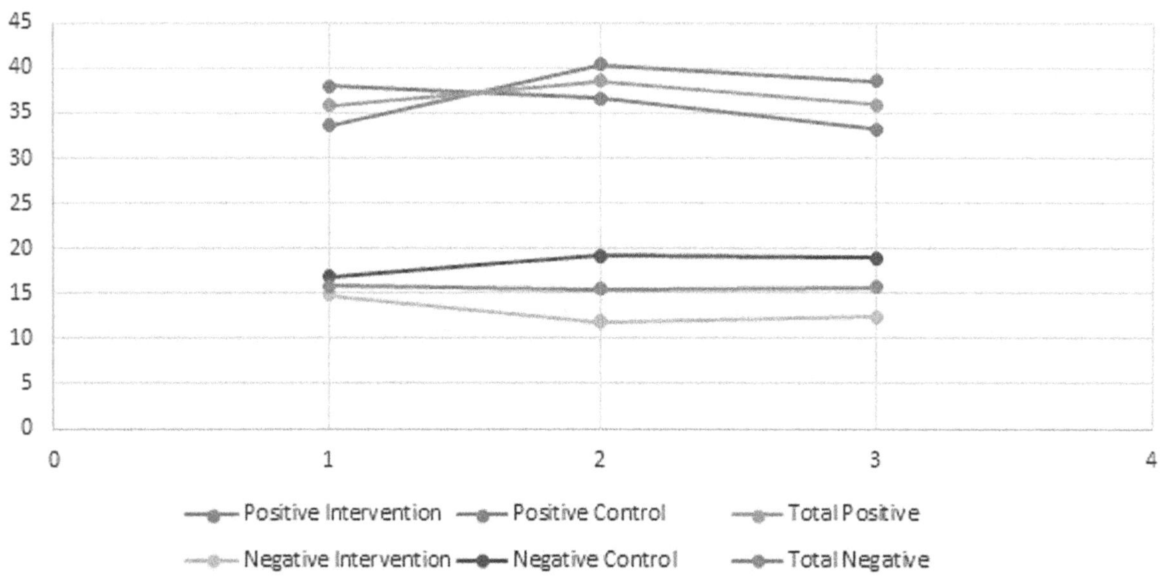

the feeling of safety. It was fascinating to learn that though their work demands that they provide safety for others, it was apparent they rarely, if ever, give thought to that which provides themselves safety.

Each participant could perceive a change in their mood that occurred during their art making session. Each was able to identify the emotion or feeling that they brought into the session and noted that emotion or feeling had either subsided slightly or was replaced with a more positive emotion or feeling. Some of the participants felt their change in mood was due to the distraction of the task, stating "this has been a good distraction from the news I received this morning" and other similar comments. These findings support previous research (Dalebroux et al., 2008; DePetrillo & Winner, 2005) that art making increases positive affect, leaving the art maker feeling more calm and peaceful, through the distraction of the task.

To draw about their personal resources took perhaps more thought and commitment to the art making than drawing a "happy" image (Dalebroux et al., 2008) or even a reaction to an event or stimulus (Drake & Winner, 2012; Henderson et al. 2007) as has been done in previous studies. As one participant shared, "before I could even begin to draw, I had to create a framework around the idea of safety. Was it a person or a place? What about that person or place made me feel safe?" It seemed that an interesting follow up to this study would be to discover how drawing something more cognitively demanding than drawing something recognized as universally positive (love, joy, happiness) as done by Henderson (2012) would affect the outcome over a longer time period.

Participants also attributed their shift in emotions or feelings to the subject matter of their mandalas. One participant, in particular, expressed how refreshing it was to turn her attention inward and onto herself. All too often, she found herself providing for others and being their resource. Reminding herself of those resources available to her, she was able to move towards a more positive state of mind. Other participants echoed this with similar remarks, feeling that the time spent focusing on those people, places, and things that offer them safety helped to reframe their mood in a positive direction. Bringing those things back into their conscious mind brought about feelings of peace, calm, and comfort despite the current events of their day.

FUTURE IMPLICATIONS AND APPLICATIONS

While the author's study supported both hypotheses, the results also present the need for additional research. This study is important not only for its implications in the field of art therapy, but also as an effective non-clinical intervention or self-care activity. To date, research involving the mandala has not tested the efficacy of drawing the mandala to capture the resources of the art maker. Future studies should carefully consider wording. Directing study participants to "draw images or symbols that represent safety" may contribute to the value of intervention because of the positive resource reinforcement.

While the author was specifically interested in developing an intervention for crisis workers in the context of vicarious trauma, this study could be easily replicated on any population to test the efficacy of its ability to alter affect. However, to better evaluate the change in affect, this study may have induced anxiety or negative affect prior to administering the intervention or control as a means to better capture and understand the change in affect as done in previous studies (Curry & Kasser, 2005; Dalebroux et al., 2008; Drake et al., 2011; Drake and Winner, 2012). Replicating the current study with the addition of the mood induction could better determine if the change in affect was directly altered as a result of the intervention and not other circumstances. Additionally, the study should be repeated with a larger study population to ensure consistency of results.

Figure 4. Participant Mandala: "These are just symbols of all of the people around me that protect me. And I protect them. It is a good reminder."

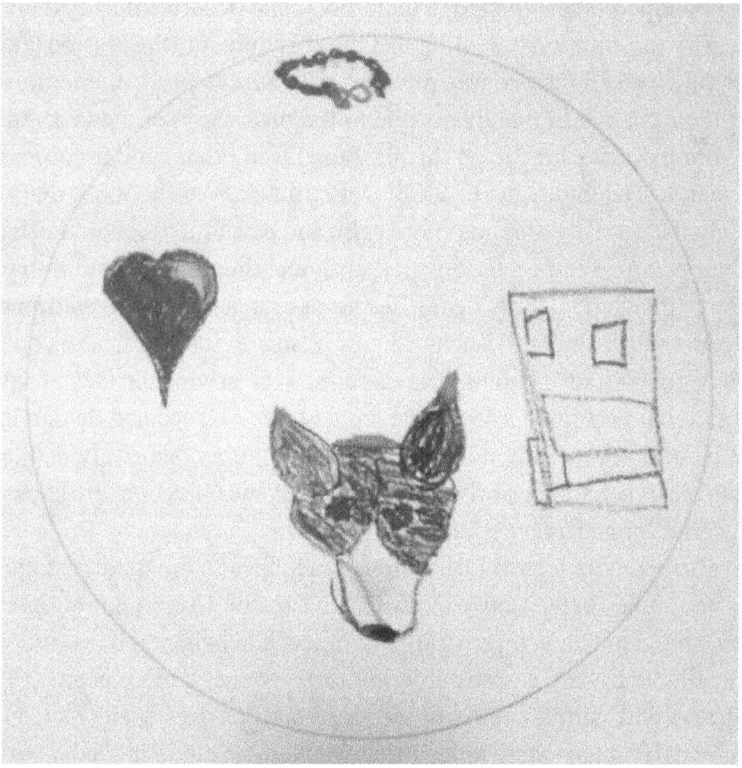

The safety of crisis workers is constantly under threat during their work and is also one of the five components of self that is affected through exposure to trauma and crisis. Therefore, safety was an obvious choice to use as the theme in the art making intervention in this context. Another valuable research approach may be to consider testing one of the other components of self that are affected by trauma: trust, intimacy, control, or esteem. Working with all five components through a series of mandala drawings may prove to significantly increase the efficacy of the intervention than focusing on any one component alone.

Additionally, considering this intervention through the lens of the constructivist self-development theory might point towards other vulnerable populations and pair them that component of self most at risk during times of adversity. Could adopted children improve attachment to their adoptive parents by connecting to resources of intimacy? Could those battling addictions improve their chances of overcoming addiction by connecting to resources of control?

This developed and tested arts based intervention could be put into practice immediately. Using mandalas to reinforce positive resource connections is an intervention based on research conducted primarily by creative arts therapists and yet, the intervention does not need to be carried out or facilitated by an arts therapist. As the intervention does not specifically delve into any trauma material therefore eliminating the risk of re-traumatization, the intervention could be facilitated in a non-clinical setting. Furthermore, after carefully researching the efficacy of other positive resource themes (intimacy, control, trust, etc.), a toolkit or field book could be compiled using the effective mandala prompts to both provide the crisis worker with an immediate distraction from the crisis situation as well as a metaphoric shield in the trauma environment.

CONCLUSION

Drawing mandalas capturing images and symbols of safety not only increased positive affect and decreased negative affect, it helped those participants who engaged in the art making reinforce their connections to resources of safety. Working in environments that continually threaten the well-being of crisis workers can take a toll on emotional and physical resources and may alter perceptions and worldview in a profound way. Interventions that support positive resource reinforcement may go far in preventing that shift in worldview or perception for crisis workers. Additionally, interventions that are easily accessible for crisis workers and are intentionally targeting the decrease of altered perceptions may significantly increase well-being and lead to a more stable state of mind that positively impacts delivery of service. Research designs such as this that are easily replicated offer vast potential for advancement in the area of trauma disorder prevention and post traumatic growth.

Kleim and Westphal (2011) suggest that trauma interventions should not be a "one size fits all" solution. Applying the same intervention to the crisis workers as to the crisis victims they serve may not provide specific kind of service needed for vicarious trauma. Their experience differs dramatically from that of the crisis victim. Crisis workers deserve more resources directed to developing interventions that relate directly to the circumstances in which the vicarious trauma is experienced. It is of critical importance and an area that has been drastically underserved.

REFERENCES

Beaton, R. D., & Murphy, S. A. (1995). Working with People in Crisis; Research Implications. In *Compassion fatigue: Coping with secondary traumatic stress disorder in those who treat the traumatized.* New York, NY: Brunner/Mazel.

Bell, H., Kulkarni, S., & Dalton, L. (2003). Organizational prevention of vicarious trauma. *Families in Society*, *84*(4), 463–470. doi:10.1606/1044-3894.131

Bober, T., & Regehr, C. (2006). Strategies for reducing secondary or vicarious trauma: Do they work? *Brief Treatment and Crisis Intervention*, *6*(1), 1–9. doi:10.1093/brief-treatment/mhj001

Bourassa, D. (2012). Examining self-protection measures guarding adult protective services social workers against compassion fatigue. *Journal of Interpersonal Violence*, *27*(9), 1699–1715. doi:10.1177/0886260511430388 PMID:22203624

Camilleri, V. A. (2007). *Healing the inner city child: Creative arts therapies with at-risk youth.* London: Jessica Kingsley Publishers.

Curry, N. A., & Kasser, T. (2005). Can coloring mandalas reduce anxiety? *Art Therapy: Journal of the American Art Therapy Association*, *22*(2), 81–85. doi:10.1080/07421656.2005.10129441

Dalebroux, A., Goldstein, T. R., & Winner, E. (2008). Short-term mood repair through art-making: Positive emotion is more effective than venting. *Motivation and Emotion*, *32*(4), 288–295. doi:10.100711031-008-9105-1

De Petrillo, L. D., & Winner, E. (2005). Does art improve mood? A test of a key assumption underlying art therapy. *Art Therapy: Journal of the American Art Therapy Association*, *22*(4), 205–212. doi:10.1080/07421656.2005.10129521

Delue, C. (1999). Physiological effects of creating mandalas. *Medical Art Therapy with Children*, 33-49.

Devilly, G. J., Gist, R., & Cotton, P. (2006). Ready! Fire! Aim! The status of psychological debriefing and therapeutic interventions: In the work place and after disasters. *Review of General Psychology*, *10*(4), 318–345. doi:10.1037/1089-2680.10.4.318

Drake, J., Coleman, K., & Winner, E. (2011). Short term mood repairs through art: Effects of medium and strategy. *Art Therapy: Journal of the American Art Therapy Association*, *28*(1), 26–30. doi:10.1080/07421656.2011.557032

Drake, J. E., & Winner, E. (2012). Confronting sadness through art-making: Distraction is more beneficial than venting. *Psychology of Aesthetics, Creativity, and the Arts*, *6*(3), 255–261. doi:10.1037/a0026909

Farrelly-Hansen, M. (2001). Nature. In *Spirituality and art therapy: Living the connection* (pp. 137–158). London: J. Kingsley Publishers.

Figley, C. R. (1995). *Compassion fatigue: Coping with secondary traumatic stress disorder in those who treat the traumatized*. New York, NY: Brunner/Mazel.

Figley, C. R. (2002). Compassion fatigue: Psychotherapists' chronic lack of self care. *Journal of Clinical Psychology*, *58*(11), 1433–1441. doi:10.1002/jclp.10090 PMID:12412153

Fincher, S. (2014). *Psychology of the mandala*. Retrieved from http://creatingmandalas.com/psychology-of-the-mandala

Fincher, S. F. (1991). *Creating mandalas: For insight, healing, and self-expression*. Boston, MA: Shambhala.

Glazer, H. R., & Stein, D. S. (2010). Qualitative research and its role in play therapy research. *International Journal of Play Therapy*, *19*(1), 54–61. doi:10.1037/a0017933

Helm, H. M. (2011). *Managing vicarious trauma and compassion fatigue*. Retrieved from http://www.lianalowenstein.com/artcile_helm.pdf

Henderson, P., Rosen, D., & Mascaro, N. (2007). Empirical study on the healing nature of mandalas. *Psychology of Aesthetics, Creativity, and the Arts*, *1*(3), 148–154. doi:10.1037/1931-3896.1.3.148

Henderson, P. G. (2012). *Empirical study of the healing nature of artistic expression: Using mandalas with the positive emotions of love and joy* (Unpublished doctoral dissertation). Texas A & M University.

Irving, M. C. (1995). *Natalistic art in therapy theory: Working with birth and prenatal issues through art*. The Union Institute.

Killian, K. D. (2008). Helping till it hurts? A multimethod study of compassion fatigue, burnout, and self-care in clinicians working with trauma survivors. *Traumatology*, *14*(2), 32–44. doi:10.1177/1534765608319083

Kivnick, H. Q., & Erikson, J. M. (2010). The arts as healing. *The American Journal of Orthopsychiatry*, *53*(4). doi:10.1111/j.1939-0025.1983.tb03405.x PMID:6638153

Kleim, B., & Westphal, M. (2011). Mental health in first responders: A review and recommendation for prevention and intervention strategies. *Traumatology*, *17*(4), 17–24. doi:10.1177/1534765611429079

Leedy, P. D., & Ormrod, J. E. (2005). *Practical research: Planning and design* (9th ed.). Upper Saddle River, NJ: Prentice Hall.

Lusebrink, V. B. (2004). Art therapy and the brain: An attempt to understand the underlying processes of art expression in therapy. *Art Therapy: Journal of the American Art Therapy Association*, *21*(3), 125–135. doi:10.1080/07421656.2004.10129496

McCann, I. L., & Pearlman, L. A. (1990). *Psychological trauma and the adult survivor: Theory, therapy, and transformation*. New York, NY: Brunner/Mazel.

McCann, I. L., & Pearlman, L. A. (1990). Vicarious traumatization: A framework for understanding the psychological effects of working with victims. *Journal of Traumatic Stress*, *3*(1), 131–149. doi:10.1007/BF00975140

McCann, I. L., & Pearlman, L. A. (1992). Constructivist self-development theory: A theoretical framework for assessing and treating traumatized college students. *Journal of American College Health*, *40*(4), 189–196. doi:10.1080/07448481.1992.9936281 PMID:1583241

Mehlomakulu, C. (2012, November 2). *Creativity in therapy: Mandalas*. Retrieved from http://creativityintherapy.blogspot.com/2012/11/mandalas.html

Metzl, E., & Morrell, M. (2008). The role of creativity in models of resilience: Theoretical exploration and practical applications. *Journal of Creativity in Mental Health*, *3*(3), 303–318. doi:10.1080/15401380802385228

Nelson, T. S. (1996). *Vicarious trauma: bearing witness to another's trauma* (Doctoral dissertation). University of Illinois. Retrieved from http://www.uic.edu/orgs/convening/vicariou.htm

Pearlman, L. A., & Saakvitne, K. A. (1995). *Trauma and the therapist*. New York, NY: W.W. Norton & Company.

Pizarro, J. (2004). The efficacy of Art and writing therapy: Increasing positive mental health outcomes and participant retention after exposure to traumatic experience. *Art Therapy: Journal of the American Art Therapy Association*, *21*(1), 5–12. doi:10.1080/07421656.2004.10129327

Pryce, J., Shackelford, K., & Price, D. (2007). Educating child welfare workers about secondary trauma stress. In *Secondary trauma stress and the child welfare professional* (pp. 51-71). Retrieved from http://lyceumbooks.com/pdf/stsch3.pdf

Rappaport, L. (1998). Focusing and art therapy: Tools for working through post-traumatic stress disorder. *Focusing Folio, 17*(1), 1-6. Retrieved from https://www.focusing.org/pdf/rappaport_focusing_and_art_therapy_tools_for_working_through_trauma.pdf

Regehr, C. (2001). Crisis debriefing groups for emergency responders: Reviewing the evidence. *Brief Treatment and Crisis Intervention, 1*(2), 87–100. doi:10.1093/brief-treatment/1.2.87

Savin-Baden, M., & Howell Major, C. (2013). *Qualitative research: The essential guide to theory and practice*. New York, NY: Routledge.

Setti, I., & Argentero, P. (2014). The role of mindfulness in protecting firefighters from psychosomatic malaise. *Traumatology, 20*(2), 134–141. doi:10.1037/h0099398

Shakespeare-Finch, J. (2011). Primary and secondary trauma in emergency personnel. *Traumatology, 17*(4), 1–2. doi:10.1177/1534765611431834

Showalter, S. E. (2010). Compassion fatigue: What is it? Why does it matter? Recognizing the symptoms, acknowledging the impact, developing the tools to prevent compassion fatigue, and strengthen the professional already suffering the effects. *American Journal for Hospice and Palliative Medicine, 27*(4), 239–242. doi:10.1177/1049909109354096 PMID:20075423

Stuckey, H. L., & Nobel, J. (2010). The connection between art, healing, and public health: A review of current literature. *American Journal of Public Health, 100*(2), 254–263. doi:10.2105/AJPH.2008.156497 PMID:20019311

Sutton, J. P. (2002). *Music, music therapy and trauma: International perspectives*. London: J. Kingsley Publishers.

Thayer, R. E., Newman, J. R., & McClain, T. M. (1994). Self-regulation of mood: Strategies for changing a bad mood, raising energy, and reducing tension. *Journal of Personality and Social Psychology, 67*(5), 910–925. doi:10.1037/0022-3514.67.5.910 PMID:7983582

University of Phoenix. (2017, April 17). *Majority of first responders face mental health challenges in the workplace*. Retrieved from http://www.phoenix.edu/about_us/media-center/news/uopx-releases-first-responder-mental-health-survey-results.html

US Department of Health and Human Services. (2005). *A guide to managing stress in crisis response professions* (SMA 4113). Retrieved from http://store.samhsa.gov/shin/content//SMA05-4113/SMA05-4113.pdf

Van Lith, T. (2014). Painting to find my spirit: Art making as the vehicle to find meaning and connection in the mental health recovery process. *Journal of Spirituality in Mental Health, 16*(1), 13–36. doi:10.1080/19349637.2013.864542

Vennet, R. V., & Serice, S. (2012). Can coloring mandalas reduce anxiety? A replication study. *Art Therapy: Journal of the American Art Therapy Association, 29*(2), 87–92. doi:10.1080/07421656.2012.680047

Watson, D., Clark, L. A., & Tellegen, A. (1988). Development and validation of brief measures of positive and negative affect: The PANAS scales. *Journal of Personality and Social Psychology, 54*(6), 1063–1070. doi:10.1037/0022-3514.54.6.1063 PMID:3397865

Yassen, J. (1995). Preventing Secondary Traumatic Stress Disorder. In *Compassion fatigue: Coping with secondary traumatic stress disorder in those who treat the traumatized*. New York, NY: Brunner/Mazel.

Young, R. (2005). *EMS stress and paramedic students*. Canadian Emergency News.

KEY TERMS AND DEFINITIONS

Arts-Based Intervention: An arts-based intervention uses an art medium or discipline to improve a process or situation, particularly one involving emotional and psychological wellbeing.

Positive Resource: Any source of support or aid that can be drawn upon when needed; contributes to a person's resilience and self-efficacy.

Chapter 4
Butterfly, Emerging:
How Trauma-Informed Services Help Survivors to Heal

Melissa Lucchesi
Voices, Inc., USA

ABSTRACT

The prevalence of traumas such as sexual violence is difficult to measure. However, it is fairly widely accepted that 1 in 5 women and 1 in 33 men will be a victim of sexual violence in her or his lifetime. Because of complicating factors to this type of trauma, survivors may not readily identify themselves as that. Healing arts and yoga help survivors to process traumatic energy and thoughts without having to delve into those dark and painful caverns. This chapter shares first person experience of sexual violence and navigating healing, as well as professional experience with other survivors, to illustrate the importance of trauma-informed healing and expressive arts when healing from trauma.

INTRODUCTION

In 2001, I was raped by someone I had dated. It was after a party in my dorm room, and my roommate had gone out to walk her boyfriend to his car. I had trusted him. He was someone my friends liked and knew. Yet, I was sexually assaulted and raped in those moments we were alone. I remember in the days that followed I would look around at the yellow and blue décor, the white painted cinder block walls, the pictures of my family and friends taped over my bed, and I felt somehow that I had watched the whole thing happen from up above. It felt like I was not entirely in my body during the assault, and instead somewhere watching helplessly as it happened.

My roommate and I had worked so hard to decorate that room, and it was touted one of the "nicest" dorm rooms in our building. We were so proud that my comforter was complementary to hers, and that we figured that we'd have enough space for a futon and breathing room if we faced our dressers towards one another and took turns using them. Yet, after I confided in my roommate about the assault, she asked if I wanted to change up the room. It struck me as such a thoughtful idea. She knew that looking at the

DOI: 10.4018/978-1-5225-5981-8.ch004

room as it was might bring everything rushing back, and that I might appreciate the change. I declined, mostly because I was angry that he had already taken so much from me and I was not about to give him our "nice" dorm room too. But a piece of me stayed trapped in that room, and remained there for years. The décor changed, the layout changed, the roommates faces too, and yet a piece of my soul that shattered that night remained stuck in the yellow and blue, and in the white painted cinder block walls.

There was very little in terms of healing when I first tried to navigate healing from rape. I sought out support groups, and there were none on campus. I was shocked to find out that there weren't campus awareness groups so I started one. I found the county's crisis center and began attending a support group there with faces and stories so similar to my own. I still felt dead inside. I felt shattered and I couldn't figure out how to put myself back together. In the spring, I attended my first Take Back the Night event on campus. The event is a movement to honor stories of people affected by sexual or domestic violence, and gives opportunities to speak out without shame. Survivors were speaking out their trauma loudly and in the middle of campus. I was in awe that so many people could relate to what I had gone through. With my dad standing strongly in the audience, I too spoke out my trauma. It was empowering, and I felt a little less broken. I continued speaking out my trauma to friends, family, my therapist, teachers, and found a path to the work I now do.

In a surreal twist of fate in 2007, I was drugged at a bar and taken to the home of a man I did not know, and I was raped. I believed I wouldn't survive that night, and I watched as my life went in a reel before my eyes. I did survive, and surviving was conflicting. I was grateful to be alive, but it was painstakingly difficult to wake up every day and live. I could not believe I did the work I did, and still this happened to me again. I was again fragmented, pieces of me this time in his home, in the different rooms I had been attacked.

A piece of me stayed stuck in the advocacy office where I spoke out what had happened and requested an advocate come with me to report the rape. A piece of me was embedded in the metal chair in the police station where I reported the rape to two male officers. A piece remained in the district attorney's office where I also had to speak it out, in the municipal courtroom where charges were pushed forward, and in the county courthouse where I sat for hours reliving my deepest trauma on the stand. Every time I spoke out my trauma, a little piece remained in that place. It is impossible to feel whole when you lose track of all of the pieces of you that have broken off.

On a very simple level, a traumatic event is anything that overwhelms our capacity to cope and respond. It leaves us feeling helpless, hopeless, and out of control. When we think about trauma we usually think about the really big ones.... but trauma lives on a spectrum. We're shaped by the big ones and the little ones. When we don't have the tools and resources to deal with traumatic events, they impact our physiology; they impact our bodies. When we're not able to get ourselves to safety or say what we need to say, traumatic energy gets stuck in the body. (Hala Khouri, 2015)

Khouri's description of trauma is powerful because it encompasses its very essence, and bears witness to the energy trapped inside; it recognizes the mind, body and spirit touched by trauma.

Trauma is unique in that it is an experience that happens to the body, affects the mind, and touches the spirit. When a trauma happens to a person, it is not easily shaken.

No experience is more one's own than harm to one's own skin, but none is more locked within that skin, played out within it in actions other than words, in patterns of consciousness below the everyday and the constructions of language. Trapped there, the violation seems to continue in a reverberating present that belies the supposed linearity of time and the possibility of endings. (Culbertson, 1995)

This mind-body-spirit experience then commands a mind-body-spirit healing and approach to healing.

Scope of the Hurt

The Center for Disease Control estimates that 1 in 5 women and 1 in 59 men will be raped in their lifetime, and 1 in 4 women and 1 in 9 men have experienced unwanted sexual contact, or sexual assault. 1 in 3 women and 1 in 8 men have experienced non contact sexual violence. The CDC also explains that this is a grave underestimate of the scope of this issue, as many people do not report sexual assault, or even identify what happened as such. (Center for Disease Control [CDC], 2017) With these estimates, and not accounting for the multitude of traumas experienced over a lifetime, it is clear we are a society of traumatized individuals.

Trauma researcher Bessel Van der Kolk explains that our current models overlook important truths.

1) our capacity to destroy one another is matched by our capacity to heal one another. Restoring relationships and community is central to restoring well-being; (2) language gives us the power to change ourselves and others by communicating our experiences, helping us to define what we know, and finding a common sense of meaning; (3) we have the ability to regulate our own physiology, including some of the so-called involuntary functions of the body and brain, through such basic activities as breathing, moving, and touching; and (4) we can change social conditions to create environments in which children and adults can feel safe and where they can thrive. (van der Kolk, 2015)

This points to the possibility that we can heal our own traumas by using voice, by understanding our histories, and that trauma-informed spaces can further trauma healing creating spaces safer for all children and adults.

Survival

It was a curvy and often times treacherous road navigating those first bits of survival after this trauma. I spoke to my therapist, and again to family and friends, and used my voice as fiercely as I could in the criminal court system, but I felt debilitated. A friend referred me to someone working with survivors through yoga. She met with me in the very early mornings before work to do yoga and process the traumatic energy I felt trapped inside. Each time that I would leave the little studio, I felt I could take a deeper breath. I also began furiously collaging shoeboxes. I ripped up magazines and catalogs and created boxes filled with anger, fear, disgust, shame, guilt, hope, self-love, and light. I had stacks of boxes and with each box I was lighter and more hopeful.

I watched as I used my voice to speak out, my body to do yoga, and my hands to create, my whole world opened up and slowly the scattered, shattered bits found their way back together. The life that had become so very small began to burst with hope that I would be able to reclaim the dreams I had before this. I founded a nonprofit, Voices, Inc., (Voices, 2017) on the premise that all people of all backgrounds deserve this access to healing and light. We offer opportunities for healing in creative ways, and creating a healing journey unique to each survivor. We also educate everyone who will listen on how to be trauma-informed and build a safer space for the survivors in our communities and in our own lives.

Healing Arts and Trauma Healing

Research suggests that becoming aware of the things going on inside of the body and the sensations felt, may help to connect survivors to themselves once again, reducing symptoms of Post-Traumatic Stress Disorder (PTSD). Building connection to the body, and helping survivors bring awareness to the present moment can help them mindfully move through a moment of triggered PTSD and help promote healing. (van der Kolk, Stone, West, Rhodes, Emerson, Suvak & Spinnazolla, 2014)

The women I have worked with in group have connected with each other, and learned to use those same skills—yoga, art, movement, voice—to find ways to heal their lives. I watch as the women so deeply committed to their healing grow their lives, and find hope in places that may have felt dark and lonely. Bessel van der Kolk suggests:

Describing traumatic experiences in conventional verbal therapy is likely to activate

implicit memories, that is trauma-related physical sensations, and physiological hyper- or hypo arousal, which evoke emotions such as helplessness, fear, shame, and rage. When this occurs, trauma victims are prone to feeling that it is still not safe to deal with the trauma. (van der Kolk, 2006)

We do not process trauma verbally. We use art based experiences to move through a trauma-informed model of healing, where survivors remain present, working through the art or movement project while connecting with each other in a safe space.

One of our themes was a series of movement sessions. Participants first created a visual journey of their lives, traumas, and growth on a poster board. They worked with a dance teacher who showed them how to put movement to the visual, creating a piece that was shared with the larger group. The group then walked with one another and moved exactly as the person did, symbolically walking with each other through those difficult moments in life. It was powerful and left everyone with the message that they were not alone in this.

At other times, the group worked with mosaic, shattering plates-- in itself cathartic-- and created art with the broken pieces, symbolizing the ability to create their lives into beautiful works of art after feeling shattered by trauma. The group has worked with song lyrics that resonate, listening to music that means something to the individual survivor, and choosing lyrics to paint on canvas as a personal mantra. One session centered on creating mandalas out of beans, rice, and lentils. Each part of the mandala meant something personal to the survivor. For example, the center represents the core of her identity, who she is and what her personal values may be. The next layer represents her trauma, the next her circle of support, and the next her healing. At the end of the session, each person took turns emptying their work into a bin, symbolic of the process of "letting go."

A common activity the group works with is collage. Each time, there is a different theme. The figure below is from a session with a crumpled paper exercise. The participants wrote down on paper or tissue paper things that they had hoped and dreamed for before trauma. Those who could not recall a time "before trauma", including those who had been victimized starting in early childhood, shifted the

Figure 1. Visual Journey Poster

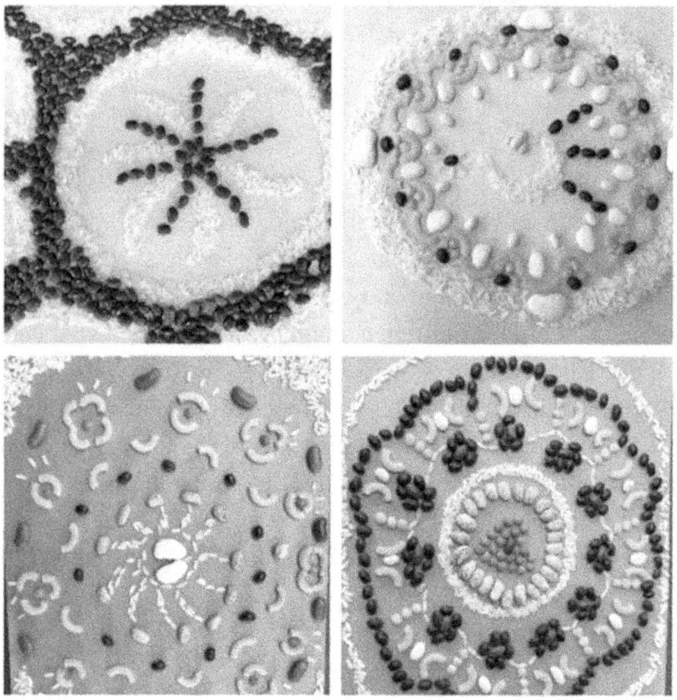

Figure 2. Mandalas

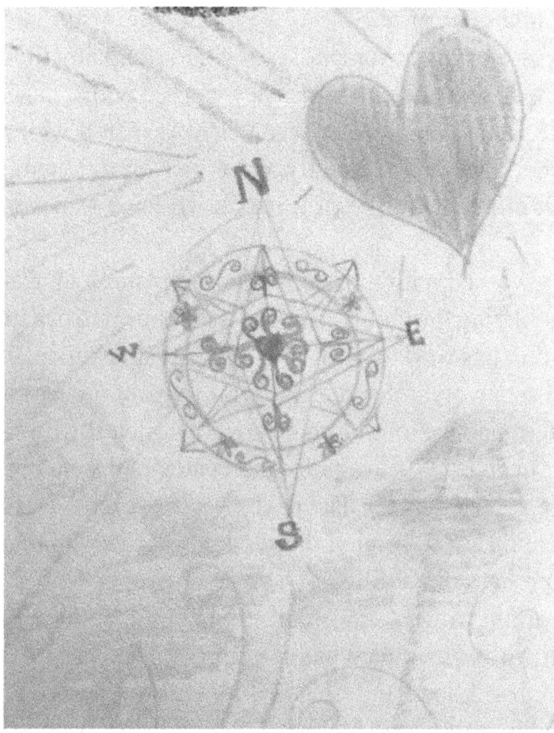

activity to work for them by writing things they hoped for before recalling trauma, or before the most recent trauma, etc. Then, they crumpled the paper up into a tight ball, and then tried to flatten it out into a straightened fresh piece of paper again. Since that cannot be done, they created a collage of their post-traumatic growth, and the things they have crafted to create beauty and light again in their lives. This is symbolic of how trauma imprints a scar on the survivor's heart, and how life is forever changed, but also how life can be beautiful and even more amazing after trauma and healing.

Other experiences include creating ornaments that open with strips of paper holding supportive messages from the group members, making sensory bracelets to touch to help them remain grounded during difficult or triggering moments, and weighted lap pads to provide comfort in stressful times. We also folded origami, a skill that can be useful for mindful distraction in tough moments.

Every group ends with a grounding technique to use when they are feeling unhinged so that they may head back into the world fully present in their bodies and minds. Each of these is another tool for the healing toolbox. Healing is as unique as the individual. The toolbox that works for one survivor, may not work for another, but having the ability to create that healing in a trauma-informed space is powerful.

Voices is committed to creating trauma-informed communities. We speak and educate on being trauma-informed wherever and whenever we can. While there is no single definition of what it means to be trauma-informed, trauma-informed services follow guidelines such as believing that victimization happens and that trauma impacts coping mechanisms. Working under an empowerment model where choices for healing are left to the survivor cultivates an environment that is respectful and safe of and for all people, minimizing the chance of retraumatization, and holding healing as the goal. (Elliot, 2005)

Figure 3. Crumpled Paper Collage

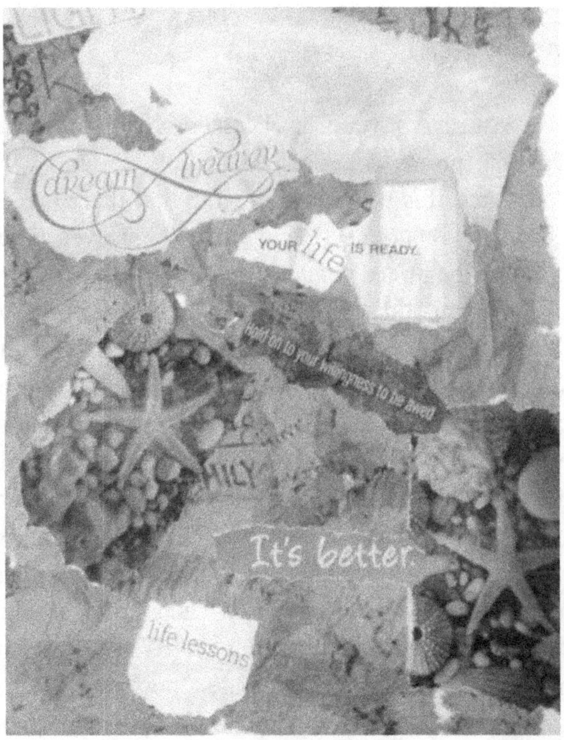

Figure 4. Origami Ornaments

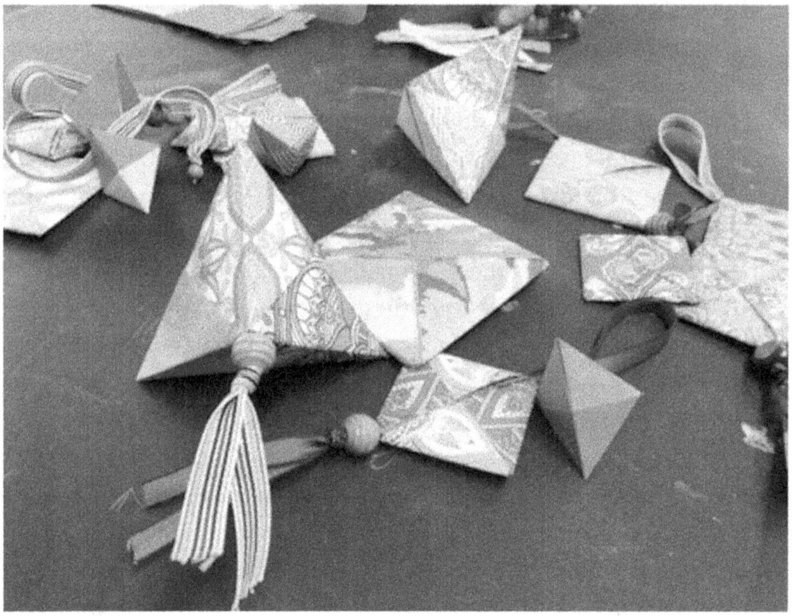

It is being mindful, *thoughtful* that trauma exists, and working to keep that idea at the forefront of one's mind. It is working to create spaces that are safe and healing, that help instead of hurt. It is truly thinking about the words and actions we as facilitators use. It isn't meant to be difficult, but is meant to become fluid in all that we do.

Trauma-Informed Lens Yoga

Part of my heart work over the last several years has been co-creating a program called Teaching Public Yoga Classes Through a Trauma-Informed Lens (Lucchesi & Soffer, 2018) with my dear friend and colleague Gwen Soffer. We created this program knowing that there are certainly survivors in every public yoga class, and that survivors do not need to identify themselves as such to hold the right to safe, healing spaces. With Gwen's knowledge as a yoga instructor and yoga studio owner (Enso Yoga, Media, PA), and my background as a survivor and someone working with trauma survivors, our program gives yoga instructors the tools to create safer spaces in every single class they teach. We believe with our whole hearts that everyone deserves the chance to experience the healing yoga can provide. Because we believe in the right to consent to touch, we teach about using permission stones. Permission stones are small stones, or whatever symbol the instructor chooses, that are available for students to *opt in* to having physical assists and adjustments in class. If someone changes their mind, they can put the stone underneath their mat or otherwise out of sight, and their change of mind will be respected. We teach simple ways to assist when someone does opt in, ways to offer verbal assists, words to consider before using, and other ways to create a trauma-informed way to teach. For example, we suggest shifting words that may hold more weight such as "bottom" or "chest" to words like "seat" and "heart center." We teach that offering suggestions instead of commands can create a powerful sense of safety and empower the student to make the practice her or his own. Everything taught is meant to be a simple *shift*, not a huge or difficult change. After completing the training, we remain open and available to participants as they work to integrate their learning into practice.

Some of the pushback we have received from some in the yoga community centers around the idea that touch is healing. The thing about touch is, it is healing unless it is not. There is a concept in yoga called Ahimsa, which simply means to cause the least harm. With this then, the yoga instructor is called to create space that will not hurt, and to instruct in ways that are the least harmful. Giving people the ability to choose touch or no touch and have that choice respected allows survivors to find healing in their own time. Shifting teaching to be trauma-informed is not meant to be difficult or entirely uproot the purpose of yoga. The goal is to allow students to make their own choices, to have their practice on their mat to be their own, and to get out of yoga what they most need and desire.

In order to gain more perspective on how important trauma-informed yoga may be, we conducted a survey for those who practice yoga and those interested in practicing yoga. We found that 97% of people surveyed had experienced one or more traumas, with 40.4% having experienced sexual assault, and 75.3% having experienced "other unwanted sexual experiences." We also found that all of the people who reported they would be less likely to attend a yoga class where they would be touched, would attend if touch was by consent only. The majority of people reported that they would sometimes like physical assists and adjustments, and sometimes would not. (Trauma-Informed Lens Yoga Survey 2, 2017) This makes the opt-in consent for touch critical. Just as we do not walk up to people on the street and touch them, and just as we are educating on the importance of gaining consent before sexual activity and assuring we still have that consent during, it is important here.

I was afforded the opportunity to practice yoga in a trauma-informed space at Enso Yoga. From the moment you walk into the studio, it feels comforting. Instructors are friendly and big-hearted, and one glace around the room and you'll see people of all ages, gender and body types. It's an open and welcoming space. Having touch be my choice completely changed what I was able to get out of my yoga practice, and how yoga has helped me to heal.

As I began, I was thinking a lot about my trauma. In part because the nature of the work I do, but also because I would find myself on my back, staring at a ceiling, and my mind drifted here and there back to my rape. I'd shoo off the thoughts and realign with my practice. At first, I didn't take a stone in any class. I just wanted the space to do my own thing and dip my toe into the deeper waters. Quickly, I felt more comfortable taking a stone in a familiar female instructor's class. Each time, I would take a stone and confidently place it at the front of my mat, signaling to her that I was ok with her touch. As she adjusted me in a few poses, I realized that I survived. I liked the information I gained through her adjustments. After a few weeks of regularly taking classes, I realized that I was thinking less and less about my trauma on the mat and elsewhere. I decided to challenge myself and take a stone in a familiar male instructor's class. Again, I survived, and I was grateful for the information and help in a few different poses.

As time went on, I longed to challenge myself physically. I liked watching what my body was capable of doing. I welcomed the help from an instructor the first time I "flipped my dog." I had never done it before because I was afraid I'd do it wrong and look silly. I also wasn't sure that I could. As I grew stronger in my practice, instructors helped me go a little bit deeper, each time only with my consent. I learned how to do fallen triangle, how to correctly do crow pose, and challenged myself successfully to do bird of paradise. I was incredibly excited that I learned to do these beautiful poses that challenged me physically as well as mentally. I gained such confidence in my practice, and it became a lovely part of my spirituality.

I fell hard for yoga as I watch it transform my life in and outside the studio. I am confident in saying that I wouldn't be where I am with my practice if I hadn't been afforded the opportunity to get there in my own time and space. Being fully supported in my practice, wherever it was each day was crucial. By being given options as opposed to commands, and ideas instead of "this way or no way," I was given a gift of a practice that is mine and no one else's. Having my boundaries respected, and allowing me to choose when I was ready to go deeper, whatever that meant for me, led me to what yoga is truly trying to achieve—being a catalyst for the journey to Self. I watched myself transform before my very eyes. Life got larger and I had tools to support the expansion. Any small remnants of trauma that were still interrupting my life got smaller. I am so grateful to this trauma-informed space for allowing me the room to get there.

Creating Sanctuary

In my early work in the victim services field, I learned about The Sanctuary Model. Sandra Bloom, a pioneer and warrior in the right to healing spaces, created The Sanctuary Model, in which everyone is informed and has the tools and language to create safe spaces and reduce the effects of trauma. Through this model, trauma histories are important, and safety while navigating the depths of that trauma is crucial. In the late 1980s, she transformed the mental health unit at a suburban Philadelphia hospital, giving self-care skills, expressive art groups, and understanding of the wounds trauma leaves behind. What doctors found was that people began to fare much better with the recognition of their traumatic pasts, and the skill building, safety, and security they were afforded as they healed (Bloom, 1992).

I spent years working in places where speaking out my trauma was discouraged. In those spaces, I watched a lot of people working with survivors while hiding their own pain. We joked how social service professionals ate too much cake and drank excessively to deal with all of the stuff we had to deal with on a daily basis. Every time we turned around, there was another cake to celebrate something else, and another happy hour to celebrate the end on the work day. No one talked about their own pain. When I did, it seemed like I was the only one working there who had been hurt. Yet, I knew this was impossible.

If people are given the opportunity to deal with their trauma histories, to have those stories respected, and given skills for nurturing their spirits, the whole workspace can heal. There would not be the need to drown out our feelings in cake, or alcohol, or whatever else dulls it in the moment. Healing spaces create healthier people.

A VISION FOR THE FUTURE

Healing arts can only be healing if they are trauma-informed. Where there is the opportunity to heal, there is also the opportunity to hurt. I go through life, mostly because of the work I do, and because I wear a permanent "trauma-informed lens", thinking of ways to make things safer for everyone. If it is safer for those who have experienced sexual violence, it cannot help but be beneficial for everyone. Training people to put on this trauma-informed lens before operating is my passion. Talk therapy is great, and traditional support groups can be so helpful, but there is a need more and more in our world for non-verbal healing opportunities. Wouldn't it be a wonderful place where someone could walk into any business or seek out any service and it would be a safe space? I imagine a world like that. The survivor in that world moves through seamlessly, finding pieces that work best to benefit her personal journey. She can choose to see a reiki practitioner, a yoga class, a massage therapist, or an art class, and she can be confident that she will feel safe and supported. She will know that she will not be thrown into the deep depths of reliving trauma, because she will have choices that are respected, and knowledge of what her experience will look like. She can try different things to create the healing journey that suits her best.

Some may question why survivors do not just seek out services that are trauma-sensitive, specific groups and classes made just for trauma survivors. Many people do not wish to speak out as a survivor every single time they do something. Typically survivors want to operate in their daily lives without directly "dealing with" their trauma. A survivor should not have to disclose personal information to a provider to find a safe and welcoming yoga class, or to get a massage, or receive reiki healing. These services should be trauma-informed at the start for all people no matter if they identify publicly as trauma survivors.

The recent social media movement where women and some men too were hash tagging "me too", speaking out their traumas, and calling out perpetrators of sexual assault and harassment is a testament to how great this need is for trauma-informed communities. Many people may have been surprised that so many of their friends and family were identifying as survivors. Others may have had their own past full of traumas triggered by everyone else's "me too," or may have felt solidarity in the movement. Some may have questioned their own actions or the actions of people in their lives, while others may have already known about the sheer number of people living in our world with histories of trauma. This movement is only highlighting what so many of us have known for years—our communities are filled with people who are hurting. Now we are being called to do something about it.

We live in a world that often wishes to brush things under the rug, which refuses to face the difficult realities before us. I, and I would venture to say most survivors, have felt the hurt of silence. There may be people who refused to believe our stories, or those who refused to listen. Those who attempt to stifle our voices when we choose to speak out are damaging to the healing process. If survivors are given the space to be listened to and believed, and the safety and security of knowing they will not be further hurt in the process of healing, I believe we can transform the world.

We have all heard the saying "hurt people hurt people." Hurt people also hurt themselves. While we are all walking around with trauma histories to some degree, where are the true healing spaces to assure we can go on living the full and brilliant lives we hoped for? If each of these potentially healing arts was truly trauma-informed, then every time a hurt person engaged in them, she or he would have another opportunity for healing.

The healing arts offer a mind-body-spirit approach to wellness. Trauma affects people on a mind-body-spirit level. Integrating the two offers a unique opportunity to individuals to heal on many levels from histories that may limit their daily lives.

For me, as I worked to craft my personal healing, I felt the fragmented, shattered bits of me that were peppered in places of hurt and speaking out, slowly come back together. I imagined these as pieces of colored glass, flying over space and time, and reconnecting as well as they could to create a mosaic before me, more intricate and complex than before. My trauma story integrated into my life, and I was able to experience post-traumatic growth. As I moved the energy in my body through yoga and healing and expressive arts, I found that the negative effects of trauma dissipated, and what was left was a strong and resilient, out-spoken, fierce survivor and thriver.

The purpose of being trauma-informed is simple— there are people who participate in the healing arts who are survivors whether they have disclosed that or not. No one has the automatic right to touch people. In yoga there is a concept called Ahimsa, which means to do the least harm possible. While yoga and other healing arts have an incredible ability to heal, they also have the potentially to do the opposite. Such beauty and human growth can come from committing to healing. But each individual should have the right to come to this in his or her own time and space. When a butterfly emerges from its cocoon, it is an incredibly painful experience. However, if a chrysalis is forced open to help the butterfly, the butterfly will die. It has to go through that painful process to become what it is meant to become.

REFERENCES

Basile, K. C., Smith, S. G., Breiding, M. J., Black, M. C., & Mahendra, R. (2014). *Sexual Violence Surveillance Uniform Definitions and Recommended Data Elements, Version 2.0*. Center for Disease Control.

Bloom, S., & Farragher, B. (2013). *Restoring Sanctuary: A New Operating System for Trauma-Informed Systems of Care*. Oxford University Press. doi:10.1093/acprof:oso/9780199796366.001.0001

Culberston, R. (1995). Embodied Trauma, Re-establishing the Self. *New Literary History*, *26*(1).

Elliot, D. E., Bejelajac, P., Fallot, R. D., Markoff, L. S., & Glover Reed, B. (2005). Trauma- Informed or Trauma- Denied: Pricincples and Implementation of Trauma- Informed Services for Women. *Journal of Community Psychology*, *33*(4), 461–477. doi:10.1002/jcop.20063

Kouri, H. (2015). *Hala Kouri's Trauma-Informed Yoga Teaching Path*. Retrieved from https://www.yogajournal.com/teach/hala-khouris-trauma-informed-yoga-teaching-path

Lucchesi, M. (2016). *Voices, Inc*. Retrieved from www.connectwithvoices.org

Lucchesi, M., Matteuchi, A., & Soffer, G. (2018). *Breaking Tradition in Favor of Consent: Results of Trauma-Informed Lens Yoga Survey II*. Retrieved from http://ybicoalition.com/breaking-tradition-favor-consent-results-trauma-informed-lens-yoga-survey-ii/

Lucchesi, M., & Soffer, G. (2015). *Trauma-Informed Lens Yoga*. Retrieved from http://www.traumainformedlensyoga.com/

Van der Kolk, B. (2006). Clinical Implications of Neuroscience Research in PTSD. *Annuals of the New York Academy of Sciences,* 1-17.

Van der Kolk, B. A., Stone, L., West, J., Rhodes, A., Emerson, D., Suvak, M., & Spinazzola, J. (2014). Yoga as an Adjunctive Treatment for Posttraumatic Stress Disorder: A Randomized Controlled Trial. *The Journal of Clinical Psychiatry*, *75*(6), e559–e565. doi:10.4088/JCP.13m08561 PMID:25004196

KEY TERMS AND DEFINITIONS

Ahimsa: A key concept in the Indian religions and yogic practice that literally means to do no harm. It is a part of the first limb of yoga from the Yoga Sutras of Patanjali.

Creative Arts: In this context, the creative arts are anything utilizing creative expression and imagination through art, crafts, movement, music, etc.

Healing Arts: In this context, the healing arts refer to holistic and complementary healing modalities that aim to help people overcome difficulties such as trauma.

Chapter 5
Learning Together:
Intergenerational Experiences for Pre-Service Art Educators

Karin L. Tollefson-Hall
James Madison University, USA

ABSTRACT

This chapter describes a 17-year partnership between the James Madison University Art Education Center and the Virginia Mennonite Retirement Community. The collaboration centers on a service-learning experience for pre-service art educators to provide art instruction to the residents of the retirement community. In 2009, the author became the coordinator of this service-learning experience and instructor for its corresponding art education course. The art education students work with independent living and memory care residents of the retirement community. Being a part of a collaborative, long-term program with the retirement community has provided tremendous learning experiences for the author, her students, the residents, and the retirement community staff regarding the power of art making in an intergenerational setting. This chapter includes a literature review, examples of artwork made in the program, descriptive observations, and reflections on the author's experience working with students and residents in the retirement community.

INTRODUCTION

Entering the auditorium, I spotted Mary across the room and quickly crossed the space to greet her. Mary is an extremely loyal artist to our classes rarely missing a day in seventeen years, and I was instantly glad to see she had returned again. Exchanging smiles and greetings I asked Mary how her summer had been. Her simple reply, "well I won 70 blue ribbons at the Fair." The astonishment must have been obvious on my face, as she humbly qualified the fact by saying, "most of them were for baking." We continued to chat a few minutes longer as she described how it is possible to bake 70 items for the County Fair in one week. Every day I spend at the retirement community my assumptions of the elderly are challenged, this was just one of those moments. (Author's personal experience)

DOI: 10.4018/978-1-5225-5981-8.ch005

The past 60 years have changed the economic structure of America. The agrarian landscape has, for the most part, disappeared and, with it, the close proximity of extended family members. Reduced frequency of contact with significant interaction has negatively affected relationships among the generations. A fear of aging, stereotypical thinking by both young and old, hostility between the generations, myths associated with aging, and deteriorations of the mind and spirit of the elderly are problems associated with segregation of the generations. (Newman, 1997 as cited in Whiteland, 2013, p. 397)

Studies have shown that ageism is common among college aged students in the United States (Fearnside et al., 2015; Knox et al., 2005; Yilmaz et al., 2012). Changes in attitude towards older adults can be fostered by common interests or experiences. Art making as a shared experience can be key to making connections between generational divides that lead to shifts in attitude and behavior (Fearnside et al., 2015). In Fearnside et al.'s (2015) study, undergraduate students enrolled in a digital photography course at Tiffin University in Ohio were given the assignment to interview residents at local nursing homes and then produce a series of photographs aesthetically representing the conversation. The students in study are not art majors and were taking the course as an elective or to fill a general education requirement including university requirements for community service. Using interview questions pre-determined by the class, students were initially fearful of the interviews, but in the course of conversation were able to find some form of commonality with their elderly partner. The photographic series were produced at the university and shared with the elderly participants at the conclusion of the course. Through analysis of class discussions, the researchers determined trends in comments indicating bias and ageism in the students. In post-project reflections, the researchers noted that students reported empathy for the elderly, surprise at what they learned about their elderly partner in the interview, or a change in the interviewees attitude to the experience once a commonality was discovered.

While we tend to focus on changing attitudes towards the elderly, it is important to recognize that biases come from both parties in an intergenerational program. Angela La Porte (2002) conducted a qualitative research study of an inner-city afterschool program connecting youth ages fourteen to eighteen with elderly persons living in their neighborhood. During a period of twelve weeks the teenagers spent six hours each week visiting a neighborhood partner who was over age 62 and who received Meals-On-Wheels services. The purpose of her study was to "investigate the development of intergenerational relationships that were encouraged through the program's three components, social service, oral history, and artmaking" (p. 54). La Porte recounts hesitations and skepticism by the elderly participants in the Harlem afterschool programs towards the teens that would be visiting them.

Universities are well suited to provide opportunities for intergenerational programs, as community outreach is a common component of university missions (Felton & Clayton, 2011). Because teacher education programs depend on hands-on teaching interactions in diverse settings with a wide range of student populations, pre-service teacher divisions are prime sites to collaborate with community centers to provide intergenerational learning experiences. Pre-service teachers, or teacher candidates, are university students who are completing a program that results in a state certified teaching license. University faculty working in the field of teacher education serve dual roles of modeling effective teaching practice and as facilitators of opportunities for their teacher candidates to practice the modeled skills in order to acquire these skills for themselves. "The literature on service-learning in teacher education indicates significant, positive correlations between in-service training and student outcomes" (Miraglia, 2017, p. 117). The goal of this chapter is to highlight the benefits of a long standing intergenerational art program for the elderly in assisted living and memory care facilities as well as for pre-service art educators.

One form of intergenerational learning programs are co-located care facilities. Co-located care facilities are non-profit or for-profit centers that combine day care for the elderly and young children in the same space, such as the program documented by Rachel Heydon (2007). The social benefits for the elderly and youth in learning together are similar regardless if the "youth" are young children or young adults. These benefits include increased self-esteem and usefulness, breaking of stereotypes, increase in understanding of other generations, increased empathy, diminished fears of aging, and increased sense of community (Heydon, 2007; Brummel, 1989; LaPorte, 1998; Grobstich, 2011; Zelkowitz, 2004; Tapley, 2004; and Larson, 2006).

In contrast to co-located care facilities, described in this chapter is an intergenerational service-learning experience for university students who are aspiring art educators (pre-service art teachers). In 2001 the Art Education Center at James Madison University (JMU) initiated a collaboration with a local retirement community, the Virginia Mennonite Retirement Community (VMRC), in order to provide art classes for the retirement community residents taught by the JMU pre-service art teachers. This mutually beneficial collaboration provides a service desired at VMRC and for the Art Education Center, opportunities for students to practice teaching in the community. One of the goals of the Art Education Program at JMU is to prepare teacher candidates for teaching all ages of individuals and to instill the value of lifelong learning. Additionally, the teaching experience at VMRC provides practice in differentiating instruction based on learning style, ability, and readiness for learning. Socially, both parties gain new friendships and connections to the larger local community, increased empathy, reduced bias, improved confidence and skills in art and teaching, and pride. Throughout this writing all names of university students and retirement community residents and staff have been changed to protect privacy.

BACKGROUND

Good teachers, like good parents, hope that the personal relations formed will enhance the likelihood that their students will live in and promote a public climate in which caring relations will continue to flourish. An important task for teachers is to connect the moral worlds of school and public life. (Nodding, 2012, p. 779)

If university faculty involved in teacher preparation desire to produce future teachers who enact an ethic of care in their teaching of youth, it is imperative for these faculty to begin by demonstrating care ethics with university students. Establishing service-learning experiences for pre-service teachers offers the opportunity to practice their developing skills in teaching by connecting to public life. Based on guidelines developed by the Alliance for Service-Learning in Education Reform, Kraft (2000) provides that service learning is a recognized method of learning that results in students' actively engaging with their community through collaborative processes. As an embedded part of the curriculum, service-learning significantly builds upon the following student-centered experiences: meeting specific needs of the community, authentic processes of self-reflection, experiencing real-world situations, and, developing a caring sense for others (p. 76). Research studies of service-learning experiences in an arts-education context have done much to encourage the reformulation of curriculum and associated practices (Taylor, 2002, 2005; Taylor & Morris, 2004; Russell & Hutzel, 2007; Buffington, 2007; Krensky & Steffen, 2008; Innella, 2010; Hutzel, Russell, & Gross, 2010). It is important to note that the cited studies support the inclusion of service-learning in general as valuable in art education. The studies are not limited to service-learning that are intergenerational or that involve pre-service teachers. For example, Russell and Hutzel (2007) define service-learning and how it relates to social emotional learning for students without describing a specific program or project. In Taylor's (2002, 2005) studies she describes two versions of service-learning programs that unite pre-service art education students with school children in afterschool programs. Strong evidence throughout the field of teacher preparation encourages the inclusion of service-learning though very few studies have been published specific to pre-service art education students and intergenerational service-learning.

Developing a sense of caring for others, one of the outcomes of service-learning, is the core of Nel Nodding's Ethic of Care. Care ethics are a feminist philosophical perspective of morality and decision making that is bound by context. As one of the first people to write a comprehensive theory of care ethics, Nel Nodding proposes that relationships are fundamental to being human, as identity is created and defined through relationships. In other words, caring relationships are the ethical basis of humanity and the volition to care is universal. Caring relationships involve the relationship between one who cares and one who is cared for that occur innately, such as between parent and child, but also those that occur out of a sense of duty such as the relationship between teacher and student or patient and caregiver (Burton & Dunn). In teacher education, the James Madison University education programs, including the Art Education Center, continually assess pre-service teachers' professional dispositions in order to predict if students will be able to perform the necessary behaviors of a successful teacher upon completion of the program. Two of the ten categories of dispositions are Respect for Others and Ethics and Fairness. Respect for others includes creating a classroom climate of respect, demonstrating the ability to act appropriately in a group of individuals with different values and perspectives, and communicating respect by listening to others and responding appropriately. Ethics and Fairness requires teacher candidates to model equity and fairness, to express empathy, and to make fair and unbiased decisions. Both of these areas are preformed successfully when a pre-service teacher utilizes an ethic of care. With regard to service-learning and care ethics, Nodding provides caution:

When children are rewarded for the caring responses we hope to encourage, the reward may displace the genuine impulse to care. Unfortunately, something like this often happens in service learning. When service learning becomes a course that must be graded, the empathic heart of it is placed at risk, and students may concentrate on the grade and its effect on their grade point average (GPA). Again, we can see that successful practice in caring depends on the caring relation between a master-carer and the one learning to care. One must learn (consciously or unconsciously) what it means to be cared for before one can learn to care for others. (Nodding, 2010, p. 148)

The James Madison University Art Education Center prepares majors in Studio Art, Design, and Art History to qualify for a preK-12 Visual Art Teaching License in Virginia. The Art Methods courses and accompanying field experiences in local schools and community settings form the core learning experiences and environments for how to be a successful art teacher. Imbedded in the Secondary Art Methods course is an intergenerational service-learning experience designed to instill the value of lifelong learning in the arts. To attempt to counter Nodding's concerns about service-learning participants' focus on grades rather than caring, the course is placed second in the sequence of art methods. Starting with the Elementary Methods course, art education, students become familiar with the art education faculty members who model a high level of support and care as they guide students through their first field experiences in elementary art classrooms. Including the intergenerational service-learning component in the second course means that students have become familiar with the program expectations and are comfortable with faculty who have worked to gain their trust before sending them into a potentially unfamiliar setting, a retirement community. The expectation that a teacher will care for her students is not a surprising or new idea to the pre-service teachers. Most students who enter a teacher licensure program do so because they had positive, and presumably caring, relationships with at least one teacher in their past that has generated their desire to become a teacher.

Even while not enjoying the course overall, students can still demonstrate caring in their field experiences. For example, in the past semester one student determined before the end of the course that he would not be continuing in the art education program. While his decision was made at some earlier point, the student did not explain his decision to leave with the faculty member until his scheduled teaching days at the retirement community had ended. He expressed not wanting to let down the residents, demonstrating a level of care even though he no longer desired to continue in the teacher education program.

COLLABORATIVE ART CLASSES AT A RETIREMENT COMMUNITY

Partners and Program History

The VMRC is home to over 800 residents. It is a non-profit continuing care retirement community, established in 1954, which provides services from independent living apartments through complete living care. Many local clubs, organizations, and university programs provide a variety of services and activities at VMRC as volunteers or for degree credit. VMRC embraces the arts in the lives of seniors with two dedicated spaces within their campus for rotating juried art exhibitions. Since the beginning of the JMU Art Education Center collaboration with VMRC, the art classes have evolved. Initially, the Secondary Art Education Methods course was only offered once each academic year. With the addition of the author as a new faculty member in art education at JMU, it was possible to teach Secondary Art Education Methods in both fall and spring semesters, doubling the amount of art class time shared with residents at VMRC.

The groups of residents that JMU pre-service art education students instruct has also grown. In the first years of the program, when the art classes were more limited due to scheduling, only residents from independent and assisted living were invited to attend. As the number of classes offered grew, memory care residents were added to the participants. Memory care, is the term used to designate units of an assisted living community that specialize in the long-term nursing care for patients with Alzheimer's disease, dementia, or other types of memory problems. The VMRC calls their specific living services Memory C.A.R.E, standing for **C**elebrating successes, **A**ffirming abilities, **R**eframing relationships, and **E**xperiencing moments of joy (http://www.vmrc.org/harrisonburg-va-memory-care). In this chapter, the more common spelling memory care will refer to the residents participating in the art class who reside in the Memory C.A.R.E facilities at VMRC.

When memory care residents were first included in the art program, the classes took the form of one mixed group of memory care and independent/assisted living residents taught the same lessons in a shared space. After two semesters, VMRC staff determined that separated classes would be preferential. From a teaching standpoint, it was not feasible to accommodate all of the residents' needs within a small activities room. This change brought the art program to the configuration it currently holds, one art activity offered within the memory care common space and a different art project taught in the activities room to independent and assisted living residents. A typical JMU semester is sixteen weeks long. The JMU art education students travel to VMRC for one hour each week during thirteen of the sixteen weeks of the semester. A semester-long session of art classes always starts with an introductory visit and ends with an art sharing gathering.

Intergenerational programs of any disciplinary focus can be beneficial for teacher candidates. The use of visual arts as the focus of study for the collaboration enhances the possible connections and benefits for residents and students. “Meaningful visual art engagement establishes social connections. It engenders empathy, reveals commonalities, and distinguishes what makes each individual unique” (Whiteland, 2013, p. 398). Working together in art making produces an opportunity for JMU students and VMRC residents to get to know each other quickly through creative expression. To maintain the focus of the art program as collaborative the art projects for each semester are mutually determined. One component that defines service-learning from community service, is that service-learning is collaborative and mutually beneficial (Felten & Colton, 2011). Nel Nodding (2012) also includes the concept of mutual understandings in the Ethic of Care. In her philosophy, she emphasizes the importance of recognizing the difference between assumed needs and expressed needs, and encourages the carer to listen attentively to what the cared-for wants rather than assuming to know the needs of others (p. 773).

In the first two weeks of the semester the students work in the classroom at JMU to prepare a project idea and an example product. The students’ first visit to VMRC is a meet-and-greet style event. Residents and students gather together in a circle for introductions. The VMRC Activities Coordinator and the author moderate the session including a welcome, introductions, and other logistical items. For the introductions, each student shares their name, art or design area of concentration, and a description of the project they want to lead. While the students are sharing, the example products are passed around the circle. Residents have an opportunity to ask questions about the projects for more clarification or to express opinions of the examples. The purpose of the sharing of examples is for the residents to select the four to six projects that will be completed in the assisted and independent living activities room. So that no one resident dominates the decision making for the group, the author brings ballots that list all of the project examples to the meet-and-greet. During the introductions, residents take notes and mark on the ballots which projects they are most interested in learning over the next eleven weeks of classes. After the introductions and voting, the JMU students are taken on a short tour of VMRC and meet with the VMRC Volunteer Coordinator for a training on policies and expectations when they are in the facility.

Back at JMU the author tallies the votes and creates a calendar of projects that is shared with the Activities Coordinator at VMRC. Rather than assuming what types of art experiences the residents will be interested in learning, the residents have an opportunity to voice their opinions for their proposed curriculum. The author encourages and welcomes the residents to tell or show ideas of projects they want to make at any time during the semester. On occasion, project ideas have come from the residents. For example, one fall Patty brought in a fabric and bead necklace that she had bought from a craft fair. After studying the necklace together for a few moments, Patty and the author determined what would be necessary to recreate such necklaces. In the following weeks, the author prepared the necessary materials for the JMU students to teach the class how to envision and create their own necklaces.

Art as Healing

In a course “Art of Necessity” Art Education Professor Emeritus from SUNY New Paltz, Alice Wexler, collaborated with Bill Richards, the Director of the Art Studio Program in the Northeast Center for Special

Care in New York. The "Art of Necessity" course engaged pre-service teachers in working one-on-one for an extended period of time as artistic mentors to persons with traumatic brain injury (TBI). The main question of inquiry for this co-taught university course was "How do the inherent healing properties of painting help to transform lives interrupted by injury?" (p. 22). This approach to using art for healing, "Art of Necessity," was developed by Richards.

Wexler (2004) describes the challenge of healing from TBI as follows:

Intention and emotional drive must be stimulated in order for the complex and interdependent function of the brain to be recovered. Brain injury affects cognitive, emotional and physical centers and results in disorientation and disconnection with self and the world. The process of recovery is, therefore, a redefinition of self. It often means leaving the previous life behind and creating a new one. With any severe injury there is a loss of orientation, body image, and place in the world. (p. 22)

But Richards' "Art of Necessity" is intentionally not art therapy. He regards art practice as healthy rather than therapeutic, differentiating his program from art therapy in several aspects. At the Northeast Center for Special Care patients are referred to as neighbors. In the art studio and through the pre-service teacher course, neighbors are paired with a mentor. The mentor is not a therapist, but rather "a friend, a parental figure, and a concerned but unprobing guide. Imagery emerges from the patient while the mentor encourages but rarely intervenes" (p. 23). The mentor is not trying to guide the neighbor to communicate specific messages as might be done by a therapist. Instead, they allow the neighbor to be deeply involved in the art materials and processes, letting messages emerge organically. Also in contrast with the practice of therapy, Richards uses art to focus on the neighbor's abilities and possibilities rather than what needs to be corrected in patients. He notes that the common practice of art therapy often utilizes physical or cognitive activities that require little or no thought. In contrast to this approach, Richards believes that art activities, such as painting, challenge TBI neighbors to use imagination and thinking (p. 34).

Carl was a particularly memorable memory care participant in the VMRC art classes. He was jovial and talkative, humorous and friendly with visitors and the art education students. When the activity was to create a small yarn weaving on a cardboard loom, Carl selected red, white, and green yarn. He shared that his color choice came from the colors of the Ethiopian flag, inspired by time he spent in Ethiopia as an adult. After sharing this fact, during the remainder of the classes in which Carl participated the author noticed that he frequently used red, white, and green even when he no longer verbally articulated why.

In the Secondary Art Education Methods Course, JMU pre-service teachers' service-learning experience has many similarities with the "Art of Necessity" course. Both courses require extensive journaling and reflection on the learning and new meanings students make as they work with disparate populations that are experiencing limitations due to age, health, or injury. Also, both courses set reflective practice as a necessary component of service-learning for recording changes in understandings, beliefs, and emotions. Students involved in service-learning need an outlet to sort through what they are actively experiencing. Felten and Clayton (2011) note that reflection is one of the core characteristics of service-learning.

While TBI is not the cause of cognitive loss for the VMRC residents who work with JMU art education students, there can be similarities in the changes in cognitive function of persons with dementia to those who have experienced TBI. Tucknott-Cohen and Ehresman (2016) researched the impact of art therapy on overall quality of life for one woman with dementia of the Alzheimer's type (DAT). Their results show that art making was valuable to DAT patients by providing an outlet for communication when verbal ability has declined. Providing an accepting space for the altered sense of reality that is a result of DAT, art making allows for time to focus on the patient's strengths and abilities, increasing emotional states, and engages complex cognitive functions such as the imagination.

A supporter of the value of including the arts in the lives of persons living with DAT, Bastings (2006) explains her findings.

Additionally, Bastings points out that studies on the direct impact of the arts on dementia patients are limited in scale with sample sizes too small to be generalizable. Also, while the arts have been recorded as beneficial for similar reasons to those found by Tucknott-Cohen and Ehresman, there are few controlled studies allowing for outside factors to be totally removed documenting the sole impact of art on dementia patients.

As non-clinicians working in the arts in a health care setting, this collaborative art program with VMRC has a similar philosophy to Richards' use of art. The JMU art education students engage with the memory care residents without goals of changing behavior or improving function. Instead the art activities are provided as a time for social gathering, a means of expression in any way the resident chooses, an exploration of materials, and a time for the students to practice universal teaching skills. Students listen attentively and converse with residents who are still verbal; they encourage and support the art making of all residents guiding them through the steps of the activity. As Wexler and Richards' students overcome fear and biases of what it means to have a TBI, the JMU art education students confront their fears and stereotypes of aging and elder care facilities. They come to understand and appreciate what residents can still do instead of only thinking about what is no longer possible.

...the arts are used to build skill (mastery), yield products in which the artists and their community can take pride, build sense of self, build social networks, and present no risk of failure. Effective arts programs are designed to go beyond keeping people with dementia busy. These programs are meant to provide access to connection with friends, family, and extended community and access to ways of giving meaning to experiences, feelings, and observations. (Basting, 2006, p. 17)

Example Scenario From the VMRC Art Classes

Henry came to our art classes in the memory care room for a little more than two years. He was a quiet but friendly face at the table. In the beginning, Henry would occasionally talk for a short time about his professional life as a golf course designer, but as time went on his verbal communication in art class slowly ended. I have observed this with many residents in memory care, as their dementia progresses the desire or possibly the capability to participate verbally diminishes.

As access to rational language is limited by the disease, people with dementia need to rely more on their emotions to connect with the world. Expression through art can foster a closer relationship between elders with dementia and others because the intimacy during the creative process can reveal the self that remains within the person with dementia that may normally be concealed in her or his daily interactions. (Lokon, et al, 2012, p. 340)

Henry was not unusual in his communication and I was just excited to see him returning to the class week after week. What I did notice about Henry was his comfort with a paint brush. He never talked about his art making experiences though I know he had artistic training in design. Every time we brought paint, he quickly took hold of the brush and would not stop painting until the class had ended.

In the beginning, he would paint some representational imagery. The use of paint varies in the memory care classes. Sometimes paint is used to simply apply decorative color, other times I bring objects for simple still lifes to inspire the residents with paint. In these open instances when, for example, I brought vases of spring daffodils cut from my garden that morning, Henry would paint something abstract but recognizable due to color or simple form to represent the flower vase on the table. With time, like his verbal communication, his use of representation faded as well. While he no longer painted recognizable images, he would paint until the paper or canvas was full. When given a square or rectangular paper, Henry would start at the bottom and fill it with lines of paint. Careful to leave little white space between the lines, changing colors often and randomly, the paper slowly filled with rows of paint. The memory care aides mentioned to me that he also exhibited this behavior during other art activities on days of the week when my students were not teaching.

For the memory care art sessions, the students and I plan a new short lesson each week. On one particular week, the lesson was to create a collaborative composition where each resident painted a circle and, if they wanted, added a silhouette of a soaring bird. Each resident was given a piece of paper with the circle drawn in the middle. Rather than requiring the memory care participants to operate within a pre-cut circle, drawing it on the paper let them paint beyond the edges, and at the end of the lesson the circles were cut out and the residents arranged them in a manner that pleased them on a large sheet of black paper. When Henry received his paper with the circle, he picked up the brush, as always, and proceeded to create concentric circles tracing the outline of the drawn circle, filling the page radially out to the edges. This was the only time I saw Henry diverge from his straight horizontal lines. Again, I noticed how comfortable Henry was when there was a brush is in hand.

There are often volunteers and visitors sitting next to memory care residents, aiding them in the art making or offering companionship. Fortuitously, one day a middle-aged woman entered the room as we were beginning to clean up the supplies, she walked over to Henry giving him a hug and addressing him as dad. While the memory care aides helped Henry clean up so that he could spend time with his daughter, I took the initiative to introduce myself and tell her how much I enjoyed her father's participation in the classes, and that he seemed to like painting. The daughter smiled, and told me that he was a recreational oil painter throughout his life. While Henry never shared his experience with me verbally, if he still remembered his oil paintings, his muscle memory knew that he had been a painter, and something inside him was still a painter. (Author's personal experience)

Student Responses to Intergenerational Experiences

In *Building Bridges Across Ages and Cognitive Barriers Through Art: College Students' Reflections on an Intergenerational Program with Elders Who Have Dementia,* Lokon, Kinney, and Kunkel (2012) collected and analyzed 300 journals written by college students in 2009-2010 at the conclusion of an art program in two retirement communities. For the study, undergraduate student volunteers spent ninety minutes each week for ten to twelve weeks working one-on-one with a dementia resident making art. The majors of the students were not included in the data so it is unclear if any of the student volunteers were studying or teaching art. From the journal reflections collected at the conclusion of the program, the authors concluded that students valued the intergenerational art program for several reasons. In general, student's attitudes towards the elderly with dementia improved, they reported increased confidence, comfort, and knowledge in their interactions with persons with dementia, and their self-esteem increased. The students generated a sense of friendship with their partners, reported decreased fear of their own aging, and in general expressed enjoyment with the experience (p. 344).

Over the eight years that the author has been directing the Secondary Art Education Methods course with its intergenerational service-learning component and reading students' journals, it is clear that students' opinions vary on the experience. All students are able to delineate value in their time with VMRC residents in memory care and assisted/independent living and indicate how it has helped them grow as teachers. For example, students frequently share that they learned to be patient and flexible in teaching. The time spent teaching in VMRC helped them better understand how to make accommodations for diverse learners' needs. Here are some sample quotes taken from student end of the semester reflections from 2010-2017.

...it's helped me retain an open mind and to not forget that no matter the age group, everyone in that group is different and will approach art individually and with different personalities.

Now I want to be more involved with my students and speak with them about their making.

[Working with the residents taught me] not to be quick to judge student ability.

[I] may have to reiterate processes multiple times before it's understood.

The most valuable thing I learned from VMRC was that learning is a lifelong process and art is a great way to reconnect to memories and to form new friendships. I was impressed with the openness to new ideas. The artmaking was not the most important part, but instead the stories that the residents told and our friendship through artmaking. I also learned that anyone, at any age can learn from someone else despite age difference, no matter how drastic.

With the description of the teaching skills learned, the students also express definite differences in the level of enjoyment in the process. Students' attitudes can change drastically based on a momentary encounter. Often the students who enjoy the experience more are those who have spent significant amounts of time with elderly family members in homes or retirement centers, those who are interested in specializing in teaching persons with exceptional needs, and a few students have parents who work in retirement communities. These students come to the first day more confident as they know what to expect. Other students are hesitant and reluctant at first due to lack of interest in the elderly, lack of time spent with older adults, or previous negative experiences with nursing or elder care facilities.

Example Scenario From the VMRC Art Classes

Lucas was one such student. He is a quiet and personally reflective student. Over the semester, I quickly learned how to recognize the small upturn of a smile and sideways glance he would get when he was thinking deeply about a comment in class, but was reluctant to add to the conversation. Lucas was always prepared on his teaching days at VMRC and knew exactly how to execute the lesson for the day. He never added comments in class beyond the practical aspects of teaching. I could see in his behaviors implementing a lesson to the group that he was nervous, but he was always successful by the end of the activity. On the last day at the art show farewell gathering, I noticed Lucas standing to the side of the group talking with Margaret, a resident from the independent living group. Margaret is relatively new to the art classes, having participated for three or four semesters. She is highly skilled in drawing and has brought me framed portraits of children that she has drawn to proudly demonstrate her past training. As Lucas and Margaret were talking, Lucas was smiling and animated. I did not go close enough to eaves drop on what they were discussing, and to this day I still do not know their topic of conversation. But the expressions conveyed attentive listening and engagement as between friends. In Lucas' final journal entry recapping the overall experience, he plainly admitted, "I didn't really enjoy working at the retirement, until the last day when I talked with Margaret." (personal communication, December 2017)

A very small moment can be impactful in shaping a student's attitude about their time teaching at VMRC. Nodding (2012) notes the importance of listening in caring, and its connection to art understandings. "Receptive listening (attention) is at the heart of caring for human others, but it is also central to hearing the messages from books, art, music and nature" (p. 775).

Art Criticism in Therapeutic Settings

Since the widespread implementation of Discipline Based Art Education (DBAE) in the early 1980s (Marche, 2002), the teaching of art criticism as a core component of art education curriculum has been accepted as good practice in the field of art education. DBAE and the National Art Education Association (NAEA) promote four content areas of learning as essential to teaching visual art: art history, art production, art criticism, and aesthetics. The first version of National Standards for Visual Art, written and distributed by the NAEA in 1994 (https://www.arteducators.org/learn-tools/national-visual-arts-standards) are formed around these four content areas. As states and school districts began generating their own standards of learning for visual art, the resulting standards were also based on art history, art production, art criticism, and aesthetics; and many sets of standards retain these four content areas today. For example, the Visual Arts Standards of Learning for Virginia Public Schools (http://www.doe.virginia.gov/testing/sol/standards_docs/fine_arts/) are broken into the following strands: Visual Communication and Production; Art History and Cultural Context; Analysis, Evaluation, and Critique; and Aesthetics. The JMU Art Education Center believes that a comprehensive art education includes all four areas of DBAE plus visual culture, meaningful self-expression, and theme-based instruction as promoted by art education scholars such as Stewart (2005), Anderson and Milbrandt (2004), Barrett (1997), Duncum (2001), and Walker (2001). Pre-service teachers in the Art Education Center are encouraged to implement comprehensive art education in their future teaching in school settings. They are also reminded that not all settings for art learning have the same goals. Art educators need to assess the goals and purposes of each learning setting to determine the most appropriate curriculum. The retirement community art classes are designed to meet the needs and interests of the residents while also providing an opportunity for pre-service teachers to teach. In VMRC the residents are most invested in art production. Our classes are short, meeting for forty minutes once a week for an average of ten weeks. Due to these constraints and the service-learning collaboration that honors the needs of all parties, the art classes at VMRC are centered around art making and self-expression. In the process of making, aesthetics and art criticism are discussed and practiced as residents make compositional and design choices. The university students not only guide technical art skills, but also talk with the residents about their ideas for the projects to push and assist expression. They ask the residents questions about their choices in color, artistic style, and composition which is a form of art criticism and aesthetic discussion. Traditional art criticism practices of talking about works of art created by professional artists have been led by other volunteer groups at VMRC outside of the art classes. Because there are other opportunities for traditional art criticism practice at the retirement community, the art classes are open to dedicating more time to art making.

Initiated by his own experiences with cancer, Terry Barrett, well known art educator specializing in art criticism, shared his life's work as a teaching artist to engage with a variety of populations of the ill, elderly, and their caregivers. Barrett (2011) writes about holding art criticism sessions in a community health center and retirement communities soliciting written and oral responses to works of contemporary art that he felt related to life, struggle, whimsy, and joy. Through the art sessions he offered his expertise in expressing ideas about contemporary art to groups of people who could benefit from a safe space to make meaning about their lives and situations in a new way, by relating it to art images. Barrett (2011) explains how he felt he was part of Nel Nodding's Ethic of Care. "We were simultaneously 'carers' and 'cared fors'." We demonstrated our caring for one another by being open about the vulnerabilities we were feeling, thus lessening isolation. We all felt cared for by the respect we felt from one another as we read our interpretations and as we listened to each other's experiences with respectful attentiveness (p. 94).

Terry Barrett (2011) explains what he feels he has gained through his art criticism sessions with the ill, ageing, and caregivers as well as the importance of art's role in the experience.

Such conversational work is a way for participants to connect with themselves in new ways, and to connect to others with whom they share their thoughts and feelings. Loneliness and isolation are lessened. The conversations and writings quickly help form communities of care… I have grown from these experiences. I am more empathetic with all people. I have less fear of aging. I have new respect for the elderly. I gained hope for future work. As a teaching artist, I am more confident and willing to take risks with people with whom I might not otherwise engage. (p.100)

Example Scenario From the VMRC Art Classes

Each semester spent working with the VMRC residents is deeply moving. Like every year, in 2013 the semester long art program finished with an exhibition of the residents' work and time for students and residents to exchange farewells.

At the social gathering one woman pulled me aside. She has participated in every art class we have offered for 12 years, and she wanted to tell me something about the class. Not sure whether she wanted to offer praise or criticism I followed her away from the group. What she told me was the best gift I have received from my experiences as a researcher. She said: "All of my life they told me I can't learn because I am dyslexic. My brother, who is an electrical engineer, came to visit me last weekend and I showed him the artwork I have made with the JMU students. He was amazed at what I had made and proud of all that I learned. I finally proved them wrong" (Personal communication, April 2013). One of the greatest benefits of our art program at the retirement communities, according to the VMRC staff, is showing families what their loved ones are capable of doing. I am honored that my students and I provide experiences for the elderly to prove us wrong. (Author's personal experience)

CONCLUSION

Throughout the collaboration with VMRC staff and directing the students' teaching of art lessons in the retirement community, patterns of statements in student journals and residents' comments at gatherings have emerged. While hesitant or anxious when first told they will be teaching the elderly, students' attitudes change by the end of the course. They recognize the teaching skills they have gained in making accommodations, patience, flexibility, and listening. Very few students express dissatisfaction with the experience since most create positive social connections with the residents. The residents show their appreciation for the program by continuing to return. While the total population of residents in the art classes is continually changing through loss and new arrivals, there has been a steady core of loyal participants. Four women have participated in every art class that the Art Education Center has offered since the collaboration began in 2001. In conversation with the residents, they share excitement about meeting new students each semester, developing greater art skills, looking forward to something new each week, and the social atmosphere of the group. Residents who have had greater amounts of art experiences in their lives bring artwork they have made outside of the student taught classes to share with the author and the students, proudly displaying their skills, requesting specific projects, or teaching the students a technique they have mastered.

Any class of students, no matter their age, will have different abilities and preferences in their art making. Based on eight years working with the residents at VMRC the author has learned how to work with the residents through trial and error, guidance from retirement community staff, and research on memory care. Here are some of the lessons learned about the types of projects that have been successful with residents.

- Higher functioning residents want to learn and improve their artistic skill. The JMU students often are reluctant to instruct the residents or directly suggest how to improve their art making. It could be assumed that this comes from an uneasiness with telling an elder what to do. The author learned to coach the students to help them feel more comfortable with giving specific directions and teaching techniques.
- Residents in both independent and memory care enjoy using all types of paint for a variety of purposes.
- Sharing visual images with residents is a helpful way to open conversation.
- All residents become easily frustrated when given blank paper and asked to come up with an idea for their artwork. Like students in school, they prefer to have some guidance for subject matter. Try to provide broad themes for students or residents to engage in their art making, giving them a source to begin an idea they want to communicate. This is a delicate balance of providing an idea for inspiration but not over directing the topic so that it does not allow students or residents choices in expression. A few examples of topics that have been successful at VMRC:

- How has music impacted your life?
- Visually interpreting a poem
- Personal stories/ identity
- Memory boxes
- Collaborative murals based on common locations or regions of the country where residents lived
- Artist books or collaborative works on family or community
- Personal connections to place
- Conservation/environmental issues
- Repurpose/recycle

- Drawing, while a desired skill, is difficult to teach. Residents want to improve but are hesitant and self-conscious of their skills. These lessons require frequent encouragement and are more successful if a very specific drawing technique is practiced and then utilized in a final work.
- While in school curricular process can be more valuable than products, the elderly tend to be more invested in the product. Provide activities that not only increase skill or introduce novel materials but also provide an attractive product. Additionally, residents have limited living space, limited income, and participate in many activities. They do not have space to save every artwork they produce, and therefore appreciate making art objects that can be given away as gifts.
- Memory care projects work best if they are completed in one class, have purposeful but limited choices, and are adaptable to a wide range of skills.
- Pre-service teachers of the classes need to practice patience and flexibility. Successful pre-service teachers are ready to repeat directions as many times as needed, rephrase choices and directions that are not understood, listen attentively, and encourage resistant or hesitant learners.
- Pre-service teachers learn to become comfortable with silence. Residents may need more time to absorb directions and questions than younger learners. Less experienced teachers can panic when they experience silence with a class. Pre-service teachers should be reminded to always allow residents ample think time and not to jump in with answers or restating questions too quickly.

ACKNOWLEDGMENT

The James Madison Art Education Center would like to thank the staff and residents at the Virginia Mennonite Retirement Community for their dedicated efforts and support of the art class collaboration. Providing a space for the classes, guidance from health care professionals, and sharing in materials have made this program successful and sustainable.

REFERENCES

Anderson, T., & Milbrandt, M. (2004). *Art for Life: Authentic instruction in art.* Columbus, OH: McGraw-Hill.

Barrett, T. (1997). *Talking About Student Art.* Worcester, MA: Davis Publications.

Barrett, T. (2011). Experiencing art with the ill, the elderly, and their caregivers. *Teaching Artist Journal, 9*(2), 90–100. doi:10.1080/15411796.2011.556565

Basting, A. (2006). Arts in dementia care: This is not the end…it's the end of this chapter. *Generations (San Francisco, Calif.), 30*(1), 16–20.

Brummel, S. (1989). Developing an intergenerational program. *Journal of Children in Contemporary Society., 20*(3–4), 119–133. doi:10.1300/J274v20n03_13

Buffington, M. (2007). The big idea: Service-learning and art education. *Art Education, 60*(6), 40–44.

Burton, B., & Dunn, C. (n.d.). Ethics of Care. *Encyclopedia Britannica*. Retrieved from https://www.britannica.com/topic/ethics-of-care

Duncum, P. (2001). Visual culture: Developments, definitions, and directions for art education. *Studies in Art Education, 42*(2), 101–112. doi:10.2307/1321027

Fearnside, L., Bereza, M., & McConn, G. (2015). Using photography to foster intergenerational understanding. *Journal of Visual Literacy, 34*(2), 70–80. doi:10.1080/23796529.2015.11674730

Felton, P., & Clayton, P. (2011). Service-Learning. *New Directions for Teaching and Learning, 128*(128), 75–84. doi:10.1002/tl.470

Grobstich, A. (2011). *Building social capital through intergenerational art participation: An analysis on trends in generational social capital* (Master of Arts dissertation). The American University. Retrieved from Dissertations & Theses. (AAT 1497652)

Heydon, R. (2007). Making meaning together; Multi-modal literacy learning opportunities in an inter-generational art programme. *Journal of Curriculum Studies, 39*(1), 35–62. doi:10.1080/00220270500422665

Hutzel, K., Russell, R., & Gross, J. (2010). Eighth-graders as role models: A service-learning art collaboration for social and emotional learning. *Art Education, 63*(4), 12–18.

Innella, V. (2010). Curriculum and the gallery space: A service-learning partnership. *Art Education, 63*(3), 46–51.

Knox, D., Kimuna, S., & Zusman, M. (2005). College student views of the elderly: Some gender differences. *College Student Journal, 39*(1), 14–16.

Kraft, N. (2000). The role of service-learning in critical thinking. In D. Well & H. Anderson (Eds.), Perspectives in Critical Thinking: Essays by Teachers in Theory and Practice (pp. 75-94). New York, NY: Peter Lang Publishing.

Krensky, B., & Steffen, S. (2008). Arts-based service-learning: A state of the field. *Art Education, 61*(4), 13–18.

LaPorte, A. (2002). Intergenerational art education; Building community in Harlem. *The Journal of Social Theory in Art Education., 22*, 51–71.

Larson, R. (2006). Building intergenerational bonds through the arts. *Generations (San Francisco, Calif.), 30*(1), 38–41.

Lokon, E., Kinney, J., & Kunkel, S. (2012). Building bridges across age and cognitive barriers through art: College students' reflections on an intergenerational program with elders who have dementia. *Journal of Intergenerational Relationships*, *10*(4), 337–354. doi:10.1080/15350770.2012.724318

Marche, T. (2002). Discipline before discipline-based art education: Federal support, curricular models, and the 1965 Penn State seminar in art education. *Arts Education Policy Review*, *103*(6), 25–33. doi:10.1080/10632910209600743

Miraglia, K. (2017). Creating authentic preservice art teacher experiences through service-learning. In L. N. Hersey & B. Bobick (Eds.), Handbook of Research on the Facilitation of Civic Engagement through Community Art (pp. 116-151). Hershey, PA: IGI Global.

National Art Education Association. (n.d.). Retrieved from arteducators.org

Russell, R., & Hutzel, K. (2007). Promoting social and emotional learning through service-learning art projects. *Art Education*, *60*(3), 6–11.

Stewart, M. (2005). *Rethinking Curriculum in Art*. Worcester, MA: Davis Publications.

Tapley, E. (2004). Seniors with cognitive disabilities: Assisting visual memory. In A. M. LaPorte (Ed.), *Community connections: Intergenerational links in art education* (pp. 45–56). Reston, VA: National Art Education Association.

Taylor, P. (2002). Service-Learning as postmodern art and pedagogy. *Studies in Art Education*, *43*(2), 124–140. doi:10.2307/1321000

Taylor, P. (2005). The children's peace project: Service-learning in art education. *International Education Journal*, *6*(5), 581–586.

Tayor, P., & Ballengee-Morris, C. (2004). Service-Learning a Language of "we.". *Art Education*, *57*(5), 6–12.

Virginia Department of Education Standards of Learning (SOL) & Testing. (n.d.). Retrieved from www.doe.virginia.gov/testing/sol/standards_docs/

Virginia Mennonite Retirement Community. (n.d.). Retrieved from www.vmrc.org

Walker, S. (2001). *Teaching Meaning in Artmaking*. Worcester, MA: Davis Publications.

Wexler, A. (2004). The art of necessity: Pictures of lives reclaimed from trauma. *Art Education*, *57*(1), 21–34.

Whiteland, S. (2013). Intergenerational visual arts programs at shared sites: A step toward sustainability. *Journal of Intergenerational Relationships*, *11*(4), 396–409. doi:10.1080/15350770.2013.839324

Yılmaz, D., Kisa, S., & Zeyneloğlu, S. (2012). University students' views and practices of ageism. *Ageing International, 37*(2), 143–154. doi:10.100712126-010-9097-5

Zelkowitz, M. (2004). Bringing the outdoors in: An intergenerational community service mural art project. In A. M. La Porte (Ed.), *Community connections: Intergenerational links in art education* (pp. 57–68). Reston, VA: National Art Education Association.

ADDITIONAL READING

Barrington, K. (2010). Creative expression for social justice with older adults. In T. Anderson, D. Gussak. K. Hallmark, & A. Paul (Eds.) Art Education for Social Justice. (91-96). Reston, VA: National Art Education Association.

Bobick, B. (2017). Promoting civic engagement through university curricula. In L. N. Hersey & B. Bobick (Eds.) Handbook of Research on the Facilitation of Civic Engagement through Community Art. (218-236). Hershey, PA: IGI Global. doi:10.4018/978-1-5225-1727-6.ch011

Bradshaw-Beaumont, H. (2017). Collaboration, teamwork and service learning within an after school community arts project: After school mural arts project. In L. N. Hersey & B. Bobick (Eds.) Handbook of Research on the Facilitation of Civic Engagement through Community Art. (36-56). Hershey, PA: IGI Global.

Carter, P., & Everitt, A. (1998). Conceptualising practice with older people: Friendship and conversation. *Ageing and Society, 18*(1), 79–99. doi:10.1017/S0144686X97006764

Cohen, G. (2006). Research in creativity and aging: The positive impacts of the arts on health and illness. *Generations (San Francisco, Calif.), 30*(1), 7–15.

Greene, M. (1995). *Releasing the Imagination.* San Francisco, CA: Jossey-Bass.

hooks, b. (1995). *Art on My Mind.* New York, NY: The New Press.

LaPorte, A. M. (2004). *Community Connections: Intergenerational Links in Art Education.* Reston, VA: National Art Education Association.

Maarhuis, P., & Rud, A. (2017). Dewey, school violence, and aesthetic response: Healing the community through arts after disaster. In L. N. Hersey & B. Bobick (Eds.) Handbook of Research on the Facilitation of Civic Engagement through Community Art. (237-266). Hershey, PA: IGI Global.

Milbrandt, M. (2006). A collaborative model for art education teacher preparation. *Arts Education Policy Review, 107*(5), 13–21. doi:10.3200/AEPR.107.5.13-21

KEY TERMS AND DEFINITIONS

Ageism: Stereotypes, prejudices, or biases based on a person's age.

Ethic of Care: A feminist moral theory based on the assumption that relationships are fundamental to human identity and moral action. Care ethics involve the relationships between a carer and a cared for that are biological or by obligation.

Intergenerational: Programs or activities that involve persons of different generations.

Memory Care: A form of living care for patients with memory related problems such as dementia and Alzheimer's disease.

Pre-Service Teacher: Students currently working towards completion of a teaching license at a college, university, or related program.

Service-Learning: An educational approach that combines course learning objectives with community service. Service-learning is connected to curriculum, based in mutual partnerships, and includes student reflections on learning goals.

Section 3
Learning Adaptive Responses

Our responses to the world around us are often informed by our past experiences. Past experiences, whether positive or negative, often hold great power in our present state of being. If left unresolved, past traumatic experiences can hinder present growth of body, mind and spirit, due to an inhibited ability to cope with the past. The following chapters provide tools for non-clinicians to utilize and teach to those they serve in order to help move away from maladaptive responses and adopt more positive, adaptive responses.

Chapter 6
The Magic of Monologue:
Healing Depression Through Drama

Sue Gauthier-Pin
Peninsula Center for Children and Families, USA

ABSTRACT

In this chapter, the author explores her personal experience with depression and the healing through applied community theater. The author discusses how her autobiographical performance is similar to aspects of drama therapy, mindfulness, and cognitive behavioral therapy. The author explores how four common treatment goals for depression can be addressed through the process of writing, rehearsing, and performing an autobiographical performance. Advice is given to non-clinical practitioners on how to address depression among their clients. Findings from this case study promote that applied community theater, in addition to traditional treatments, can serve as catalyst for furthering the healing of depression.

INTRODUCTION

Depression. It is that deep well of despair that many people suffer with silently and struggle to find relief from without some kind of professional intervention. It can sneak into our lives without us even realizing it, making us feel listless, lonely and longing for hope and the person we used to be. This chapter proposes that in addition to seeking professional clinical services, depressive symptoms can further be healed through the experience of engaging in an autobiographical community theater performance.

In 2017 I experienced a relapse of what some might call, "high functioning" depression, and found that performing with my local community theater was an incredibly healing experience. By high functioning, I mean that I was still able to go to work and show up for my clients, but the moment I came home, I would crawl into bed and cry and "beat myself up" mentally. I had stopped hanging out with friends, and sludged through the paperwork required for my job, often crying while typing. I was living with the phrase, "I'm a terrible person," on repeat every day and the "shoulds" were deafening. I have struggled with depression since I was young, but, for a time, I had managed to be in remission. In late 2016, however, when a swift wave of grief and life transitions changed the tide, I was knocked back into a familiar hole of excruciating pain. It was subtle at first, and I began noticing that I was more

DOI: 10.4018/978-1-5225-5981-8.ch006

tired than usual and was struggling to concentrate on tasks. Then came the plummet in self-esteem and my "inner critic" began to tell me the most heinous things about who I was and how I was completely unworthy of my existence. Every bump in the road felt disheartening. Every move felt laborious. The fear of disappointing others and the threat of failure loomed constantly. There were stretches of days where I did not want to get out of bed and thought about taking my own life; doubting the whole time that I would ever recover.

I would tell myself, "you should have known better," because in the thick of it, this was the most embarrassing part: I am a trained mental health professional. I have a master's degree in Counseling Psychology with a specialization in Expressive Arts Therapy. I am a registered Marriage and Family Therapist Associate in the state of California. I work in schools, at an addiction treatment facility, and see clients in a group private practice. I work with people struggling with depression everyday. Yet there I was, in the middle of an exceptionally hard season of life, feeling like the biggest imposter. I often worried about what people would think if they found out that I was struggling, too. I was in the deep end of a depressive "spiral of shame."

Many of the thoughts, emotions, and behaviors I have described in my narrative fit within the clinical criteria of depression set forth by the American Psychiatric Association (2013) in their Diagnostic and Statistical Manual of Mental Disorders (p. 155). The DSM-5, which is the manual used by mental health professionals to diagnosis mental health disorders lists nine different types of depression and views depressive symptoms on a spectrum ranging from mild to severe. I will expand on the two types that I have identified in my own experience, Persistent Depressive Disorder (also known as Dysthymia) and Major Depressive Disorder.

In the beginning of my narrative, the characteristics of my depression were that of Dysthymia. The DSM-5 (American Psychiatric Association, 2013) characterizes it by a "depressed mood for most of the day, for more days than not, as indicated by either subjective account or observation by others, for at least two years," and must include the experience of two or more of the following symptoms: "poor appetite or overeating; low energy or fatigue; low self-esteem; poor concentration or difficulty making decisions; feelings of hopelessness" (p. 168). My Dysthymia gradually worsened and eventually I met the criteria for Major Depressive Disorder (MDD), which is characterized by having symptoms over a two week period that represent a noticeable change in functioning. One of the symptoms is either a "depressed mood" or a "markedly diminished interest or pleasure in all, or almost all, activities most of the day, nearly every day", and must include four of the following symptoms: significant weight loss or gain; insomnia or hypersomnia; psychomotor agitation or retardation; fatigue or loss of energy; feelings of worthlessness or excessive inappropriate guilt; diminished ability to think or concentrate or indecisiveness; and recurrent thoughts of death, suicidal ideation, or suicide attempt (American Psychiatric Association, 2013, p. 160).

In this narrative, I used the term "high functioning" depression. This is a new term coined by popular culture that to some might mean Dysthymia, but to me, the term feels like it fits my experience with a milder form of MDD. Annie Wright (2017), a psychotherapist and contributor to the mental health blog site The Mighty, explains that the term was created as a way for people to delineate between the stereotypical "crippling depression" and the lived experience of those who are still able to go to work, spend time with friends, are in romantic relationships, etc., yet are struggling to "keep it together" and are "gripped with a challenging set of symptoms invisible to those of us who love and know them" (Wright, 2017). Wright (2017) warns that even though "high functioning depression doesn't look like the stereotype of depression most of us hold in our heads, this diagnosis nevertheless carries significant risks if left untreated."

Unfortunately, depression does not resolve on its own, and clinical treatment is recommended in order to resolve it. The two most effective evidence-based treatments for depression are psychotherapy and/or medication management. Wright (2017) cites "The Canadian Psychological Association," saying, "Psychotherapy is as effective as mediation in treating depression and is more effective than medication in preventing relapse. For some patients, the combination of psychotherapy and mediation will be more beneficial than either treatment on its own." Recognizing my descent into the abyss, I chose to go back to therapy with my old therapist who had helped me in the past and introduced me to expressive arts therapy many years ago.

Soon into our work together my therapist, Marilyn, gently offered the idea that "perhaps your depression is your soul grieving its loss of connection with you" (M. Owen, personal communication, 2017). Gob smacked, I knew that she was onto something. The last time we worked together I produced a piece of mixed-media art that moved me out of my depression and into the light of the living. Once again, she suggested I go back to the basics for any creative person; to re-engage in a life-giving arts practice. A few days later, my dear friend, Ann Wellman, the creator and director of the Long Beach Community Theater in Long Beach, CA, posted an advertisement that she was accepting submissions for her next show, and that she needed performers. Remembering the sage advice from my therapist, I pushed myself to courageously submit a piece and it was accepted.

The Long Beach Community Theater (LBCT) is a grassroots, storyteller theater that serves to "inspire and lift up" individuals in the Long Beach and Greater Los Angeles community (Wellman, 2018). This small theater focuses on performers presenting a five-minute piece on a specific topic that must be a true autobiographical story. Performers can tell their stories through any art form, not just acting. Performances are similar to that of a variety show centralized on one theme. Topics range from hard-hitting and deeply moving, to light-hearted and fun. Ann states on the LBCT's website that,

All are welcome to participate - from children and youngsters, to adult dreamers and senior citizens. Male, female, transgender, gay, straight, happy, sad, experienced-on-the-stage to never-been-on-the-stage-before-in-my-whole-life-but-I-always-wanted-to-get-on-the-stage – diversity is not only welcomed, it is encouraged. (Wellman, 2018)

Ann's aim is to provide a safe and supportive space, "to empower artists and audiences to make Long Beach a more conscious and compassionate community and [to] generate dialogue" (Wellman, 2018). With this being the goal of the LBCT, it is considered an "applied" theater experience. Applied theater is a term used to describe, "forms of dramatic activity that primarily exist outside conventional mainstream theater intuitions, and which are specifically intended to benefit individuals, communities and societies" (Nicholson, 2005, p. 2).

In this chapter, I share my story of depression and redemptive healing through my personal experience of an autobiographical performance with the LBCT on the theme of "…The Magic of Music." I acknowledge that my perceived transformative experience is in part due to my knowledge of the clinical underpinnings of the healing power of the arts, and that not all participants in the LBCT will see or have seen their experience in the same light. I will compare my community theater experience to that of models of drama therapy; specifically a branch of Self-Revelatory Performance, the "Embodied Life Stories Process." I will discuss how my theatrical experience inadvertently addressed five of the typical psychotherapeutic goals for someone seeking clinical treatment for depression, including socialization, improved self-esteem, self-expression, shame resilience, and improving the mind-body connection. My intention is that this chapter will serve to educate and empower arts-based, non-clinical practitioners with the clinical knowledge of how their work is serving to heal the individuals in their communities on a mental, emotional, and behavioral level.

My Experience With Therapeutic Theater

The autobiographical performance that I reference throughout this chapter was entitled, "Finding My Voice: A Musical Montage," and took place on November 4, 2017 with the LBCT in Long Beach, CA (Gauthier-Pin, 2017). I was one of twenty-four performers that took the stage that night to share our stories on "…The Magic of Music." My piece focused on my experience of being a very shy child who found her voice through musicals. In my piece of work, I take the audience through moments of my life when I was able to express myself through singing. The piece included snippets of music from *Aladdin*, *Newsies*, *The Sound of Music*, *Fiddler on the Roof*, *Moana,* and *Les Misérables*. The piece was funny, heartwarming, and concluded with me sharing about my grief surrounding the death of a friend. My dream for the piece was to take the audience on an emotional journey, and to allow my shy inner six-year-old child the opportunity to shine on stage. The entire process of writing my piece, rehearsing it, and eventually performing it took a tremendous amount of courage. I was terrified throughout the entire journey. It felt like I was taking a huge leap of faith, but I did it and my piece was well received by the audience. This process felt like therapy, a spiritual awakening, and a "homecoming" back to myself. Even though I was receiving psychotherapy, I pinpoint this experience as the catalyst that catapulted me out of my depression.

Clinical Approaches

Being a clinical expressive arts therapist, I draw many comparisons of my healing journey to forms of drama therapy, mindfulness, and cognitive behavioral therapy. First, I will discuss what I feel is a similar clinical approach from drama therapy, Self-Revelatory Performance. Self-Revelatory Performances (Self-Revs) were born out the movement of autobiographical theater that began in the second half of the twentieth century and was influenced by "the embrace of the memoir in literature, sociopolitical and feminist visual art, solo performance art, and autobiographical performance" (Pendzik, Emunah and Johnson, 2017, p. 1). Autobiographical performances were noted for their novelty of sharing honest and raw portrayals of the actors' personal lives. As a first time autobiographical performer, historic actor Spalding Gray shared that his experience had culminated in a cathartic release by appearing on stage as himself, and sharing a piece of his story with others (Snow, 2017, p. 29). From this, Renée Emunah was inspired to create the drama therapy process of Self-Revelatory Performance, which is differentiated from other autobiographical performances, because " in addition to being based on one's real life, it presents issues whose exposure demands a high level of risk-taking, partly because they are current issues, rather than past issues which have already been resolved" (Snow, 2017, p. 31). The aim of Self-Revs is to help clients or students work through a current issue with the intention of performing their piece for a carefully selected and empathetic audience. Emunah (2017) explains that "the piece grows alongside the person's life, and the person's life is influenced by the work on the piece" (p. 42). The performers' work culminates with one performance in front of a participatory audience that the performer can interact with in order to enhance the healing potential of the piece. When the performance has finished, the performer talks about their experience with the audience, and the audience is able to share with the performer how they were moved by their personal narrative. Thus, providing a corrective emotional experience of being seen, heard, validated and accepted through the performer's courage to be open and vulnerable with themselves and the audience.

LBCT's approach to storytelling theater is similar to that of Self-Revs in that Ann goes to great lengths to insure that her performers feel supported and uplifted. She also encourages her performers to dig deep and leave their hearts on the stage. Vulnerability is of the utmost value, because it has the power to transform the performer and the community at large. Ann wants to give her performers the opportunity to be seen, heard, and celebrated for who they are and for them to revel their own theatrical brilliance.

Secondly, I found aspects of the advice that Ann gave me to be similar to that of Cognitive Behavior Therapy (CBT). CBT is a type of psychotherapy in which negative patterns of thought about oneself and the world are challenged in order to change unwanted behavioral patterns or treat mood disorders such as depression. CBT has even been studied and found to be effective with actors who struggle with performance anxiety (Clason, Johansson, and Mortberg, 2015, p. 1). Approaches that were similar to CBT were utilized at rehearsals and through communication with Ann throughout the process leading up to the performance.

Thirdly, I found that the practice of mindfulness was included in my process with the LBCT. Mindfulness has been combined with CBT to form Mindfulness-Based Cognitive Therapy (MBCT). This approach is "a modified form of cognitive therapy that incorporates mindfulness practices such as meditation and breathing exercises" (MBCT, 2018). Research has found that by utilizing mindfulness, psychotherapy clients can "break away from negative thought patterns that can cause a downward spiral into a depressed state so they will be able to fight off depression before it takes hold" (MBCT, 2018). In my experience, mindfulness practices were explored during rehearsals. Performers were encouraged to practice mindfulness any time they were practicing their performance, on the stage or at home.

Clinical Implications

Reflecting back on my experience with depression, I noticed two main aspects that stand out to me. The first being the insurmountable shame that I felt as a therapist who was supposed to be helping people struggling with depression and yet, somehow, found myself in the throws of it myself. The second aspect being the slippery slope of isolation that ultimately was affecting my identity and my sense of worth. These two overarching themes impacted my well-being of feeling worthy of being around others, contributed to a significant drop in my self-esteem, bound me by the inability to be honest about my depression with others, and created an experience of a mind-body split during this time. In this section, I will examine four common clinical therapeutic goals for treating depression and how my experience with the LBCT addressed these goals.

Shame Resiliency

Often times when I am working with someone struggling with depression, one of the primary goals is healing the underlying shame contributing to their depressive symptoms. Many folks experience shame as a deeply rooted cognitive distortion of "not being enough" and "not being loveable." The director of the LBCT, Ann, took great care to treat my journey from writing my piece to the culminating performance with incredible tenderness and respect for the sacred and courageous act of sharing my story. Rubin (2017), the creator of the Self-Rev "Embodied Life Stories Process," states that one of her first goals in working with clients is to build attachment as the foundation of the therapeutic process in order to counteract shame (p. 129). Attachment can be summed up as the connection we have with others that makes us feel safe and secure in the world. Beginning in childhood, we form attachments to our caregivers, which can help or hinder us in developing trust and our sense of self. As adults, when we experience excruciating vulnerability, our struggles with early attachment can arise. In my case, my depression had begun to distort my perception of myself and what I was capable of accomplishing, making me feel wildly insecure. In many ways, my interactions with Ann were similar to that of early attachment in childhood when children need to be "mirrored" in order to feel safe and secure. Through working closely with Ann, I came to trust her insight and that she had my best interest at heart. More importantly, she was able to mirror back to me that my story was worthy of being shared, which began to change my inner dialogue to "I am good enough to share my story," thus beginning to soften the hold that my shame had over me. Rubin (2017) states, "The experience of seeing oneself through another's eyes can be deeply shaming or profoundly healing" (p. 129). In my case, my experience of working with Ann, as my director, served as the foundation of my healing experience.

Another way in which Ann fostered "counter-shaming" experiences is how she facilitated the traditional "critiquing" process with the cast (Rubin, 2017, p. 132). Ann was clear about making this a positive experience for everyone involved. She set boundaries for the members of the cast by asking cast members to share "comments, compliments, and questions." After performing my piece for the cast for the first time, I was slightly checked-out or "dissociative," meaning that it felt as if part of me had left my body and was observing from afar. I was nervous about the feedback that I would receive. My depression told me that "I was terrible and sounded like a dying bird," but to my surprise and relief, I was met with beautiful compliments, positive comments, and very insightful questions aimed not to tear me down, but to lift me up and expand my piece's potency. This experience provided me with evidence that I could use to tell myself the truth about my performance, that I indeed was "good enough" to be a part of the show.

Another unintended intervention that helped my depression was Ann's encouragement to practice positive self-talk. This is a common intervention used in Cognitive Behavioral Therapy, similar to that of "thought stopping" and "thought replacement." Thought-stopping is an intervention utilized to stop the vicious cycle of negative thoughts that produces negative feelings, which lead to negative actions or behaviors. Thought replacement interrupts the cycle of negative self-talk by interjecting positive statements into our thoughts, to create positive feelings, that then lead to positive outcomes. From the first rehearsal to the night of the performance, Ann encouraged the cast to think positively and urged us to actively choose to change our inner dialogue to be more positive in the service of our confidence on the night of our performance.

Socialization

The second goal that is addressed in the treatment of depression is to increase socialization. This goal was addressed in a number of ways through the LBCT. The first way in which Ann facilitated socialization in the group was by taking great lengths to help the cast feel comfortable with one another. Ann began each rehearsal by centering the group by reviewing the mission, vision, and philosophy of the LBCT to remind us of our common goals. That was followed by leading us through group drama games such as "Zip Zap Zoom," a friendly competition of saying tongue twisters, and working with a partner to foster deeper connections and relaxation with one another through the "Rag Doll" exercise. These games promoted group cohesion through mirroring, consistent eye contact, and greater physical intimacy between cast members, cultivating safety and trust among the group. Through these activities I was able to interact with everyone in the cast, making me feel more comfortable opening up and sharing my story. I was also able to develop deeper rapport with at least one person in the cast who became my safe person that I would check in with throughout the process.

Another way in which a sense of connection with others was created was through performing for an audience. In Self-Revs the audience is aware that they are witnessing the performers' intimate process and are asked to "soften their hearts to receive their stories" (Rubin, 2017, p. 137). In the same way Ann reminds the audience of the LBCT that the performers are courageous for sharing their stories, and she requests that the audience hold the performers and their stories with the deepest respect. As a performer, taking the stage felt like an initiation rite, like being presented in front of my community for a coming of age ritual; moving from a place of feeling hidden to highly visible (Volkas, 2017). My hope was that my story would resonate with at least one other person and that it would help them to make meaning of their own personal narrative. Sajnani (2017), a drama therapist, contributes this emotional interplay between the performer and the audience to be the relational aesthetics of performance. Relational aesthetics call the audience to lean in and create "a shared world or a conduit for [a] relational experience" (2017, p.87). This phenomenon of a shared experience reminds me of the quote by Marianne Williamson: "As we let our light shine, we unconsciously give other people permission to do the same. As we are liberated from our own fear, our presence actually liberates others." In this way, "the role of the audience as witness can repair a vital link, bringing the person back into community from isolation" and can help audience members tap into their own meaningful experiences, creating deeper connections with one another (Rubin, 2017, p. 129).

The Mind-Body Connection

The third clinical goal addressed by my experience was cultivating a mind-body connection through mindfulness and the embodiment of emotions. Mindfulness is the practice of being "present", and is often achieved by engaging one's awareness of the physical body in order to feel more grounded. A key component of mindfulness is to "just notice" how you feel without judgment, then to let go of the thought or feeling, bringing your awareness back to your physical body (Mendez-McLeish, 2017). Ann encouraged us to practice deep breathing in order to achieve a sense of relaxation. I vividly remember using this technique right before taking the stage on the night of our performance and attribute mindfulness to feeling more centered during my performance.

Practicing mindfulness also made it easier to embody my emotions on stage. Part of depression is the struggle with emotional regulation and quickly becoming overwhelmed. Mindfulness allowed me to feel emotions without judging them. In a sense, I gave myself permission to feel again, without becoming overwhelmed (Rubin, 2017, p. 136). This practice was important in order to be able to authentically convey emotion on stage. Without mindfulness I would have struggled to feel present enough to explore the embodiment of my story. By being able to remain present, I was able to tap into the excitement of my 6 year old self, feel confident while punching the air, courageous by making large circles with my arms, and pausing to allow my tears to well-up while looking at the picture of my friend who had passed away. The embodiment of emotions gave me the gift of being able to access more positive emotions that

I had not felt in awhile, thus reminding me that "hope is real and recovery is possible" (Tworkowski, 2015, p. 45). Through performing, my body, mind and emotions became more integrated and my inner dialogue shifted to, "you can feel this joy again" and "you're allowed to tell your story." By having Ann encourage me to have bigger, more dramatic movements and pausing to take a moment with my grief, it strengthened my connection to my emotions and gave me hope again. This experience evoked fear, anxiety, and shame, but also taught me that I can tolerate feeling my emotions and have the tools to bring them into balance.

Self-Expression

The fourth goal addressed through my experience with the LBCT was self expression. The story I performed was autobiographical and exposed the audience to a range of emotions. I shared vulnerable parts of my narrative of being shy, living with shame, and the depths of my grief. Social work researcher Brené Brown, has found that vulnerability is the birthplace of connection. She says in her TedTalk (Brown, 2011), "In order for connection to happen we have to allow ourselves to be seen, really seen", and in doing so we can begin to have a sense of belonging. Therefore, the process of writing and performing an autobiographical performance, that was able to be received by an empathetic audience, gave me what is known as a "corrective emotional experience." In the past, vulnerability has meant that I would feel shame, embarrassment and would want to hide. This experience made me feel differently, in that I could trust others with my tender heart. I could be seen, heard, validated, accepted and even celebrated. Instead of being torn apart, I was lifted up by my community, which began to change my association with vulnerability from one of fear to one of trust. Brown (2011) says that when we own our story and live in our truth, we have the capacity to change the power it holds over us. We can be redeemed.

DISCUSSION

It is my goal that by sharing my personal experience with "applied" community theater that arts-based non-clinical practitioners will feel empowered in their work as change agents in their communities. My story is not an isolated case. According to The National Institute of Mental Health (2017), "16.2 million adults in the United States have had at least one major depressive episode," representing "6.7% of all U.S. adults." Based off of the case study of my experience, applied therapeutic theater programs are making a difference in the lives of both individuals and communities, and can be a valuable resource to those struggling with depression.

The beauty of communities cultivating "applied" community theater and other therapeutic arts programs is that it provides a free platform for those who lack access to psychotherapy or are unaware that psychotherapy could be beneficial for them. Out of the many Americans experiencing depression, 37% will not receive treatment due to the many barriers preventing them from getting help (NIMH, 2017). One of the barriers to receiving mental health care is the unfamiliarity with the symptoms of depression. Many folks may not know that they are struggling with a mental health issue. They may just say, "I'm not feeling well," but do not recognize and interpret their symptoms to be that of a depressive episode

(Gulliver et. al, 2010, pg. 5). Another barrier is that depression in many communities is still stigmatized and misunderstood. There is still the sentiment that if someone wanted to feel better that they could "pull themselves up by their bootstraps." This belief is incorrect and perpetuates harm to those struggling with depression. It is shaming, counter-productive, and has the tendency to drive those who are struggling into even more isolation. This kind of stigma can worsen one's distressing internalized belief that reaching out for help will make them a burden on their families, friends, and communities. Financial limitations are another barrier to seeking treatment. Therapy can be expensive and many insurance policies cover limited amounts of psychotherapy sessions. Unfortunately, many creative arts therapies are also not covered by insurance policies, which means those seeking help will have to pay out-of-pocket. These barriers are particularly concerning considering that depression does not go away on its own. It requires some form of healing intervention in order for it to be alleviated.

The Do's and Don't

Although depression needs to be addressed by a clinical professional, non-clinical practitioners can be tremendously helpful in companioning someone struggling with depression on their journey. First, you can help others by knowing the signs and symptoms of depression. If you feel that someone you are working with might be struggling with depression or confides in you that they are struggling, meet their vulnerability with empathy, understanding, and non-judgment. Be prepared and have a list of local mental health professionals and hotline phone numbers available to give to those who are struggling. Mental health providers want to be of service and most are happy to provide you with a free consultation if you have questions or need clarity on when to refer your participants for clinical treatment.

If you are considering facilitating an autobiographical performance, know that "heavy" emotions can be triggered in the process. To avoid this, encourage your participants to share "scars, not wounds." Consider creating a consent form that explains the emotional and social risks of sharing one's story with a public audience. Also, consider having some kind of informed consent for your audience, so they are aware of the depth of material being shared and how it might impact them. Please be mindful that the drama therapy approach shared in this chapter, Self-Revs, is a form of therapy. If you want to create a performance where the actors explore their current issues, like a Self-Rev, I strongly suggest collaborating with a drama, creative arts, or expressive arts therapist in order to provide more safety and containment for your participants.

Through this case study of my own experience, I found that non-clinical arts-based programming can aid participants in their recovery from depression by fostering a sense of belonging through forming secure attachments between facilitators and participants, by building safety and trust within the group, and by offering a reparative experience of empathetic witnessing. Facilitators can prioritize helping their participants reduce their sense of shame by promoting vulnerability and setting boundaries in order to create containment. Facilitators can also promote the performance of autobiographical material for participants to be able to embody and process their emotions. It is also helpful to intentionally nurture your participants by teaching them to practice mindfulness and positive self-talk, which will inspire a more calm and supportive environment.

From the evidence proposed in this chapter, applied community theater can provide an inspiring platform for individual and social change. Applied theater that utilizes autobiographical performances creates a supportive environment for participants to explore their personal narratives and helps connect them to others in their community. By participating in this type of program, performers can begin to have a sense of purpose for their pain, and are able to alchemize their negative experiences into something life-giving that has the potential to heal themselves, the witnesses in the audience, and those in their greater community. Sajnani (2017) offers that "performing one's life on stage…involves giving aesthetic expression to lived experiences in the service of healing for both actors and audiences" (p. 85). Applied theater, including the LBCT, has the potential to transform the cultural narrative of depression from one of secrecy and shame to one that promotes a culture of vulnerability and whole-hearted living.

REFERENCES

American Psychiatric Association. (2013). *Diagnostic and statistical manual of mental disorders* (5th ed.). Arlington, VA: American Psychiatric Publishing.

Brown, B. (2011, January). *Brené Brown: The power of vulnerability* (Video File). Retrieved from https://www.youtube.com/watch?v=iCvmsMzlF7o

Clason, J., Johansson, F., & Mortberg, E. (2015). Individual cognitive therapy for professional actors with performance anxiety. *Ann Depress Anxiety*, *2*(6), 1066.

Emunah, R. (2017). From behind the scenes to facing an audience in self-revelatory performance. In S. Penkzik, R. Emunah, & R. J. David (Eds.), *The Self In Performance: Autobiographical, Self-Revelatory, and Autoethnographic Forms of Therapeutic Theatre* (pp. 37–53). Palgrave Macmillian.

Faigin, D. A., & Stein, C. H. (2015). Community-based theater and adults with psychiatric disabilities: Social activism, performance and community engagement. *American Journal of Community Psychology*, *55*(1-2), 148–163. doi:10.100710464-014-9695-6 PMID:25520209

Gauthier-Pin, S. (Writer/Performer). (2017, November 4). *Finding my voice: A musical montage* (Video File). Live performance in St. Thomas of Canterbury Church, Long Beach, CA. Retrieved from https://www.youtube.com/watch?v=Dq_r7ODbj2U

Gulliver, Griffiths, K. M., & Christensen, H. (2010). Perceived barriers and facilitators to mental health help-seeking in young people: A systematic review. *BMC Psychiatry*, *10*(1), 113. doi:10.1186/1471-244X-10-113 PMID:21192795

Mendez-McLeish, S. (2017). *The art of arriving* (Video File) Magnolia Moon Healing Arts. Retrieved at https://youtu.be/RnlZSsVIZ_Q

Mindfulness-based cognitive therapy. (2018). *Psychology Today*. Retrieved from https://www.psychologytoday.com/us/therapy-types/mindfulness-based-cognitive-therapy

National Institute of Mental Health. (2017). *Major depression*. Retrieved from URL https://www.nimh.nih.gov/health/statistics/major-depression.shtml

Nicholson, H. (2005). *Applied drama: the gift of theater*. New York: Palgrave. doi:10.1007/978-0-230-20469-0

Pendzik, S., Emunah, R., & Johnson, D. R. (2017). The self in performance: Context, definitions, directions. In S. Penkzik, R. Emunah, & R. J. David (Eds.), *The Self In Performance: Autobiographical, Self-Revelatory, and Autoethnographic Forms of Therapeutic Theatre* (pp. 1–18). Palgrave Macmillian.

Rubin, S. (2017). Embodied life stories: Transforming shame through self-revelatory performance. In S. Penkzik, R. Emunah, & R. J. David (Eds.), *The Self In Performance: Autobiographical, Self-Revelatory, and Autoethnographic Forms of Therapeutic Theatre* (pp. 129–139). Palgrave Macmillian.

Sajnani, N. (2017). Relational aesthetics in performance of personal story. In S. Penkzik, R. Emunah, & R. J. David (Eds.), *The Self In Performance: Autobiographical, Self-Revelatory, and Autoethnographic Forms of Therapeutic Theatre* (pp. 85–95). Palgrave Macmillian.

Snow, S. (2017). Influences of experimental theatre on the emergence of self-revelatory performance. In S. Penkzik, R. Emunah, & R. J. David (Eds.), *The Self In Performance: Autobiographical, Self-Revelatory, and Autoethnographic Forms of Therapeutic Theatre* (pp. 21–35). Palgrave Macmillian.

Volkas, A. (2017). Autobiographical therapeutic performance as individual therapy. In S. Penkzik, R. Emunah, & R. J. David (Eds.), *The Self In Performance: Autobiographical, Self-Revelatory, and Autoethnographic Forms of Therapeutic Theatre* (pp. 113–127). Palgrave Macmillian.

Wellman, A. (2018). *Long beach community theater*. Retrieved from http://longbeachcommunitytheater.com

Wright, A. (2017, May 17). *What are the signs of 'high functioning' depression and could you have it?* Retrieved from https://themighty.com/2017/05/signs-of-high-functioning-depression-or-dysthymia/

Chapter 7
Embroidery, Resilience, and Discovery:
Embroidery as Healing in the Guajira Peninsula

Sarah Joy Baker
Eastern University, USA

ABSTRACT

This chapter explores how embroidery as a visual mapping tool can address situations of historical trauma and increase community resilience through a process of conscientisation and grassroots organizing. The author will draw from her fieldwork with a group of indigenous Wayuu women in the Guajira Peninsula in northern Colombia, a region that has been significantly affected by climate change and decades of armed conflict. The women created embroidered maps of their daily lives, analyzed these maps for common themes and challenges, identified the root causes of the oppression they experience daily, and discussed action steps to address these power disparities. The author suggests that embroidery is a powerful healing tool for engaging indigenous women in a dignified manner by illuminating their narratives of resilience in order to address historical trauma.

INTRODUCTION

Embroidery is an effective tool that can be used to help indigenous women around the world reflect critically on their daily lives, and discover the inherent resilience they possess that allows them to navigate historical and ongoing trauma from a grassroots level. The author will draw from her fieldwork with a group of Wayuu indigenous women in northern Colombia who suffer multiple traumas as a result of poverty, climate change, large-scale development projects, and a decades-long civil war. This uncertain future is a subtle and ongoing form of trauma that challenges community autonomy, produces feelings of isolation and helplessness, and threatens their traditional way of life. Despite all of this, the Wayuu women remain resilient in the face of complicated macro pressures present in their territory.

DOI: 10.4018/978-1-5225-5981-8.ch007

In the following chapter, the author will explain how an embroidery mapping project was used to create a safe space for the participants to address their historical trauma by constructing a collective story through art. As they shared their embroidered maps with each other and analyzed them for common themes and challenges, the women entered into a time of critical reflection regarding the conspiring systems and structures that impact their unique way of life. This awareness-raising process forged new relationships among the women, and increased their sense of solidarity. Ultimately, they unearthed a reservoir of resilience to take action and address ongoing community needs using their local strengths and resources.

HISTORICAL TRAUMA AND RESILIENCE

Historical Trauma Among Indigenous Communities

Although indigenous people groups make up six percent of the world's population, they are disproportionately affected by historical trauma as compared to their non-indigenous peers (Lauderdale, 2008, p. 1840). Historical trauma (HT) refers to a cumulative and collective "emotional and psychological wounding, over the lifespan and across generations, emanating from massive group trauma experiences" like colonization, massacres, genocide, displacement, and dispossession (Kirmayar, Gone, & Moses, 2014, p. 311). Mass trauma, on the other hand, is the result of a frightening, life-threatening event experienced by many people at one time. (Boyd Webb, p. 4). While HT includes some sort of mass trauma, mass trauma does not necessarily result in HT.

Research shows that the effects of historically situated traumas can accumulate over time and across generations. This means that family members who did not experience the original trauma may still suffer symptoms of that trauma generations later. A study by Sotero (as cited in Beltrán & Begun, 2014) reveals that indigenous communities often teach their offspring "to share in the ancestral pain of their people and may have strong feelings of unresolved grief, persecution, and distrust". These memories are exacerbated by contemporary suffering that continues to plague indigenous groups such as the exploitation of their lands for natural resource extraction, displacement, forced relocation, poverty, structural inequality, and racial discrimination (Beltrán & Begun, 2014).

The Colombian Context

The general violent conditions resulting from Colombia's ongoing 60-year internal armed conflict and its spillover into neighboring countries, especially at the borders, have had a direct and disproportionate impact on the lives of indigenous peoples. Exacerbated by drug cartels, armed groups, and multinational companies pursuing the rich natural resources in their territories, this serious humanitarian situation has resulted in displacement, extreme marginalization, and environmental degradation in indigenous communities.

According to Tovar-Restrepo and Irazábal (2013), 28 percent of indigenous peoples in Colombia live in conditions of extreme poverty (p. 46). This reality is intensified by a decades-long civil war that has been internationally recognized as one of the "most severe internal conflicts in terms of displacements and killings" (Tovar-Restrepo & Irazábal, 2013, p. 45). Because indigenous communities have refused to take part in the conflict, they have found themselves at odds with all armed groups. In their attempt at neutrality, they have made themselves more susceptible to human rights abuses and killings. From 2002 to 2009, more than 1,400 indigenous men, women, and children were murdered as a result of the conflict (ABColombia, 2010, p. 9).

Displacement is another symptom of the armed conflict. Demographics show that those displaced are disproportionately women, children, and indigenous populations living in areas where the fighting is most severe. Of the 3.5 million people displaced due to the war by 2009 (which is a conservative estimate), 71 percent are estimated to be women and children (Tovar-Restrepo & Irazábul, 2013, p. 46). A study conducted by the Inter-American Court of Human Rights estimates that four out of ten families displaced are female-headed and of those, 49 percent by indigenous women (Tovar-Restrepo & Irazábul, 2013, p. 46).

Megaprojects that exploit indigenous territories rich in natural resources further aggravate the trauma caused by the armed conflict. These projects, which include mining, oil extraction, and agro-industry, are often implemented without regard for the environmental or social impact they have on indigenous communities. A report written by ABColombia, in conjunction with Oxfam (2010), explains that these projects bring with them "increased militarization of indigenous territories and greater risk of attacks by guerrilla groups" (p. 4). There is a direct link between the presence of extractive industries and the occurrence of violence and displacement.

In Colombia, the new Constitution of 1991 ratified international agreements that put much stronger emphasis on the rights of indigenous peoples to genuine participation in the decisions that affect their communities and lands. However, due to coercive tactics used by companies such as "misinformation and lack of information in appropriate indigenous languages, failure to consult with the communities directly affected by their activities, the forging of signatures, and bribery, as well as the co-opting of leaders", and a lack of political will from the Colombian authorities, these recently achieved rights are rarely experienced by indigenous communities (ABColombia, 2010, p. 4).

The Wayuu People of Northern Colombia

The author conducted her fieldwork in the semi-arid Guajira Peninsula in northern Colombia with a group of women from the Wayuu indigenous group. The Wayuu are an Amerindian ethnic group that inhabits the arid Guajira Peninsula straddling the Venezuela-Colombia border, on the Caribbean Sea coast. The Wayuu are the largest indigenous group in both Colombia and Venezuela, with an estimated population of 300,000 and 400,000, respectively (Silva 2008). According to Robles (2008), the Wayuu are a matrilineal society. They live on dispersed settlements, or *rancherías*, with extended family members and organize themselves socially and geographically according to female lines of descent. There are 27 matrilineal clans in the territory whose ancestry is marked by distinct burial grounds (Robles, 2008, p. 7).

The Wayuu have a shared history of conflict and resistance as well as acceptance and exchange with *arijuna*, or non-Wayuu. For more than five centuries, the Wayuu have both preserved their tribal identity and adapted to the changes taking place around them. Though they are one of the only indigenous groups throughout the Western Hemisphere to have effectively resisted European control, they have embraced outside influences when deemed beneficial to their survival. A clear example that shaped their economic identity was the appropriation of pastoralism in the 16th century from early European settlers. This adaptation and others are survival strategies that have allowed the Wayuu to maintain a balance between long-standing cultural traditions rooted in their semi-subsistent lifestyle and the adoption of Western practices, such as marketing and commercialization (Robles, 2008).

Unfortunately, the Wayuu are facing new macro pressures that are harder to resist and pose new challenges to their autonomy and traditional way of life. According to Riaño-Alcalá (2015), La Guajira has for centuries been a "land coveted by settlers, soldiers, missionaries, smugglers… and more recently, by the state, multinational mining companies, environmentalists, tourism, and drug and arms traffickers" (p. 288). Among many, two growing threats to the Wayuu community that exacerbate one another are a decrease in rainfall due to climate change, and the growing presence of water-intensive extractive industries. The largest above ground coal mine in the world, *Cerrejón*, operates in the region and uses approximately 2,700 cubic meters of water per day.

Article 17 of the United Nations' Universal Declaration on the Rights of Indigenous Peoples requires that both the state and transnational corporation must consult with indigenous groups prior to the commencement of any large-scale development project in order to anticipate any adverse economic, social, environmental, or cultural effects. This process also requires that fair compensation be provided for any such negative consequences felt by the community (Zapach, 1997). Unfortunately, because the *Cerrejón* mine was initiated 16 years before these stipulations were required by Colombian law, the potential social and environmental impact of the project was not considered prior to its implementation, "nor were provisions made for the Wayuu to function and to survive the inevitable negative impacts of pollution, increased population pressures in the area, depletion of their subsistence base, shortages of land, and changes in their social systems" (Zapach, 1997, p. 12). No attempt was made to study how the mining operation would affect the land use patterns or their cultural traditions that have enabled the Wayuu to survive for centuries in such a harsh environment (Zapach, 1997).

Two major rivers flow through this mostly harsh environment; the Rancheria River in Colombia and the El Limón River in Venezuela, representing the main sources of water. With very little or no consultation of the general public, *Cerrejón* was able to privatize, dam, and deviate the Rancheria River in order to use the scarce water resources in its operation. These actions, coupled with a drastic decline in rainfall over the past 20 years, have contributed to rapid rates of desertification, which threatens the biodiversity in the region and makes it increasingly difficult for the Wayuu to continue their pastoralism and horticulture practices. According to Uriana (2008), the mine's presence in the territory is directly linked to environmental degradation, health concerns such as increased infant mortality rates, and tenuous access to clean water (p. 117). Infant mortality rates in the region have climbed to 32 percent in recent years as compared to the national average of 18 percent (UNICEF Annual Report, 2013). There is no doubt that a large-scale development project of this kind, in a delicate desert environment like that of the Guajira, contributes to an atmosphere of vulnerability for human and natural life in the region.

The instability created by a growing extractive industry and worsening climate change has generated feelings of isolation and helplessness. With the advent of a new post-conflict period in Colombia, the resource-rich Guajira Peninsula will likely see an increase in large-scale development operations (Riaño-Alcalá, 2015). In a region already facing severe water shortages, an increase in the presence of water-intensive megaprojects will only further endanger the Wayuu's tenuous way of life. The author posits that this unwelcome situation perpetuated by external actors is a subtle and ongoing form of trauma. When this present-day challenge is combined with the historical trauma of armed conflict and displacement, disruption of traditional practices, and the undermining of community autonomy, it produces an "unresolved and ambiguous sense of loss and grief" (Kirmayar, Gone, & Moses, 2014; Grant, 2008, p. 127). This sense of loss, in turn, generates feelings of isolation and helplessness, and clouds a community's ability to envision a brighter future.

Resilience

Although the Wayuu face an uncertain future, their experience can be defined as one of survival and resilience. Resilience is the ability to "thrive under adverse circumstances" (Cameron, Pinto, & Tapanya, 2014, p. 457). According to Masten (2009), resilience does not require an abundance of resources but instead is the result of "ordinary magic" (p. 29). 'Ordinary magic' can be fostered by many internal and external factors, which include strong and meaningful relationships, positive-thinking, problem-solving skills, and a sense of purpose (Chavkin & Gonzalez, 2000; McCartney, Harris, and Farrow, 2012; Ng, Ang, and Ringo Ho, 2012). Following a traumatic event, resilient individuals and communities are better equipped to envision and take practical steps towards a more positive future.

The literature characterizes resilience in many different ways. In a study of resilient youth in a context of violence, Jain and Cohen (2013), posit that resilience is dynamic and can change according to one's developmental stage or context (p. 652). Heise (2013) highlights the cumulative nature of resilience. He explains that positive adaptation to adversity can actually help individuals confront stressful or tragic events later in life. In other words, coping with adversity fosters and instills future coping mechanisms. Heise calls this the "steeling effect" (p. 3). Finally, resilience is a "reciprocal transaction" that is co-constructed by individuals and their contexts (Theron, 2013, p. 528).

An individual's ability to overcome hardship is also impacted by their context and culture. This ecological resilience framework is important to take into account when working cross-culturally and has been the focus of recent research. A study of two black South African university students revealed that their Afrocentric worldview, with its emphasis on interconnectedness and harmony, enhanced their ability to adapt to situations of poverty and discrimination. The students expressed the importance of being rooted in a "larger harmonious whole" that gives meaning to all life events. In this way, setbacks are reframed as opportunities for growth instead of personal failure (Theron, 2013, p. 534).

The Latino culture, which is the backdrop for the Wayuu indigenous culture, is characterized by values of *familismo* and *personalismo*. *Familismo* places importance on the family unit above the individual. The family is obligated to provide for each other economically, emotionally, and relationally. *Personalismo*, emphasizes personal goodness or the ability to get along well with others. This value contributes to resilience because when faced with adversity, Latino youth seek to serve others in positive ways (Reyes & Elias, 2011, p. 729). A study on resilience factors among Mexican American youth shows that after experiencing discrimination, they are likely to exhibit helping behaviors as a means of coping with their negative feelings (Brittian et al., 2013, p. 336).

Art and Resilience

Art making is an additional tool that can help cultivate greater resilience. A study by Macpherson, Hart, and Heaver (2015) found that "visual arts can foster a safe space, helping people connect, and develop a sense of belonging through verbal and non-verbal means" (p. 11). The process of art making can help externalize difficult feelings in a positive way, develop creative problem solving skills, and instill flexibility and resourcefulness, all of which have been described as protective factors in resilience theory.

The Artists Collective, an inner city community arts center in Connecticut, is one of many examples of how art is being used to foster resilience among marginalized communities. According to Rhodes and Schecter (2012), the center "promotes resilience by creating a refuge from the surrounding poverty and violence…and strengthens youth's personal and social resources" (p. 826). The Artists Collective is a safe space for at-risk youth that offers a different narrative about life in the neighborhood to that of the local drug culture. It is also a "cultural oasis" that celebrates African American heritage and is a space that students can feel proud of and call their own (Rhodes & Schecter, 2012, p. 827).

The Artists Collective has also sought to cultivate healthy relationships and promote cultural education through the arts. Music and dance, the main art forms taught at the center, instill social skills, community responsibility, ethnic pride, self-esteem, and self-awareness (Rhodes & Schecter, 2012). Engaging in group dance activities, for example, can help students overcome traumatic experiences by reducing the sense of isolation reinforced by their trauma. Through collective rhythmic movement, students become aware of their own bodies and connect corporally to others. Reestablishing this sense of connection to self and others is an essential component of resilience and contributes to the healing process (Rhodes & Schecter, 2012, p. 843).

A qualitative study conducted by Reynolds and Prior (2006), explored the impact art making has on women diagnosed with cancer. The study found that engaging in the arts promotes flow, a "psychological state characterized by intense concentration and full involvement in an activity" (Reynolds & Prior, 2006, p. 256). This "extended presence" during the art making process gave participants a reprieve from intrusive thoughts and fears surrounding their condition. As they learned to respond to the limitations of their art materials, individuals were able to foster the internal resources necessary to deal with adversity. For many of the women, making art became an antidote to the helplessness they felt in the face of their illness. They described art making "as a journey with its own momentum…they could not predict exactly what would happen on this journey, nor could they fail" (Reynolds & Prior, 2006, p. 260).

EMBROIDERY MAPPING PROJECT

Participants

(all names used in this chapter are pseudonyms)

Two years ago, a group of Wayuu pastors formed an association called ASPEWA to address ongoing needs in the territory, like environmental degradation, mining, climate change, and illiteracy. Luis, one of the founders of ASPEWA, explained that, "because of macro forces, the social fabric of our communities is beginning to tear. Our vision is that the church take the lead on defending life in our God-given territory" (personal communication, 2016). The three-fold aim of the association is: 1) to strengthen the Wayuu church as an organization working for the collective wellbeing of the Wayuu people; 2) to promote the holistic training and formation of Wayuu leaders and pastors; and 3) to become a "gatekeeper" or controlling authority that interacts with local, regional, and international actors with presence and influence in the Wayuu territory and that channels the resources and support coming from the outside in a more orderly, strategic, and dignified manner.

As is often the case for organizations with a religious bent, the representation of women within ASPEWA is minimal. Without taking into account the perspective of women connected to the association, the male leadership of ASPEWA identified community needs and opportunities. This provided the framework to develop the association's objectives and action plans. In addition to not being representative of the Wayuu people as a whole, this is particularly problematic because the research shows that the success of grassroots organizations largely depends on the participation of the women. For this reason, with the endorsement from ASPEWA's leadership, the author sought to create a space for female voices to be heard as well.

The mechanism employed to create this space was a three-day workshop in the town of Uribia. With logistical support from ASPEWA, 13 Wayuu women, representing five different church denominations and ranging in age from 18 to 54, gathered together to embroider and analyze representations of their daily lives. To understand the impact of the workshop, the author conducted a concluding focus group interview with the participants. There were two other co-facilitators present during this process.

Observations of Trauma-Related Behavior

Although they did not discuss trauma specifically during the course of the workshop, the author did observe several common signs of trauma during the embroidery activity. First, the women made several references to feeling lonely or isolated. One woman, for example, explained that although she is married, she often feels like a single mother. Another participant expressed her frustration with rarely being able to visit the neighboring town due to her responsibilities at home. This space for sharing with other women, therefore, was special for her. A second observed indicator of trauma was the difficulty that the women had in expressing future desires. The participants were so focused on daily survival that they had trouble communicating their dreams for the future.

The author also noticed several indicators of HT, especially with regards to cultural and family identity. According to Grant (2008), "a key element of historical trauma is [an] unresolved and ambiguous sense of loss that is associated with damage to culture… and cultural identity" (p. 127). Listening to the participants' stories revealed a deep sadness regarding their inability to maintain their autonomous, traditional way of life. The women explained that because of water shortages, they often split their time between the *rancherías* and the cities. As a result, they are continually forced to make a choice between their language, culture, worldview, and values and those of mainstream society. This "struggle for acceptance carries a high price [because] they must loathe and reject everything about themselves to become 'acceptable'" (Lawson-Te Aho, 2014, p. 184). Additionally, many of the participants' children spend their week in the city at school and return to the *ranchería* on the weekends. A Wayuu pastor observed that these students often experience deep spiritual and emotional distress as a result of being disconnected from their cultural values and family members. This fragmentation is likely rooted in a history of colonization and dislocation that undermines cultural continuity and challenges a community's purpose, vision, and voice.

Context

The interplay of numerous macro and micro pressures make daily traditional life challenging for most Wayuu women living in the Guajira Peninsula. The declining rainfall in the region, a product of climate change and water-intensive extractive industries, has put added stress on the already precarious Wayuu economy centered on the raising of goats and seasonal agriculture. In years with normal weather, the Wayuu plant twice annually following the rain patterns in the region. The harvests are used for family consumption and to feed their herds of goats. Though life is by no means easy, with the harvests they eat well enough and are able to maintain their traditional way of life. However, having not been able to plant for five years due to an ongoing drought, the Wayuu are being forced once again to adapt to the changing conditions around them. In fact, many Wayuu families are migrating to urban centers.

In the cities, finding a steady job is extremely difficult due to lack of education and nepotism within the socio-economic landscape. Those in power often give jobs to family members or people from the same clan. Juan, one young pastor, explained, "In the villages we knew how to survive by raising goats and maintaining our gardens, but in the cities, we cannot do this. We do not know how to survive in this new environment" (personal communication, March 30, 2017). Increasingly disconnected from their land and villages, the women must grapple with their sense of purpose and identity in a new context. Like many immigrants forced from their homelands, they may experience discrimination, which contributes to feelings of alienation and invisibility. This, in turn, "fosters feelings of insecurity, fear, and shame in majority group interactions" (Yeh et al., 2008, p. 39).

Life outside of the villages makes the women acutely aware of their inadequacies in a modern, westernized context. In the *rancherías*, the participants' worth stems from their ability to maintain their households, their mothering skills, and the quality of their handmade bags and hammocks. In the cities, however, worth is derived from education, workplace title, and financial achievement. For the women, this produces feelings of sadness, shame, and powerlessness as reflected in the following statement, "The majority of us know that we are not professionals because we did not have the chance to study. This leads to more difficulty and more need" (personal communications, February 18, 2017). Unlike their male counterparts, the women have less opportunity to study because of family responsibilities and lack of resources. If there is money for education, it is often given to the males first.

METHODOLOGY

Communities plagued by persistent poverty and trauma are often understandably wary of initiatives conducted by outsiders. The Wayuu are no exception. Their resource-rich land is a continual target for megaprojects that are driven by economic interests with little or no concern for the human and environmental impact. For this reason, the author approached her work using a Participatory Action Research (PAR) lens. Indigenous communities often think of traditional forms of research as another form of colonization in which their local knowledge is co-opted by external actors. PAR, on the other hand, seeks to create horizontal power dynamics based on trust and equality, and recognizes that knowledge generation is a collaborative process in which the skills and expertise of participants is crucial to the outcome of the work (Brydon-Miller, et al., 2011).

The heartbeat of PAR is *conscientisation*. According to Freire (1974), *conscientisation* implies making and remaking the world through reflection and action. Freire posits that the very act of knowing, and the power ascribed to this act, must be reframed and reconsidered so that "there is no longer one who thinks, who knows, standing in front of others who admit they don't know… Rather, all of them are inquisitive learners, avid to learn" (Freire, 1974, p. 27). In the context of action research, this means that knowledge is co-created between investigator and participant. Vertical power dynamics, therefore, are challenged as both parties assume the responsibility of learning from one another.

One of the most important processes involved in *conscientisation* is the movement from awareness to action. Critical reflection allows people to better understand their world and transcend their own experiences in order to recognize the larger social, political, and cultural forces that impact their lives. In doing so, marginalized individuals who have been conditioned to see themselves as *objects* of a dehumanizing society can become *subjects* who are free to shape their own lives (Kirylo & Boyd, 2017). In other words, *conscientisation* implies that individuals can not only liberate themselves from oppression but can also transform unjust structures. Critical reflection sparks critical action as communities unlearn the destructive myth that their disenfranchisement is either their fault or linked to fate (Kirylo & Boyd, 2017).

Over the course of the three-day workshop, the author sought to foster an environment of deep listening between the Wayuu participants in order to learn from their lived experiences as indigenous women. She wanted to explore how embroidery could be used as a tool to facilitate a process of *conscientisation*, in which participants could share openly and honestly with one another, understand how systems of oppression impact their daily lives, and translate this new knowledge into grassroots action.

As an outsider, the author was particularly sensitive to her ascribed power and did everything she could to create horizontal relationships between herself and the women. This is one of the main reasons she chose an arts-based approach. Art is a universal language that can be used to create an environment where all participants are given a voice and the opportunity to express themselves. By embroidering alongside of the women, the facilitators both received their stories and shared their own personal narratives. This lessened vertical relationships by allowing mutuality and reciprocity to flourish. Embroidery was chosen as the artistic medium because it is a traditional art form that the Wayuu women use to decorate their dresses. Also, it is portable, inexpensive, and all of the necessary materials can be found locally.

Explanation of Embroidery Process

Opening Ritual

The workshop began with an opening ritual that represented the creation of a safe space. Each woman was given a tent stake and pounded these stakes into the ground to form a circle. This was a symbolic gesture that marked their commitment to the process as well as to each other. With a ball of yarn in their hands that was passed around the circle, each woman said their name and expressed one expectation they had for their time together. Before tossing the ball to someone else, they wrapped it around their stake. This secured the spider web and allowed them to return on Day Two and Day Three with a different color of yarn and a different question. Adding to the web each day represented their increased unity and learning as a result of their time together.

Making and Sharing the Maps

After the ritual activity, each participant was given an embroidery hoop, cloth, a needle, and a variety of embroidery floss. The facilitator asked them to consider the following questions about their typical day: What chores do you do on a daily basis? Where do you walk to on a daily basis? Who do you interact with every day? What are the challenges you face? The women spent the first day embroidering their stories.

On Day Two, the discussion amongst the women turned to the analysis of their embroidered maps. The women were divided into two groups to explain their maps to each other. This was a rich time of sharing that created a much-needed space for the women to recognize their commonalities, which heightened their sense of emotional connection to one another. Marcela, a shy middle-aged woman, pointed to the kitchen she embroidered on her map and said, "This is my office" (personal communication, February 17, 2017). Understanding her sentiment, the women in her group responded with hearty laughter. As the women discussed the different aspects of their embroidered maps, a group identity began to emerge.

Figure 1. Wayuu woman embroidering her map. (photo by Lauren Jones, 2017)

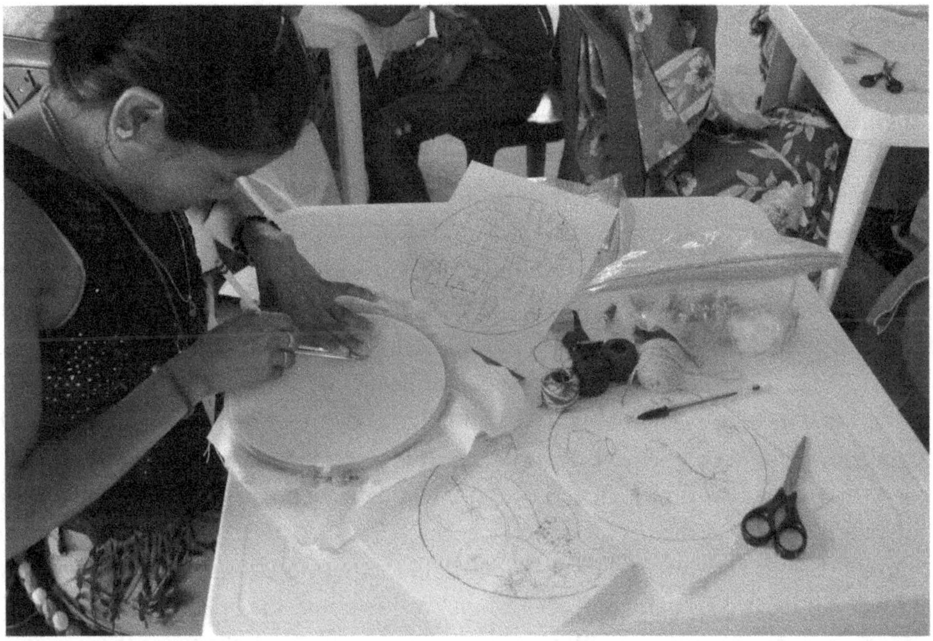

Figure 2. Women discussing their maps. (photo by Lauren Jones, 2017)

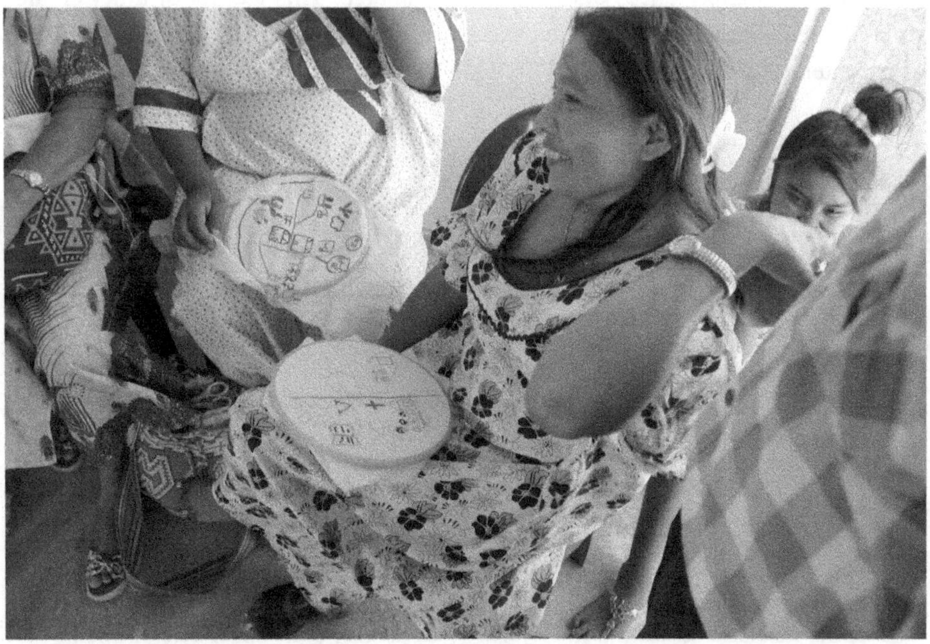

Analysis and Critical Reflection

After the time of sharing, the women taped their maps to the wall to create a collective gallery. The facilitators invited the participants to approach the wall and look closely at the collection of maps with the aim of identifying the common themes and challenges revealed by the embroidered images. During this time, the women generated a list of their commonalities, as seen in Figure 3. What followed was an unplanned time of sharing about the difficulties that each woman faced in their daily lives. For the participants, it seemed important to share these struggles with one another. It was a cathartic moment in which their individual stories of hardship became a collective story of survival. Lorena, the wife of the president of ASPEWA, shared the difficulties she faces as a mom and medical student. She explained that she often feels pulled in two different directions and is rarely able to spend quality time with her young daughters. When Lorena expressed that she often feels like a single mother, several other participants nodded in agreement. Another woman explained that many of her family members are sick and that she does not have the money to get them the medical help they need. Her feelings of desperation also resounded throughout the group. Seven of the 13 women identified lack of money as one of their most pressing needs.

Once common themes and struggles were identified, the participants selected the themes that were most urgent for them to discuss and analyze further. At this point, the space became one of reflection and dialogue, centered on the question, "Why is this happening?" To probe these themes more fully, the women conducted a *problem-tree* analysis, as indicated in Figure 4. As they identified the root causes and consequences of each challenge, they were better equipped to talk about solutions. This activity also projected their individual experiences onto a communal stage. This feeling of unity created a stronger platform to talk about resilience. What ensued was an animated conversation regarding their most urgent need- access to water.

Figure 3. Common themes and challenges, as identified by the women

Commonalities Identified in Narrative Form

- Our main form of income is making *mochilas* (crocheted bags)
    - This is a sporadic form of income; we are often taken advantage of by middlemen who enter our communities and buy our bags at a very low cost
    - Because of need, we are forced to *regalar* (or give away) our bags
- We are all Christians
- All of us have a *rancheria* (remote, traditional village)
    - Many of us split our time between the *rancherias* and the city, which affects our way of life
- We all have goats and other animals
    - It is more difficult to maintain our goats and gardens because we do not have water; this leaves our households in disarray
- Our water sources depend on the *jagüey* (dug pools to capture rain water) as well as windmills that draw the water up from wells
- We all have similar chores and responsibilities like cooking, making handmade bags and hammocks, collecting firewood, and caring for our children, etc.
    - We spend more time looking for water and firewood, which means we have less time to crochet our *mochilas*
- We all love coffee

Figure 4. Problem-tree analysis of lack of water

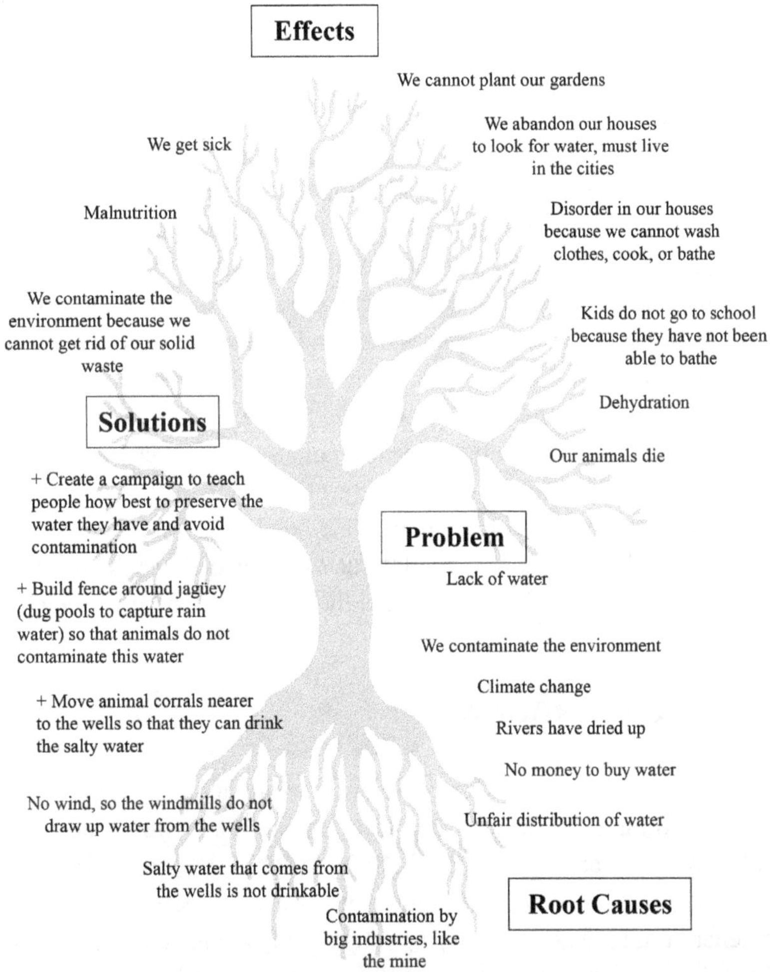

As the women discussed their limited access to potable water, they identified both macro and micro pressures that play a role in creating their present situation. The presence of *Cerrejón* mine, for example, was widely identified as a macro pressure while lack of care for the environment was recognized as a micro pressure contributing to the shortage of water in the region. The consequences of this issue revealed complicated realities that threaten their traditional way of life. Without water, the women cannot maintain their traditional gardens. This leaves their households in disarray and makes feeding their children a more challenging and time consuming activity. The scarcity of water has also taken its toll on their traditional economy, especially goat herding. Goat herding is a primary economic activity that carries great cultural significance in Wayuu culture. Due to drought, many families have abandoned this practice and sought other alternative sources of income in the cities, like selling their handmade bags and hammocks to intermediaries, who in turn sell them to tourists. The women expressed their exasperation about the irony of having less time to make artisan goods because they have to spend more time looking for water and firewood.

Identifying Solutions

In a group session, the women drafted and analyzed a list of the complex factors that contribute to the daily challenges they face. In doing so, the women were better equipped to address their feelings of trauma caused by these factors. According to Lawson-Te Aho (2014), "consciousness produces a capacity to choose" between giving up or fighting back (p. 189). In this case, the process of *conscientisation* empowered the women to act. They moved "beyond being a passive recipient of whatever life dishes out, to becoming an active participant with other oppressed persons in shaping and changing their world" (Kirylo & Boyd, 2017, p. 80). Through this participation, the women identified solutions to their challenges that ranged from changes in personal behavior to the need for more systemic political change.

One response that emerged from the group was the need to work together as artisans in order to help ensure a fair price for their bags and hammocks. They went as far as electing a female pastor to help them organize. They also identified the need to preserve their existing water sources. One woman explained that they should build fences around the *jagüeys*, man-made pools that collect rainwater, to keep their goats and other animals from contaminating this water source. These responses, proposed by the women themselves, helped to assuage their trauma-related feelings of powerlessness and helplessness. The women were empowered by the common realization that they do have the resources and power with which to respond and mitigate some of the challenges they face as Wayuu women.

IMPACT ON HISTORICAL TRAUMA

Traumatic experiences can shatter a person's worldview, creating feelings of isolation, helplessness and uncertainty regarding the future. The lack of ability to envision a positive future "is one of the most profound losses following a situation of trauma" (Boyd Webb, 2003, p. 9). Historical trauma, on the other hand, weakens cultural identity and continuity, and creates a deep spiritual wounding that can be passed down from generation to generation. Symptoms of HT include depression, an unresolved sense of grief, a learned helplessness, as well as maladaptive behaviors such as substance abuse. To create a productive space for healing to occur, a sense of safety must be restored, connections to self and others reestablished, and cultural values reaffirmed and celebrated. This enables communities to become stronger together and take practical steps towards a meaningful future following a traumatic event.

Art and creativity are important tools that can be catalysts for this healing process. Art making emphasizes possibility, persistence, and vision, thus shifting "the focus from trauma to sources of joy and strength. It helps transform thinking from victim to survivor… and encourages strength and positive thinking that may help in future challenges" (Heise, 2014, p. 3). For a group of indigenous Wayuu women facing an uncertain future, the artistic process of embroidering maps of their daily lives allowed them to begin to address their historical trauma. By constructing a collective story and alternative narrative, they were able to question their current reality. This strengthened the unity and consciousness of the group, which created a platform to talk about resilience. Ultimately, this new narrative allowed the women to envision a more hopeful future characterized by solidarity and action. What ensues is a discussion on how the embroidery project fostered healing, empowerment, and community resilience.

Creating a Collective Story

According to Tulinius and HØlge-Hazelton (2011), collective stories are "a liberation narrative of the disempowered… by situating their lives in a larger social and historical context and by directing energy toward changing the social structures that perpetuate injustice" (p. 44). These narratives bind people together emotionally and therefore, can overcome feelings of isolation and alienation that trauma produces. Furthermore, collective stories instill a "language of possibility" in which social action and societal transformation are possible (Gore, 1993, p. 96). Recent research shows that storytelling is a dynamic mechanism for healing historical trauma because it is a form of indigenous resistance that gives voice to narratives of oppression and corrects inaccurate histories as told by outsiders (Lawson-Te Aho, 2014). According to Beltrán and Begun (2014), "the process of creating and sharing narratives is a transformational tool for reclaiming knowledge and highlighting resiliencies despite legacies of colonization and ongoing discrimination (p. 162).

The women created a collective story by making and sharing their embroidered maps with each other. Figure 3 highlights the collective story co-constructed by the participants. Creating this narrative was an important process that bore witness to the women's struggles, illuminated their collective resilience, and offered them encouragement to persevere.

Critical Reflection and Action

After constructing a collective story, the women were tasked with reflecting on the micro and macro pressures that affect their traditional way of life, families and communities. This was done with a *problem-tree* analysis. While discussing challenges related to their lack of income, the women expressed that one of the main reasons they struggle to find work is because of their lack of education. Many of the women shared that they were unable to complete a basic education because they were married at a young age, grew up in rural villages where access to schools for girls is minimal, or their parents did not have the necessary money. Reflecting on the root causes helped the women to situate their challenges within a larger socio-economic context.

The identification of the root causes perpetuating the challenges faced by the women was an important step in the healing process in two main ways. First, it helped the women to become more aware of their personal histories and "created new understandings about the dynamics of culture within the complexities of contemporary life" (Beltrán & Begun, 2014, p. 162). Second, it created a much-needed space for the participants to consider how they can respond to these pressures. One of the consequences of HT is a learned helplessness that may lead to psychological and spiritual submission. The critical reflection and action components of *conscientisation*, therefore, gave the women a choice to either surrender or resist the effects of trauma. This choice carried with it the potential for psychological and spiritual empowerment and as such, was a small a step towards healing (Lawson-Te Aho, 2014, p. 189).

Solidarity: From Cliques to Unity

With the intention of creating a more organic environment that would lend itself to conversation amongst the women, the facilitators set up the chairs in a circle rather than the default classroom-style arrangement. As the women entered the room, however, they moved the chairs around and sat in small groups, according to family and church connections. Throughout the embroidery activity, the room was consistently quiet, perhaps indicating a level of shyness or discomfort among the participants.

This dynamic shifted radically by the end of the Day Two. The women were sitting together in a large group and had broken out of the noticeable cliques that marked the first day's activities. Lorena expressed passionately during the focus group interview, "In this group, what we have in common is that we are sisters in Christ, even though we come from different churches, different municipalities, and different villages. This sense of connection is what I long for the most when I meet other women" (personal communication, February 17, 2017).

The simple act of coming together and sharing was a powerful experience for these women. According to Luis, a Wayuu pastor and president of Aspewa, the women are often isolated in their rural *rancherías*. Their time is spent rearing children, maintaining the household, raising goats or other animals, and making crocheted bags and hammocks. Add in the time they are required to spend procuring the day's water needs in an increasingly water scarce region, and they are left with little or no time to create friendships outside of the family unit, which compounds their feelings of isolation.

The new connections made during the embroidery activity increased the participants' sense of solidarity and became a pathway for healing. During the activity, the women expressed on multiple occasions that they were grateful for the opportunity to come together and form new relationships. During a focus group interview, Alejandra said that she felt closer to the other women after the embroidery exercise, and that making the maps together gave her the confidence she needed in order to share her experiences with the group. She developed a sense of trust that allowed her to be vulnerable.

Marcela, one of the most timid participants who remained quiet for most of the group interview, finally shared her perspective. Her words capture the sensation of moving from isolation to solidarity:

I am so grateful that God brought me to this group, to share with my sisters. Sometimes, I go to the nearest town, but only for a moment. I have too many responsibilities at home. In this group, I learned something new about the roots of my problems and the consequences. I have solved something here in this group because of each of you and because God brought me here to share. (February 18, 2017)

Marcela's words capture what many women experienced in the course of the workshop: that as a result of sharing with one another about their common challenges, they found new emotional strength to envision change going forward. As individuals bond emotionally around shared trauma or difficulties they develop more faculties for practical action. According to Goleman, Boyatzis, and McKee (2013) this emotional capital 'drives people to do things together that no individual could or would do" (p. 475).

Resilience and Hope

During the embroidery activity, stories of pain and struggle were reframed as narratives of resilience and hope. Hope "is the expectation, dream, and belief that healing is possible… [it] is a psychological emancipation" (Lawson-Te Aho, 2014, p. 191). Several women, for example, expressed a shared concern and commitment to helping each other despite their own challenges. Erica, one of the youngest participants, expressed:

Sometimes, we don't know our neighbors. We don't know the needs they have because we are isolated, closed in. Maybe, we can resolve our problems by getting to know our neighbors and sharing with them. (personal communication, February 18, 2017)

Erica intuits what the literature shows and what was observed in the workshop, that resilience, or the ability to push through hardship, is increased through solidarity. In a concluding group session, for example, Liliana expressed that, "Each one of us can find the solution. The capacity that we have can help us find the solutions to our difficulties" (personal communication, February 18, 2017). Having heard from other women express similar struggles and disappointments, she was emboldened to seek healing and change.

Another way that the embroidery process instilled hope was by transforming personal stories from something mundane into something important. Lorena explained, "Embroidering my life made me wake up. Before, I didn't think the things that I do are important, but now I know that they are" (personal communication, March 30, 2017). These words demonstrate that the power of narrative lies in its ability to restore self-determination and foster the courage necessary to see beyond the grief of historical trauma.

A Mastery Experience

Mastering a new skill, like embroidery, can increase resilience because it helps develop confidence and the ability to focus (Macpherson, Hart, & Heaver, 2015). In this way, the embroidery workshop was a mastery experience for many of the participants. For those that did not know how to embroider, learning a new art form increased their confidence. For the women that had embroidered before, applying this art form in a new way helped them to see their lives from a new perspective. One participant stated, "I knew how to embroider but I had never embroidered these things before, like where I walk to or my daily chores. I discovered something through this process of creating the map, these drawings mean something" (personal communication, February 18, 2017).

The Healing Spiral: An Explanation of Growth and Resilience

In Figure 5, the healing impact of the embroidery project is highlighted in a visual form. The inward swirl represents a process of narrowing in on a shared identity, which requires the presence of *conscientisation*. Many of the women came from different villages and church communities and did not know each other before the workshop. The invitation to embroider a map of their daily experiences, therefore, was an invitation to become vulnerable with the rest of the group. Together, they created a collective story of survival in the face of overwhelming pressures that threaten their indigenous way of life, which led to an increase in the solidarity of the group. As the participants recognized their own stories in the maps of their peers, this generated a new and profound understanding that they were not alone in their challenges to meet the severe demands of daily life. The act of creating a collective story produced group solidarity and strengthened their shared identity as Wayuu women. This new identity empowered the women to address their trauma-related feelings of isolation and learned helplessness, two consequences of HT. As their awareness grew regarding the mix of micro and macro pressures that negatively impact their lives, they were better equipped and informed to respond to a broken, oppressive system, albeit in small ways.

The outward spiral represents a burgeoning movement towards collective action and is dependent upon the formation of a shared identity through collective storytelling and solidarity. An increased awareness regarding the complicated nature of poverty and oppression in the region resulted in individual empowerment. The participants began to identify their own capacity to confront their problems, which would not have been possible without the first step of naming and witnessing their struggles. This, in turn, generated collective action. The women recognized that their welfare is intimately wrapped up in the wellbeing of their peers and neighbors. Individual struggles turned into the community's fight for survival, an anthem of hope and resilience.

The author posits that a process of *conscientisation*, which requires both an inward journey of critical reflection as well as an outward journey of critical action, is essential for healing to occur. During the inward journey, community members begin to create a collective identity by naming their inner strengths and resources and identifying the systemic pressures that compound their experiences of historical trauma. This inward process increases a community's sense of solidarity and binds them together emotionally. Once these critical social ties are created, strengths and resources are identified, and micro and macro pressures are named, the outward journey of restoration can begin. Every step in this process facilitates healing because they make the community stronger, more resilient, and better equipped to envision a brighter future following a legacy of historical trauma.

FOLLOW-UP WITH THE WAYUU WOMEN PARTICIPANTS

After the excitement of the initial three-day workshop, the author and her team felt a strong desire to accompany the Wayuu women as they build resilience and hope in their communities. They did not want to contribute to the all-too-common narrative of loss and solitude that occurs when researchers extract

Figure 5. The healing process resulting from the embroidery workshop

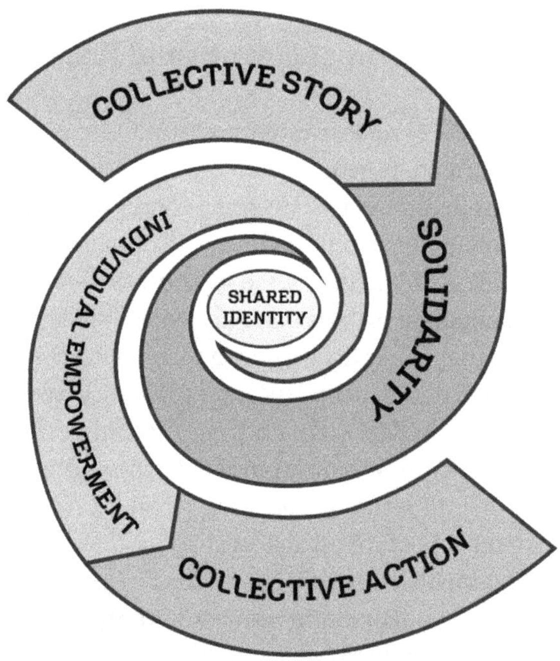

information and leave without a word. In fact, for many indigenous communities, this has exacerbated feelings of HT.

The author has returned to the Guajira on two separate occasions to continue to walk alongside the Wayuu women. This work is ongoing and the team is currently developing a three to five year community development plan to connect the participants to external markets where they can sell their bags and hammocks for a just price, as well as provide them with additional trainings to increase their knowledge of business skills, management, and quality control. The author and her team conducted two additional workshops to learn more about the process of making a crocheted bag, from the sourcing of materials to the final sale. Much of this time was spent training the female pastor that the women elected to be their leader. The author and her co-workers feel strongly that the work cannot depend on their presence in the territory. Instead, they wish to see the women empowered as leaders and change-makers, protagonists of their own story.

In these workshops, several important conversations emerged regarding the cultural significance of the Wayuu bags or *mochilas*. The women discussed strategies to preserve the cultural value of their crocheted bags despite increasing pressures to make changes in order to sell them to tourists. For example, many women are now sewing sequins to the bags to make them more appealing. They have also changed their weaving style, digressing from the traditional way of weaving in order to produce their artisan products more quickly. Additionally, the women talked about how to price their bags consistently and fairly, taking into account their labor and material costs. They even came up with a minimum price for their small, medium, and large bags, realizing that if they accept anything less than this price, they would be devaluing their work and time.

These conversations are tedious but also worthwhile. As the women continue to meet and make connections with one another, they are more equipped to face the future together, which contributes to a stronger, more resilient community. The participants remain enthusiastic about the creation of shared spaces and have expressed a deep desire to continue to gather together. Without this spirit of unity, it would be impossible to carry out community building in a dignified, just, and sustainable manner.

IMPLICATIONS OF EMBROIDERY PROJECT

The use of embroidery as a mapping tool to address HT within marginalized communities has profound and far-reaching implications for activists, community artists, and development workers. Embroidery is a universal, affordable, and portable option that has the power to facilitate *conscientisation*, or an increased awareness regarding oppressive systems and structures that perpetuate poverty as well as the commitment to act against such forces. This awareness addresses feelings of isolation, powerlessness, and helplessness by reframing personal struggle as communal resilience. This new narrative is an empowering one that creates a dynamic space for communities to address their trauma together and is reflected in the observations of a coworker:

> *Each participant was able to identify their challenges and daily difficulties but they thought these difficulties only pertained to them. When they came together as a group, however, they realized that they all pass through the same challenges and that as a group it is easier to find solutions to their problems. (personal communication, February 21, 2017)*

CONCLUSION

The embroidery mapping project created an important space for healing and post-traumatic growth to occur. By constructing a collective story characterized by *conscientisation*, the women moved from isolation to solidarity as they recognized their personal stories in the narratives of the other women in the group. Their courage to be vulnerable with one another catalyzed important friendships and created a safe space for critical reflection. Together, the participants identified many of the colluding structures that negatively impact their indigenous way of life, such as climate change and the presence of extractive industries. As their awareness of these oppressive structures increased, the women were better equipped to confront these power disparities. Through this journey, the women unearthed a reservoir of resilience to address ongoing community needs using their local strengths and resources. Each embroidered map embodied this hope through the possibility of resistance and change. Compelled by this common identity as strong and resilient Wayuu women, they took a small step towards a shared vision of a thriving community that can weather any storm.

REFERENCES

ABColombia. (2010). *Caught in the crossfire: Colombia's indigenous peoples*. Retrieved from www.abcolombia.org.uk

Amsden, J. & VanWynsberghe, R. (2005). Community mapping as a research tool with youth. *SAGE Publications*, *3*(4), 357-381. DOI: 10.1177/1476750305058487

Beltrán, R., & Begun, S. (2014). 'It is medicine': Narratives of healing from the Aotearoa Digital Storytelling as Indigenous Media Project (ADSIMP). *Psychology and Developing Societies*, *26*(2), 155–179. doi:10.1177/0971333614549137

Boyd Webb, N. (2004). *Mass trauma and violence: helping families and children cope*. New York: Guilford Press.

Brittian, A. S., O'Donnell, M., Knight, G. P., Carlo, G., Umana-Taylor, A. J., & Roosa, M. W. (2013). Associations between adolescent's perceived discrimination and prosocial tendencies: The mediating role of Mexican American values. *Journal of Youth and Adolescence*, *42*(3), 328–341. doi:10.100710964-012-9856-6 PMID:23152074

Brydon-Miller, M., Kral, M., Maguire, P., Noffke, S., & Sabhlok, A. (2011). *Jazz and the Banyan tree: roots and riffs on participatory action research. ResearchGate*. Retrieved from ResearchGate.

Cameron, C. A., Pinto, G., & Tapanya, S. (2014). Scaffolding one Thai youth's drawing toward resilience. *Culture and Psychology*, *20*(4), 453–476. doi:10.1177/1354067X14551293

Caxaj, S.C. (2015). Indigenous storytelling and participatory action research: allies toward decolonization? Reflections from the People's International Health Tribunal. *Global Qualitative Nursing Research*, 1-12. DOI: 10.1177/2333393615580764

Chavkin, N. F., & Gonzalez, J. (2000). Mexican immigrant youth and resiliency: Research and promising programs. *ERIC Digests*. Retrieved from www.eric.ed.gov

Corbitt, J. N., & Nix-Early, V. (2003). *Taking it to the streets: Using the arts to transform your community*. Grand Rapids, MI: Baker Books.

Freire, P. (1970). *Pedagogy of the Oppressed*. New York, NY: Bloomsbury Academic.

Freire, P. (1974). Conscientisation. *Cross Currents*, *24*(1), 23–31.

Goleman, D., Boyatzis, R., & McKee, A. (2002). *Primal Leadership: Unleashing the Power of Emotional Intelligence* [Kindle DX Version]. Retrieved from Amazon.

Gore, J. M. (1993). *The Struggle for Pedagogies: Critical and Feminist Discourses as Regimes of Truth*. New York: Routledge.

Grant, H. (2008). American Indians: Working with American Indians and historical trauma. *Illness, Crisis & Loss*, *16*(2), 125–136. doi:10.2190/IL.16.2.c

Heise, D. (2014, May). Steeling and resilience. *Art Education*, 26–30.

Jain, S., & Cohen, A. K. (2013). Fostering resilience among urban youth exposed to violence: A promising area for interdisciplinary research and practice. *Health Education & Behavior*, *40*(6), 651–662. doi:10.1177/1090198113492761 PMID:23818463

Kirmayar, L. J., Gone, J. P., & Moses, J. (2014). Rethinking historical trauma. *Transcultural Psychiatry*, *51*(3), 299–319. doi:10.1177/1363461514536358 PMID:24855142

Kirylo, J., & Boyd, D. (2017). *Paulo Freire: His Faith*. Boston, MA: Spirituality and Theology. doi:10.1007/978-94-6351-056-1_7

Lauderdale, P. (2008). Indigenous peoples in the face of globalization. *The American Behavioral Scientist*, *51*(12), 1836–1843. doi:10.1177/0002764208318934

Lawson-Te Aho, K. (2014). The healing is in the pain: Revisiting and re-narrative trauma histories as a starting point for healing. *Psychology and Developing Societies*, *26*(2), 181–212. doi:10.1177/0971333614549139

Macpherson, H., Hart, A., & Heaver, B. (2015). Building resilience through group visual art activities: Findings from a scoping study with young people who experience mental health complexities and/or learning difficulties. *Journal of Social Work*, *0*(0), 1–20. doi:10.1177/1468017315581772

Masten, A. S. (2009, June). Ordinary magic: Lessons from research on resilience in human development. *Education Canada*, 28–32.

McCartney, C., Harris, S., & Farrow, V. (2012). Experiences of secondary Hispanic immigrant students: Their stories of challenge and triumph. *Journal of School Leadership*, *22*(1), 26–54.

Ng, R., Ang, R. P., & Ringo Ho, M. H. (2012). Coping with anxiety, depression, anger, and aggression: The meditational role of resilience in adolescents. *Child and Youth Care Forum*, *41*(6), 529–546. doi:10.100710566-012-9182-x

Powell, K. (2010). Making sense of place: Mapping as a multisensory research method. *Qualitative Inquiry, 16*(7), 639–555. doi:10.1177/1077800410372600

Reynolds, F., & Prior, S. (2006). Creative adventures and flow in art-making: A qualitative study of women living with cancer. *British Journal of Occupational Therapy, 69*(6), 255–262. doi:10.1177/030802260606900603

Rhodes, A. M., & Schecter, R. (2012). Fostering resilience among youth in inner city community arts centers: The case of the artists collective. *Education and Urban Society, 46*(7), 826–848. doi:10.1177/0013124512469816

Riaño-Alcalá, P. (2015). Emplaced witnessing: Commemorative practices among the Wayuu in the Upper Guajira. *Memory Studies, 8*(3), 282–297. doi:10.1177/1750698014563970

Robles, D. A. (2008). *Beyond assimilation vs. cultural resistance: Wayuu market appropriation in Riohacha, La Guajira, Colombia* (Master's thesis). Retrieved from www.kuscholarworks.ku.edu

Silva, E. (2008). *Conociendo a mis hermanos Wayuu*. Author.

Theron, L., Cameron, C. A., Didkowsky, N., Lau, C., Liebenger, L., & Ungar, M. (2011). A 'day in the lives' of four resilient youths: Cultural roots of resilience. *Youth & Society, 43*(3), 799–818. doi:10.1177/0044118X11402853

Theron, L. C. (2013). Black students' recollections of pathways to resilience: Lessons for school psychologists. *School Psychology International, 34*(5), 527–539. doi:10.1177/0143034312472762

Tovar-Restrepo, M., & Irazábal, C. (2013). Indigenous women and violence in Colombia. *Latin American Perspectives, 41*(1), 39–58. doi:10.1177/0094582X13492134

Tulinius, C., & Holge-Hazelton, B. (2011). When the spiral of action research collapses: Using the arts to interpret and continue the process in collective research dialogues. *Action Research, 9*(1), 42–64. doi:10.1177/1476750311398307

United Nations International Children's Emergency Fund. (2013). *UNICEF annual report 2013 - Colombia*. Retrieved from www.unicef.org

Uriana, G. M. (2008). Impactos ambientales de la extraccion de recursos naturales y el rol de la mujer wayuu frente a los cambios climáticos en el departamento de la Guajira, Colombia. *Mujeres Indígenas y Cambio Climático: Perspectivas latinoamericanas*, 120-131. Retrieved from www.bivipas.unal.edu.co

Yeh, C. J., Pituc, S. T., Kim, A. B., & Atkins, M. (2008). Poverty loss, and resilience: The story of Chinese immigrant youth. *American Psychologist Association, 55*(1), 34–48. doi:10.1037/0022-0167.55.1.34

Zapach, M. D. (1997). *The sociocultural impact of El Cerrejon Coal Mine on the Wayuu of the Southern Guajira, Colombia* (Master's thesis). Retrieved from www.era.library.ualberta.ca

KEY TERMS AND DEFINITIONS

Conscientisation: A term influenced by Paulo Freire that refers to raising the critical consciousness of an individual or group in order to understand root causes of oppression and poverty and then act to address the root causes identified.

Chapter 8
Narratives of Writing as Healing

Jennifer Lynne Bird
Oxbridge Academy, USA

ABSTRACT

Writing as an art form helps people heal physically, emotionally, and spiritually. This chapter uses the theory of narrative inquiry to present a first-person case study of the author's writing life dovetailed with research illustrating how writing helps people heal. Writing methods will help educators, patients, people experiencing struggles, and anyone who wants to transfer thoughts to the page. Writing helps people cope with adversity, reframe situations to show a more optimistic attitude, and feel safe because the written page will not judge its author. Journal prompts serve as resources for the reader to begin or continue a writing practice.

INTRODUCTION

How can writing help people heal? This question served as the motivation for research and also led to discoveries in my roles as a high school English teacher, Stephen Minister at my church, and health coach. While writing cannot take the place of an evaluation by a trained medical expert, it can help the healing process. When a patient writes about symptoms in a journal to share with a medical professional, a high school student writes about the day's events in a journal to deal with emotions, or an adult writes a prayer in a journal to cope with uncertainty, the process of writing serves as a valuable resource. Regardless of the circumstances which motivated the writer to pick up a notebook and pen or type at a computer, writing releases thoughts and emotions from the mind to the page. When people transfer ideas to paper, stressful emotional events in the mind and physical tension in the body often improve. Writing can therefore become a catalyst for healing.

Narrative Inquiry

This chapter uses first person and the method of narrative inquiry to share stories and apply artistic methods, such as writing in journals, to the practice of healing. The theory of narrative inquiry invites writers to own their writing voices and make stories accessible. Clandinin and Connelly (2000) explain,

DOI: 10.4018/978-1-5225-5981-8.ch008

"questions of form for a narrative inquirer are with us from the outset of an inquiry. Even as we tell our own research stories prior to entering into the midst of the field stories, there is a tentative sense of plot. As we engage with research participants and live and tell stories with them, the plotlines under composition are restoried, that is, they are relived and retold. All of these tellings and livings prefigure the narrative forms of our research texts" (p. 165). Narrative inquiry, as a qualitative interpretive form of research, focuses on stories and the finding of narrative threads, or themes, in the stories. Narrative inquiries may include objective data, such as a tally of the number of times events occurred; however, a narrative inquiry also includes subjective data, such as the stories of participants. Consequently, the researcher in the field of narrative inquiry can choose to participate as a participant observer instead of only observing other people. If the researcher chooses the role of a participant observer, attention must be paid to the dual roles. Heifetz (1994) describes the dual roles by using the extended metaphor, "consider the experience of dancing on a dance floor in contrast with standing on a balcony and watching other people dance" (pp. 252-253). Narrative inquirers alternate between the balcony perspective of observation and the dance floor perspective of interacting with participants.

My research into writing as healing began with studying the stories of others during my doctoral dissertation, but expanded when the death of my mom caused me to unexpectedly find myself in the same position as the research subjects I interviewed. My research transformed from just another topic to study to having a larger purpose. My own experiences of how I used writing as healing mean as much to me as the stories of others. The research for this chapter exists as observational research and reflections of previous research projects. It serves as a qualitative interpretive analysis as well as an introduction to writing as healing for anyone looking to explore the concept in their lives.

PROLOGUE: BACKGROUND OF WRITING AS HEALING

My stress level felt worse. Reflection reminded me that life became busy, leaving me with little time to write. I feel happiest when I can immerse myself in the research and writing process, where I discover new ideas and share them with others. I knew what I needed to do: Return to writing. Writing helped me through difficult situations by bringing clarity to my life. As a National Board Certified Health Coach, I advocate a holistic approach to healing. Writing helps me manage my stress most of the time, but it does not exist as the only option or a magic cure. A couple times in my life, losses such as the death of my mom caused my stress to transform into anxiety; I needed therapy and medication, and no shame exists in either option or in asking for help. So, if you find yourself reading this publication, I hope you understand the disclaimer that none of my words can become a good alternative for a conversation with your doctor if you experience anxiety or any other health issue. When everyday stress does not cross the line into anxiety, however, writing can help.

Research exists to support the theory of writing helping people heal, beginning with the work of psychologist James Pennebaker. Pennebaker and Smyth (2016) discuss Pennebaker's original study, which led to the discovery, "people who wrote about their deepest thoughts and feelings surrounding traumatic experiences evidenced enhanced immune function compared with those who wrote about superficial topics" (p. 21). They continue with the observation that improved health continued after the writing experience and elaborate, "people who wrote about their deepest thoughts and feelings related to stressful or traumatic experiences had reliable improvements in health in the two to three months after writing" (p. 25). Additional studies on wellness and writing followed. Evans (2010) summarizes the literature and reports, "wellness and writing are connected in ways yet to be fully researched and exploited, but the literature of several disciplines declares that for many people wellness and writing are connected in ways useful for emotional, physical, and spiritual health" (p. 3). In the years since Evans reported that the connections had yet to be fully researched, Sandberg and Grant (2017) report, "more than a hundred experiments have documented the therapeutic effects of journaling. It has helped medical students, patients with chronic pain, crime victims, maximum-security prisoners, and women after childbirth" (pp. 62-63). They continue, "writing about traumatic events can decrease anxiety and anger, boost grades, reduce absences from work, and lessen the emotional impact of job loss. Health benefits include higher T-cell counts, better liver function, and stronger antibody responses. Even journaling for a few minutes a few times can make a difference" (p. 63). Furthermore, people do not have to write about traumatic events to receive the benefits of writing. Brown (2015) described the participants in her research as, "many of them worked through their emotions in letters they knew they would never send but needed to write" (p. 87).

The writing process can help anyone who feels willing to explore self-discovery. Mindfulness expert Cameron (2018) explains, "whether you write for five minutes or 60 minutes a day, journaling helps you gain perspective and deepen self-awareness – revealing your thoughts, habits, strengths, and ways of interpreting the world" (p. 45). She continues, "although journaling is an excellent practice for self-awareness, insight, and clarity, it has also proven to be a tremendous tool for navigating times of change, uncertainty, and dealing with difficult emotions" (p. 45). She encourages anyone interested in practicing journaling to use either prompts to explore ideas, or to open a notebook and put pen to paper as an act of mindfulness. I include examples of writing prompts at the end of this chapter for readers who wish to write.

As a high school English teacher, I witness my students report that writing helps them calm their minds and organize their thoughts. Life as a high school student can be difficult. The words English teacher Johnson (1998) wrote twenty years ago remain true today when she gives teachers the advice, "don't belittle your student's concerns. Acknowledge their feelings, accept their right to have a bad day or a worry, just as adults do" (p. 174). Students appreciate when teachers treat them with respect. Journal writing can provide an outlet for describing feelings when students may not want to discuss something. I tell students that if they write something which concerns them to discuss it with me, their parents, or the school counselor. I share the belief of English teacher Erin Gruwell (2007) who writes, "I, like my students, realized that it would take more than just writing to feel better – but at least it was a start" (p. 148). I shared parts of this chapter in progress with some of the high school students I teach to confirm I painted an accurate portrait with my words of how they felt in my English class as they began their writing practice. If you want to begin a writing practice, you do not need a medical credential to pick up a pen or open a blank document on your computer to receive the benefits of writing. Journal writing changed my life numerous times. I share my story while encouraging you to write the next chapter in your own story.

PART I: WRITING AND TEACHING

As soon as the bell rings, my students and I have a ritual: We reach for our journals. At the beginning of most of the high school English classes I teach, I allow about five minutes for journal writing time. I give students three options: Write about the quote I have on the board, write about the current work of literature we are reading, or write about whatever happens to be on their minds that day. At the end of each quarter, I hold individual conferences with each student where I flip through the journals to make sure they are writing, but I do not read their writing unless they request it. While I look through the journals, I ask students how they felt about writing. The majority of students tell me it helps them process thoughts and feelings. Several students tell me it helps manage stress. Students also describe that journal writing serves as practice, or warm-ups for formal essays. According to Carter (2015), "shoot for a perfect first draft and you are screwed, though; most people are paralyzed by the impossibility of that task" (pp. 204-205). I don't believe there is such a thing as a perfect first draft, but the imperfect first drafts that may not meet the requirements for a formal essay work perfectly for expressive writing in journals.

Journal writing encourages the writer to complete expressive writing. Writing teacher Romano (2013) describes, "expressive writing is where we start when we pour forth first words, seeking to make meaning from fragmented, chaotic inner speech. Expressive writing is writing closest to our speaking voice, the seedbed from which all other writing grows" (p. 189). Expressive writing focuses on the first thoughts before the voice of the internal censor starts questioning the words on the page. I want my students to feel like Lamott (1994) when she describes her process as, "so I'd start writing without reigning myself in. It was almost just typing, just making my fingers move" (p. 24). Some students prefer to type their journals, and they receive just as much as benefit as they process day to day issues in their writing. Sandberg and Grant (2017) believe, "turning feelings into words can help us process and overcome adversity" (p. 62). When adversity appears in the lives of my students, it becomes essential for me to honor their stories.

Student stories can lead to transformation. I love the work of teacher Erin Gruwell and her students, The Freedom Writers. My classes read *The Freedom Writers Diary* and discuss the philosophy of Erin Gruwell (1999), who describes of her students, "the students continued to write and began to forge stronger identities and to create a sense of community and an outlet for expression" (p. 275). My classes develop into strong communities when students care about each other and support each other. While I do not require them to share their writing during group discussions, when students do choose to share their writing with their classmates or me, they learn that others in the class share their feelings and they are not alone in their experiences.

While I choose not to share the writing of my students in this narrative to maintain the confidentiality I promised them, to give you an example of student writing I include a journal entry I wrote as a junior in high school. I keep my old journals and occasionally revisit them to reflect on my experiences.

Okay, I'm a junior. Let me see…what does that mean….more cafeteria food for one thing. Just kidding. For one thing, I'm not afraid of the school now, I know my way around (for the most part). I don't have to worry about graduation for another year. I guess I'm somewhere in the middle. I'll probably take ACTs and SATs this year, but I'm good at standardized tests so I'm not too worried. I do worry a lot though.

While it seems that my sixteen year old self wrote about surface things, at the end of the entry I started to process my thoughts and emotions about worrying. That insight comes from the writer years later after research and experience; my teenage self just enjoyed writing!

Before I returned to teaching high school students at Oxbridge Academy, I taught college students at Florida Atlantic University. The college students I taught participated in a research study to find connections between writing and healing (Bird and Wanner, 2015). We discovered, "students who demonstrated a more positive writing voice showed lower anxiety" (p. 281). Students who used more positive words in their writing samples reported lower anxiety on the Health Related Quality of Life Survey (HRQOL).

Medical doctor Rankin (2015) describes, "anxiety is an emotional feeling of nervousness, unease, dread, or apprehension" (p. 11). As someone who has experienced anxiety, I can relate to the students and feel grateful that writing helps me sort out the stress in my life. Writing becomes part of a balanced wellness plan including exercise, nutrition, and perspective. As I write these words, in a few hours all the students at my high school will attend an assembly on anxiety. Discussing issues makes a difference, because unlike the novel *The Scarlet Letter* students read, anxiety should never feel like a scarlet letter worn by anyone who experiences it. Szabo and Hall (2007) offer the encouragement, "it's time we all learned that each of us has a right – and a responsibility – to face our issues, be honest about our needs and emotions, and most importantly, to ask for help when we need it" (p. 221). Tomorrow, I plan to ask my students to write about the assembly in their journals to process their thoughts and feelings. Each day the bell rings and my students pick up their journals, I know the writing process helps them.

The Process

If you are a teacher or other educator and want to use journals in your classroom:

- Give students a choice of whether to write in a notebook or type their journals.
- Allow time for writing. A minimum of five minutes works well. Less than five minutes means students may not have the time to process their ideas.
- Maintain silence in the classroom so students can be alone with their thoughts and not distracted by classmates.
- It is your choice whether or not to read the writing, but make sure students know in advance if you will be reading their writing. Students do not want to be surprised if you tell them later you will be reading their personal writing.
- I recommend either not grading the writing or taking a participation grade. Students write differently when they know the content will be graded.
- You may have administrative tasks to complete, but take the time to write in your own journal when students are writing so they can see you as a writing role model.

PART II: WRITING AND EMOTIONAL PAIN

I first studied the field of writing as healing for my doctoral dissertation at Miami University in Oxford, Ohio. The topic of writing helping people heal emotionally became my purpose in life due to unexpected circumstances. In addition to helping other people, I also helped myself. My mom died in the middle of my graduate program, transforming me into not only an observer in my research study, but also a participant. Whenever my thoughts started racing or I missed my mom with an intensity which made me want to curl up on the floor and not get up again, I reached for my journal or my computer. My personal experiences with the transformative power of writing redefined my career and my life. I would trade all I have learned about writing as healing to be able to pick up the phone and call my mom again, but since I can't I choose to use my own experiences to help others.

While interviewing teachers about how they used writing to process their experiences, I also used writing to help me through the grieving process. Zimmermann (2002) believes, "writing allows you to access your wider mind, a wiser, more encompassing place deep within. Your story will unfold and through the writing of it, you will honor and embrace your sorrows, grow from them, and arrive at a place where life is more full and more joyful than you ever thought possible" (p. 19). Some days it became hard to feel when the emotional pain became too intense, but writing became my coping mechanism. Looking back at the writing, I can see my anger, devastation, and even moments of hope. This is an excerpt from my journal six months after my mom died when I traveled from Ohio to Delaware and Florida to visit my aunts, uncles, and cousins.

If the life you want isn't possible because of various circumstances, how do you piece together another life that may not be what you want but can still provide you with a little happiness? I think of all my dreams and my future plans that involved my mom. As I return from two weeks of visiting different cities and flying across the country on planes, I can't help but think that she would have been the first person I would have told of my adventures. I told her anyway; I know she was still part of my trip even though not in the way I wanted her to be.

After graduation, I decided to move from Ohio to Florida to make a new start and live closer to my family. Conner (2008) explains, "writing works amazingly well. If you want to engage in a vibrant conversation with the wisdom that dwells just a hair below your conscious awareness, write" (p. 57). In addition to helping me process my grief, writing helped me set new goals and dreams. By getting everything from my mind to the page, I gained clarity about my experiences. Sometimes when thoughts swirl around in a person's mind, the truth of the narrative becomes distorted. Social worker Brown (2017) elaborates, "the brain's self-protection mode often ramps up the stories we tell ourselves about what's happening, creating stories that are often not true or exaggerate our worst fears and insecurities" (p. 55). For days after my mom's death, I existed in survival mode and my subjective perspective of my life didn't always match my objective reality. My mind attempted to protect itself by processing pieces of the traumatic event at a time and when my thoughts couldn't focus, writing became a lifeline. Writer Heard (1995) believes, "a first memory is the first story embedded on the soul" (p. 72). Through a combination of writing and therapy, I refocused the first memory of the trauma and remembered the happy memories of my mom. I do not want to give the impression that writing solved everything for me during this difficult time; I also saw a therapist once a week to talk about my experiences and took an antidepressant at the advice of my doctor. Nevertheless, writing helped me on the days between therapist visits and especially the nights when I couldn't sleep and had already woken up my friends with phone calls. My journal and computer became reliable and constant companions who never gave advice and let me vent my emotions.

I could have stopped there; I did enough work on myself to not only survive but thrive. Still, perhaps because of my role as a teacher, I wanted to do more. Handler (2013) writes, "the passage of time between the event that caused grief and when the writer feels ready to pick up a pen or open the laptop is one place where your story is found. The person you were then, and the person you are now, create the voices that combine to tell the story" (p. 165). Immediately after the experience, my main focus was of course helping myself, but as time passed, I realized I wanted to share my story to help others. Along my journey I met people who cared about the topic as much as I did and we wrote together (Bird, Wanner, Urenda, and Perry, 2015). We wrote, "and we can save other lives too. While there is research that shows writing helps the author heal, can it help readers of the author's words heal?" (p. 4). I don't know the answer to that question. I don't know how many people read those words then and are reading these words now, but I have to believe my words make a difference. That is my mom's legacy, and my legacy too.

The Process

If you are going through a difficult time emotionally and want to write about it:

- Remember no one has to see your writing except you.
- Stop writing if it is too difficult.
- Your writing and computer won't judge you, so don't judge yourself for anything you write.
- If you would be upset if someone else read your writing, keep your journal in a locked file cabinet or other safe place.
- If you find yourself writing about something that disturbs you, it's time to share with a trusted friend or professional therapist.
- It is not a sign of weakness if you need therapy or medication. Don't be afraid to ask for help if you need it.

PART III: WRITING AND PHYSICAL PAIN

While I knew writing could help people heal emotionally, another serendipitous moment on my journey led me to research how writing helps people heal physically. I found myself in physical therapy for neck pain and kept a journal to try to make sense of why I felt little pain one minute and intense pain the next. I couldn't make any sense of it, but fortunately for me my physical therapist used expert knowledge to interpret my writing, make a diagnosis, and help me heal. I felt grateful for his compassion and creative thinking, since not all medical practitioners would feel enthusiastic about a new idea. After my treatment ended, we continued to work together and research how writing helps patients heal (Wanner and Bird, 2017). We designed a survey featuring both numerical subjective questions and short answer questions. Our research discovered, "patients who used more positive language when responding to short answer writing prompts on the survey we designed showed higher objective improvements on existing physical therapy measurements" (p. 663). An enjoyable interdisciplinary collaboration led to research results that made a difference in the lives of patients.

When we asked patients to respond to short answer survey questions, we asked for their first impressions. Writing teacher Goldberg (2013) shares, "practice is not for something else. Practice is the practice of being here with your life and pen now. Go, across the page – or your computer screen – what are you thinking of? Put your life on the line" (p. 22). The process of trusting first impressions in writing not only works for high school English students in a classroom, but also physical therapy patients in a clinic. When I designed my pain journal, I needed to share my first impressions in order to have the most accurate information to share with my physical therapist. When patients responded using their first impressions, they shared the most accurate impression of what they felt before the self-censor could take over their thoughts. As Bernstein (2010) writes, "let your pen flow across the page and allow your mind to release its thoughts" (p. 23). When I shared my journal, I needed to trust my physical therapist to keep my information confidential and also use it to help me. I'm sure at times my writing entertained him while he read my thoughts about my neck pain!

Most of us will be patients sometime in our lives. While writing cannot heal physical pain on its own, it can contribute to healing. When people write and release their emotions, the decrease in emotional stress can lead to a decrease in muscle tension. Enayati (2015) argues, "in a way, extreme stress is self-fulfilling. The key is to switch the focus of both our perceptions and stories to post-traumatic growth" (p. 72). Even if the patient has no control over the physical pain, the patient does have control of how he or she feels about the pain. Writing can bring clarity and perception to the pain narrative and switch the mental focus from helplessness to achieving growth about this experience. Duckworth (2016) defines, "it was this combination of passion and perseverance that made high achievers special. In a word, they had grit" (p. 8). While this definition of grit applies to a variety of situations, passion and perseverance become important during the recovery process from physical pain. Pain can lead to frustration, but a positive attitude makes a difference. Beck (2008) explains, "in other words, the negative reaction cluster – the stress reactions, the emotional pain, and the physical weakness that are wired together in your brain and body – can be rewired. The associative learning that makes us feel depressed, anxious, and old can be unlearned" (p. 11). Writing holds us accountable by revealing our thought patterns. Once we illuminate our thought patterns, we can change them. This helps not only patients experiencing physical pain, but also anyone who experiences daily stress. Dalebout (2016) observes, "journaling allows you to stop identifying with your negative beliefs or thought patterns and instead see yourself as separate from them. You start to move from judging yourself to simply witnessing your thoughts, cozying up with them, learning from them, and ultimately letting them out" (p. 12). Letting out thoughts in the form of journal writing allows the page to worry about an issue while simultaneously serving as a stress release. A positive perspective won't make life stressors disappear, but it can make life more manageable.

Another way writing can help with physical pain is by creating a journal to show medical professionals. How many times does the best question get thought of as soon as the doctor leaves the room? A pain journal or symptom journal ensures that all questions are asked and all information is conveyed to the person in charge of the patient's care. The most important quality of a pain or symptom journal is honesty. A doctor can best help a patient when he or she has all the information. Brown (2015) believes, "we can't get to our brave new ending if we start from an inauthentic place. So give yourself permission to wade through the sometimes-murky waters of whatever you're thinking and feeling" (p. 88). At times it may feel difficult to act vulnerable and authentic in front of someone in the medical field. Remember, most clinicians are compassionate professionals who will walk with you on your health journey. Medical doctor Rankin (2013) explains, "being unapologetically who we are – not just at work, but at home, in the schoolyard, at church, wherever – soothes the mind, halts the stress response, induces the relaxation response, and heals the body. Authenticity, in work and in life, can be medicine for the body" (p. 117). Not only can authenticity have health benefits by causing relaxation, when a person demonstrates authenticity, clinicians appreciate knowing all the information so an accurate diagnosis can be made. If we demonstrate a willingness to show vulnerability and articulate what we need, we lower the need for self-protection and can reach out to others when we need help.

Despite my love of television medical dramas, I have no desire to observe a surgery. I did, however, have a desire to learn more about the health care field, so I earned my health coach certification from Duke University Integrative Medicine. According to Caldwell, Gray, and Wolever (2013), "health coaching entails a specific structure and provider relationship that reinforce each other. The coach-patient relationship is specifically centered on the patient's health goals and supporting the patient in those goals" (p. 55). Health coaches partner with the patient's medical team to align the patient's personal goals with the treatment goals and help the patient achieve the goals. Beck (2001) advocates, "today, take one turtle step toward your goal. Just one" (p. 323). A turtle step is a little step that, taken with numerous other little steps, leads to success. Health coaches help patients stay motivated to reach their goals. From a health coaching perspective, writing does not eliminate pain, but can become part of the health plan. Writing down moments of success or challenge can help determine the next best steps, as well as illustrate progress. Whether writing down goals, keeping a pain journal, or processing feelings about pain, writing exists as a resource for the healing process.

The Process

If you are sick or in pain and want to write about it:

- Obviously, if you have severe pain or illness, don't write. Seek medical help immediately.
- Be honest in your writing. Your medical team can best help you if you tell the truth about your symptoms and feelings.
- Members of your medical team want to help you. Don't fear that they will judge you for writing the truth.
- Try to keep a positive attitude. Healing is a journey, and small steps still equal progress. A great lesson my physical therapist, Dr. Eric Wanner, told me when I wanted my neck pain to heal immediately is to "think like a turtle" and make slow and steady progress. Turtles travel at a slow pace, but eventually reach their destination.
- An excerpt of my pain journal is below; feel free to use it as a model for your own pain journal.

PART IV: WRITING AND SPIRITUALITY

On a beautiful Florida winter afternoon, my students and I sit outside by the lake on the high school's campus. We discuss the poetry of Walt Whitman. Whitman (1855) writes in his poem *O Me! O Life!* "That you are here – that life exists and identity, that the powerful play goes on and you may contribute a verse" (p. 341). This leads to a conversation about the difference between spirituality and religion. The sophomores in my English class give insightful answers. In their words, religion is what people practice while spirituality is how people feel. I explain that everyone has a right to his or her own religious beliefs, yet together as a class we have a spiritual moment sitting by the water in silence as we write in our journals and read poetry.

Table 1. The author's neck pain journal

Fri 3/30	Right Side Pain Low = 2, High = 4, Average = 3	Best right after leaving physical therapy. Worst when looking down at notes and stressing about summer teaching schedule. Spend time with family today which leads to laughter.
Sat 3/31	Right Side Pain Low = 2, High = 4, Average = 3	Best when doing exercises. Going for a mellow experience and listening to Taylor Swift this time.
Sun 4/1	Right Side Pain Low = 3, High = 5, Average = 4 Was going to play an April Fool's joke on you and make the numbers really high so laughed thinking about that.	Best when out to lunch with cousins and laughing. Worst when trying to hold Grandma back and prevent wheelchair escape. Epiphany of day: This is a journey. Keep thinking like a turtle. You'll get there!

Religious institutions may choose to use writing with members of their congregations. Also, anyone may choose to use writing as a reflection and form of prayer. Niequist (2016) believes, "whatever it is that you clutch onto with angry fists, that you grab like a lifeline, when you release that thing, when you let it go, that's when you'll hear the notes between the music" (p. 97). Reflection and prayer allow for silence so the noise of a busy life becomes silent. Sometimes when life seems uncertain, people turn to destructive habits; writing serves as a healthy alternative to coping with a situation and provides a reminder that a lifeline to internal strength provides more power than external distractions Enayati (2015) explains, "adversity may or may not be out of our control, but we do have control over our stories: what we tell ourselves and others about our circumstances, and how we choose to respond to them" (p. 51). When we can't control the outcome of a situation, we can still control how we react.

Whatever your religious or spiritual practices may be, the act of writing can be viewed as universal and accessible to all who choose to pick up a notebook and pen or reach for a computer. Does the story you tell yourself about your life and current situation reflect your reality? Is an obstacle a roadblock or an opportunity to learn? Brown (2015) explains, "the most dangerous stories we make up are the narratives that diminish our inherent worthiness" (p. 82). Putting thoughts on paper in the form of journal writing can clarify the difference between the actual truth of a situation compared to our interpretation of it. We remind ourselves of people and things we have for which we can show gratitude and determine what needs to change. Detours taken on the road of life can lead to new goals and opportunities.

In addition to my roles as high school English teacher and health coach, I serve as a Stephen Minister at my church. Haugk (2000) defines, "Stephen Ministers are lay Christians carefully recruited, selected, trained, commissioned, and supervised for lay caring ministry" (p. 17). With my role as a Stephen Minister, I use the same skills of reflective listening and partnering with people on their healing journeys as I do as a health coach. The difference with Stephen Ministry is that people may be experiencing a spiritual crisis instead of a health crisis, and I also have prayer as a resource. While I write about Stephen Ministry from the perspective of my experiences, the writing practices I describe are not meant to be seen only from the perspective of Christian faith.

Regardless of a person's views on religion and spirituality, the practice of self-compassion can lead to reflection and kindness toward oneself. Often people criticize themselves more harshly than other people ever could. While self-compassion can take place by thinking kind thoughts, writing can serve as an affirmation of thoughts of kindness. Neff (2011) suggests, "try keeping a daily self-compassion journal for one week (or as long as you like). Journaling is an effective way to express emotions and has been found to enhance both mental and physical well being" (p. 103). A daily self-compassion journal can remind the author to practice kindness and self-forgiveness. Whenever life seems challenging, we can enjoy the journey more by showing ourselves and others kindness and compassion. Mistakes happen as part of life, but since we cannot recapture the past like the main character in *The Great Gatsby* longs to do, writing can help us move forward. Germer (2009) shares, "keeping a journal is itself a contemplative practice and a self-compassion exercise" (p. 242). Contemplation shares characteristics with the practice of mindfulness, which promotes self-awareness and living in the present moment. Tindle (2013) explains, "the main difference between mindfulness and contemplation is that at its core, contemplation is a practice in which the contemplator seeks to come closer to a higher spiritual power" (p. 108). Some people may choose to practice mindfulness and remind themselves to refocus their attention to the present moment, while others may choose to pray as a form of contemplation.

While prayer exists mainly through spoken words, they may also appear in the forms of thoughts or written ideas. Cameron (1998) states, "it is my belief that all of us are naturally intuitive and that writing opens an inner spiritual doorway that gives us access to information both personally and professionally that serves us well" (pp. 206-207). Often, when a decision needs to be made, writing can provide guidance to the solution which makes the writer feel most at peace. Clarity appears on the page and offers valuable insight. Matousek (2017) believes, "like all forms of awakening practice, writing requires mindfulness. Just as we bring our attention back to the breath during meditation, you learn to observe the wandering mind without excessive control, and gently return your focus to the question at hand" (p. 5). Whatever question may bring the writer to the page, writing about it may provide the answer.

While Stephen Ministry provides one on one care between the Stephen Minister and care receiver, at times I find myself giving short prayers. When I visit someone in need in the hospital or pray with someone at church after the service, I may not know much about the person. During such times, I begin speaking and trust I will say the words the person needs to hear. Bernstein (2016) believes, "we change the world when we shift spiritually – when our attitudes become more loving, when we forgive, when we heal our wounds from the past, and when we embrace the present moment" (p. 172). Just like it helps people heal emotionally and physically, writing can help people heal spiritually. The journal can be a place to explore thoughts and feelings for self-forgiveness, or a place to work through a difficult conversation if it would help to forgive someone else. If the person who needs forgiveness is not willing to have a conversation or longer alive, forgiving can still take place for the writer in journal pages. Bernstein (2018) explains, "putting pen to paper is a prayer. It's an offering. You humbly look at your judgment, choose again, and then pray for that judgment to be replaced with love" (p. 186). By writing, we acknowledge our pasts, remind ourselves to remain mindful in the present, and share hope for the future.

My research and writing became part of my life's purpose. By writing about my experiences, I saw the connections between the moments that happened to me (Wanner and Bird, 2015). After completing research and writing, it helped to take time to reflect, "because research and writing feels like a larger purpose instead of just work, it translates into appreciating the moments when the puzzle pieces of ideas click into place to form projects that will help people" (p. 219). It's a magical feeling when ideas weave together like threads of a tapestry. I loved when two separate research studies to which I contributed yielded similar results. (Bird and Wanner, 2015). The writing as healing discoveries showed, "college students who used a positive writing voice demonstrated lower anxiety and stronger emotional health, just like physical therapy patients who used a positive writing voice throughout their treatment interventions demonstrated higher recovery gains for objective measures on pre-existing physical therapy surveys. The results illustrate that a strong positive writing voice can help people heal both physically and emotionally" (p. 281). Consequently, writing makes a difference in the lives of people who need healing. If my mom hadn't died, would I still feel that research and writing exist in my life as part of a larger purpose? I do know that helping other people makes me feel that I can use the pain of my life experiences to make a meaningful contribution to the world. I understand that some people may see everything as coincidences, but my spirituality leads me to believe in what Rushnell and DuArt (2017) call Godwinks, which they define as, "Godwinks are those little events that defy human understanding. In the beginning you were tempted to call them coincidences, but inwardly you sensed there was something more going on – and that God had something to do with it" (p. ix). Whatever you may believe, I hope writing helps you discover your personal gifts. I then encourage you to share your gifts with others who may benefit from the knowledge.

The Process

If you are a church leader or anyone who wants to use writing as a spiritual resource:

- If you are contemplating a question or need to make a decision, start writing and see what answers your intuition discovers.
- If you find yourself being your own worst critic, practice self-compassion and write about your strengths in your journal.
- Create a gratitude journal and make a list of things for which you are grateful. Use daily, weekly, or as often as you need.
- If you feel discouraged by acts of hate in the world, shift the focus to love and create an observation journal of random acts of kindness that you practice or witness others practicing throughout the day.
- Write a prayer for yourself or someone else.

PART V: THE ART OF WRITING

Throughout this narrative, I cited research studies illustrating the healing benefits that can happen with writing. Even with the technical dimensions of research, creativity drives the artistic writing process. I view writing as an art form, where self-expression becomes essential for the writer. Writing provides a safe space for expression, since the page will not judge the author. Even sharing the story with oneself in the pages of a journal can provide healing benefits. Sharing writing with a supportive reader can build trust and provide additional support for the writer. Romano (2015) describes of sharing stories, "it's been good to write about it and give it to readers" (p. 21). The writer decides who to trust; finding the right reader leads to a source of encouragement and helps the writer build resilience. Writing serves as a coping mechanism for life's fragile moments and can transform negative thoughts into positive ones by reframing the stories.

Just as a painter glides across a blank canvas with a paintbrush, the writer glides across a blank page with a pen. Heard (1995) writes, "when I return to writing, the lessons from art guide me. Painting and writing are both about relationships. In painting, paint thickness, brush strokes, image, canvas texture, color, and outline all work together. In writing, the words, images, rhythm, voice, and meaning must work together as well. (p. 119). In the stories captured in the pages of a journal, the writer may search for meaning instead of starting with a specific destination in mind. Journal writing focuses on the journey. During the process, the writer's voice, as unique as a speaking voice, shines through on the page. Trusting first impressions gets the writer closest to the truth of what is on the mind and in the heart. Cameron (1998) explains, "yes, writing is an art, but 'art' is part of the verb 'to be' – as in 'Thou art truly human.' To be truly human, we all have the right to make art. We all have the right to write" (pp. 232-233). Writing means connecting with the self. Take my words and paint a picture with your own words. I leave you with a review of points to ponder as you begin your writing journey.

The Process

If you want to begin your own writing story:

- Use writing to illuminate your narrative. Trust the words that appear on the page to capture the truth of your thoughts and feelings.
- Show yourself some compassion. No one is perfect. It's okay to feel what you feel.
- Take turtle steps. Whatever your personal journey may be, change takes time.
- Be authentic. No one else is you. Don't feel you need to pretend to be someone else on the page. It won't comment on your writing.
- Show grit. Passion and perseverance will help you achieve goals you set for yourself.
- Track progress. You do not have to reread previous writing, but it can help you see patterns and appreciate accomplishments.
- Share your story. You do not have to share your story, but a supportive reader can offer support and encouragement on your journey.

EPILOGUE: YOUR STORY

Practicing the art of expressive writing can lead to emotional, physical, and spiritual healing. Cameron (2018) shares, "you direct your attention to the page, open your mind, and make the invisible visible by seeing what comes through on the page" (p. 45). She adds, "the greatest discoveries of your life could appear on those paper or on-screen pages" (p. 48). To begin your writing practice, here are some ideas for prompts:

- Choose a quote that inspires you and write about it.
- Look around the room and choose an object to describe.
- Think of a favorite memory and capture it on paper.
- Free write about whatever is on your mind.
- Complete the sentences, "I am," "I want," "I believe."

I recommend the writing books *Writing Down the Bones* (1986), *Wild Mind* (1990), *and Old Friend from Far Away* (2007) by Natalie Goldberg, *The Right to Write* (1998) by Julia Cameron, *Bird by Bird* (1994) by Anne Lamott, *Writing toward Home* (1995) by Georgia Heard, and *Let it Out* (2016) by Katie Dalebout. All of the authors list a series of writing prompts which inspired me to write and develop writing prompts to use in my classroom and in my personal writing. Sharp (2000) offers anyone wanting to write the encouragement, "someone who takes the time to sit down, perhaps with pen or pencil in hand, and express themselves in their own words – this is a person who has something to say and the commitment to say it". (p. 133). Everyone has a unique writing voice, so let your writing voice shine. Goldberg (1996) provides the reminder, "when you finish a piece, you're refusing to be silenced or ignored. Writing is brave" (p. 201). I encourage you to find the courage to share your story, whether you share it with yourself or a larger audience.

While my story will continue, it becomes time for this chapter to end. I lean back in my chair and study my writing. I feel calm after my writing session. I enjoyed sharing a chapter in my life story with you. I hope reading it helps you in some way. The next chapter in your life is yours to write. Each day offers a chance to fill another blank page with hopes and dreams. May you make the most of it.

REFERENCES

Beck, M. (2001). *Finding your own North Star*. New York, NY: Three Rivers Press.

Beck, M. (2008). *Steering by starlight*. New York, NY: Rodale.

Bernstein, G. (2010). *Add more –ing to your life*. New York, NY: Harmony Books.

Bernstein, G. (2016). *The universe has your back*. Carlsbad, CA: Hay House.

Bernstein, G. (2018). *Judgment detox*. New York, NY: North Star Way.

Bird, J. L., & Wanner, E. T. (2015). Research as curriculum inquiry: helping college students with anxiety. In V. C. X. Wang (Ed.), *Handbook of research on scholarly publishing and research methods* (pp. 273–295). Hershey, PA: Information Science Reference. doi:10.4018/978-1-4666-7409-7.ch014

Bird, J. L., Wanner, E. T., Urenda, R., & Perry, R. (2015). Multigenre medicine. In J. L. Bird (Ed.), *Innovative collaborative practice and reflection in patient education* (pp. 1–19). Hershey, PA: Information Science Reference. doi:10.4018/978-1-4666-7524-7.ch001

Brown, B. (2015). *Rising strong*. New York, NY: Spiegel & Grau.

Brown, B. (2017). *Braving the wilderness*. New York, NY: Random House.

Caldwell, K., Gray, J., & Wolever, R. Q. (2013). The process of patient empowerment in integrative health coaching: How does it happen? *Global Advances in Health and Medicine: Improving Healthcare Outcomes Worldwide*, *2*(3), 48–57. doi:10.7453/gahmj.2013.026 PMID:24416672

Cameron, J. (1998). *The right to write*. New York, NY: Tarcher/Putnam.

Cameron, L. (2018). *The mindful day*. Washington, DC: National Geographic.

Carter, C. (2015). *The sweet spot*. New York, NY: Ballantine.

Centers for Disease Control and Prevention. (2011). *"Health Related Quality of Life." Health Related Quality of Life Surveillance Program*. Retrieved from http://www.cdc.gov/hrqol/hrqol14_measure.htm

Clandinin, D. J., & Connelly, F. M. (2000). *Narrative inquiry*. San Francisco, CA: Jossey-Bass.

Conner, J. (2008). *Writing down your soul*. San Francisco, CA: Conari.

Dalebout, K. (2016). *Let it out*. Carlsbad, CA: Hay House.

Duckworth, A. (2016). *Grit*. New York, NY: Scribner.

Enayati, A. (2015). *Seeking serenity*. New York, NY: New American Library.

Evans, J. F. (2010). Introducing wellness & writing connections conference papers. In J. F. Evans (Ed.), *Wellness & Writing Connections* (pp. 3–10). Enumclaw, WA: Idyll Arbor, Inc.

Fitzgerald, F. S. (1925). *The great Gatsby*. New York, NY: Scribner.

Germer, C. K. (2009). *The Mindful path to self-compassion*. New York, NY: The Guilford Press.

Goldberg, B. (1996). *Room to write*. New York, NY: Tarcher/Putnam.

Goldberg, N. (1986). *Writing down the bones*. Boston, MA: Shambhala.

Goldberg, N. (1990). *Wild mind*. New York, NY: Bantam.

Goldberg, N. (2007). *Old friend from far away*. New York, NY: Free Press.

Goldberg, N. (2013). *The true secret of writing*. New York, NY: Atria.

Gruwell, E. (2007). Teach with your heart. New York, NY: Broadway.

Gruwell, E., & the The Freedom Writers. (1999). The Freedom Writers diary. New York, NY: Broadway.

Handler, J. (2013). *Braving the fire*. New York, NY: St. Martin's Griffin.

Haugk, K. C. (2000). *When and how to use mental health resources*. St. Louis, MO: Stephen Ministries.

Hawthorne, N. (1955). The scarlet letter. New York, NY: Washington Square Press. (Original text published 1850).

Heard, G. (1995). *Writing toward home*. Portsmouth, NH: Heinemann.

Heifetz, R. A. (1994). *Leadership without easy answers*. Cambridge, MA: The Belnap Press of Harvard University Press.

Johnson, L. (1998). *Two parts textbook, one part love*. New York, NY: Hyperion.

Lamott, A. (1994). *Bird by bird*. New York, NY: Anchor Books.

Matousek, M. (2017). *Writing to awaken*. Oakland, CA: Reveal Press.

Neff, K. (2011). *Self compassion: the proven power of being kind to yourself.* New York, NY: Harper-Collins.

Niequist, S. (2016). *Present over perfect*. Grand Rapids, MI: Zondervan.

Pennebaker, J. W., & Smyth, J. M. (2016). *Opening up by writing it down*. New York, NY: The Guilford Press.

Rankin, L. (2013). *Mind over medicine*. Carlsbad, CA: Hay House.

Rankin, L. (2015). *The fear cure*. Carlsbad, CA: Hay House.

Romano, T. (2013). *Fearless writing*. Portsmouth, NH: Heinemann.

Romano, T. (2015). *Write what matters*. Lexington, KY: Zigzag.

Rushnell, S., & DuArt, L. (2017). *The Godwink effect*. New York, NY: Howard Books.

Sandberg, S., & Grant, A. (2017). *Option B*. New York, NY: Knopf.

Sharp, C. (2000). *A writer's workbook*. New York, NY: St. Martin's Press.

Szabo, R., & Hall, M. (2007). *Behind happy faces*. Beverly Hills, CA: Alegra.

Tindle, H. (2013). *Up: How positive outlook can transform our health and aging*. New York, NY: Hudson Street Press.

Wanner, E. T., & Bird, J. L. (2015). Strength from spirituality. In J. L. Bird (Ed.), *Innovative collaborative practice and reflection in patient education* (pp. 218–232). Hershey, PA: Information Science Reference. doi:10.4018/978-1-4666-7524-7.ch014

Wanner, E. T., & Bird, J. L. (2017). Incorporating a new technology for patient education. In Information Resources Management Association (Ed.), Healthcare ethics and training (pp. 662-675). Hershey, PA: Information Science Reference. doi:10.4018/978-1-5225-2237-9.ch030

Whitman, W. (1993). O Me! O Life! In *Leaves of Grass* (p. 341). New York, NY: Random House. (Original work published 1855).

Zimmermann, S. (2002). *Writing to heal the soul*. New York, NY: Three Rivers Press.

KEY TERMS AND DEFINITIONS

Anxiety: Different clinicians have different definitions of anxiety, and a person who lives with anxiety will describe it from a different point of view than a clinical definition in a textbook, but the general definition of anxiety is chronic fear or stress that can result in panic attacks and a person feeling an inability to cope with life's stresses.

Expressive Writing: Writing that is exploratory and focuses on meaning and first impressions.

Journal Writing: The process of responding to prompts and writing about thoughts and feelings. While journal writing is typically associated with writing classrooms, writing teachers including Julia Cameron and Natalie Goldberg advocate that journal writing can be done by anyone, anywhere.

Medical Professionals: People in the medical profession such as primary care doctors, specialists, physical therapists, and emotional therapists. Medical doctors Hilary Tindle and Lissa Rankin discuss that patients experience improved health when they have a positive outlook and a willingness to share their stories with their doctors.

Narrative Inquiry: Described by F. Michael Connelly and D. Jean Clandinin, narrative inquiry is a qualitative interpretative form of research which focuses on the telling, retelling, and sharing of stories.

Pain Journal: A journal describing symptoms designed to be shown to a medical professional.

Self-Compassion: The act of demonstrating the same kindness for oneself that one would demonstrate for other people.

Spirituality: Regardless of religion, spirituality and a belief in a higher power can lead to increased health and provide both hope and strength.

Writing as Healing: Numerous studies have been conducted investigating the influence of writing on physical and emotional health. James Pennebaker is a leader in the field which explores the health benefits of writing.

Writing Prompts: Questions used as starters to encourage writers to develop ideas.

Chapter 9
Storytelling Through Dance and Movement

Jenny Bopp
Westtown School, USA

ABSTRACT

Everyone has a story to tell, but because of trauma, not everyone can use words to tell it. The purpose of this chapter is to demonstrate an arts-based, trauma-informed, hope-infused movement and storytelling curriculum for adults (ages 19+) who are in recovery from various addictions or traumatic experiences. The curriculum was implemented with a group of five people selected by the supervising agency (Kingdom Recovery) to assess whether or not it proved beneficial to the participants. Assessment methods included before/after class experiences, a movement assessment checklist, and an evaluation survey. The curriculum consisted of seven lessons lasting 90 minutes each, and the goal of the curriculum was to promote life-skill building, healing, and hope. At the end of the seven-week time period, subjects performed pieces they choreographed throughout the sessions as a celebration of their accomplishments and hard work. The goals of the curriculum were accomplished successfully and 100% of the participants noticed an increase in their confidence, empathy, and creativity.

INTRODUCTION

Since ancient civilization, dance has been a form of expression and storytelling containing deep traditions and meaning in many cultures (Kreitler & Kreitler, 1972). Dance therapist David Harris (2007) says, "Dance therapy offers unusual potential for advancing [the] critical healing process in innovative ways" (p. 204). While this chapter is not about clinical dance therapy, it is about the ways in which dance can be used to facilitate healing in an everyday environment. Often, those who have experienced trauma find verbal communication about their experience difficult and potentially re-traumatizing. Dance and movement, among other art forms, offer opportunities for someone to tell their story without having to find words. In this context, movement opens the door for empathy, honest self-expression, and the release of physical tension (catharsis) which can be held in the body for years after a traumatic experience (Dayton, 2007).

DOI: 10.4018/978-1-5225-5981-8.ch009

Developing a therapeutic movement-based curriculum that is trauma-informed and hope-infused provides a holistic outlet for healing to those suffering from abuse, addiction, and physical, emotional, and mental disabilities. In order to create an effectively trauma-informed curriculum, it is necessary to first understand the effects of trauma upon the brain, the body, and the spirit, and to explore what types of experiences provide therapeutic releases (SAMHSA, 2014).

An effective therapeutic movement curriculum is informed by the understanding of trauma's effect on the body, mind and spirit, and the outward manifestation of those effects. The author developed this curriculum in hopes of providing an outlet for therapeutic release through dance by becoming informed about trauma and its effects upon the whole person. She simply watched, listened, guided the curriculum's experiences, and became a witness for the people participating in her study.

Providing safety, opportunities to build healthy relationships, and the development of coping skills (Bath, 2008), are all elements that shape the curriculum's arts-based experiences. This movement curriculum is designed to give survivors of trauma a way to reconnect with their bodies, and to build empathetic connections with other people in a safe environment. Future-oriented thinking and creativity are re-established through the curriculum's experiences, fostering new or revitalized hope for a future that could be.

Trauma's Effect on the Mind, Body, and Spirit

Trauma affects every part of a person's being. While there are many treatments for trauma survivors, most involve only one or two elements of the whole person. Holistic treatment involves the entire person, not solely the body, the brain, or the spirit. Trauma often disconnects these three parts, creating challenges that interfere with the holistic healing process. Mental illness is often viewed as a disorder in the brain alone, and rarely is a spiritual aspect taken into account. When physical trauma happens to a body, the mind and spirit are often left out of the healing process. Sometimes counselors, pastors, and therapists focus solely on spiritual healing while the lasting effects of the body and mind's reactions to trauma are not addressed. The disconnections between body, mind, and spirit are detrimental to true healing, because these three elements are so intricately connected.

The Mind

The mind is a powerful tool that must be protected and nurtured. The fascinating science behind the effect of trauma and resilience on the mind has shed light on the inner workings of the brain, and the reasons why people respond to traumatic events differently. When the brain is affected by trauma, especially for a child, a disconnect forms between the logical, decision-making right hemisphere and the emotional left hemisphere which inhibits Broca's Area (the expressive language area) from functioning properly (Crenshaw, 2006). Muteness and the inability to speak clearly about a traumatic experience is due to an imbalance of norepinephrine, a hormone released from the amygdala that attaches to a piece of information before it is sent to the hypothalamus where the information is then processed and the flight/fight/freeze response is determined (Behrens, 2014). This is an important issue; because talk therapy is a very common method used by therapists, but, unfortunately, can easily cause re-traumatization in their clients (SAMHSA, 2014).

People with healthy, well-developed brains are able to regulate their emotions, their reactions to experiences, and respond with appropriateness to new or stressful situations. A traumatized brain, however, gets stuck. Development is stunted, resulting in a lack of healthy coping mechanisms and an inability to move past an experience. The disconnect creates a block in communication among the processing parts of the brain, causing an individual's communicative abilities to become disjointed, inappropriate, or virtually non-existent (Behrens, 2014). Dr. David Servan-Schreiber (2003) calls this an "emotional short circuit" (p. 28).

In his book *The Instinct to Heal,* Servan-Schreiber (2003) recognizes two examples of emotional short-circuiting. The first is posttraumatic stress disorder (PTSD), or overly emotional reactions to situations: "After a serious trauma… the emotional brain acts like a loyal and conscientious sentry that has been caught off guard. PTSD sets off the alarm much too often, as if the emotional brain cannot be sure that everything is safe" (p. 28). This hypervigilant state keeps a person's body and mind on constant guard, and prevents him from being able to regulate his emotions and physical reactions. The constant state of stress in which the individual lives, not only creates social and mental disconnects, but potentially results in long-term physical disabilities and diseases as well.

The second way a brain may respond to trauma is "cognitive smothering" by suppressing emotions completely (Servan-Schreiber, 2003, p. 29). Denial - "an unconscious defense mechanism" (Henderson, 2000, p. 77) - is one symptom of cognitive smothering, and it creates a disconnect between the body and brain called dissociation. Dissociation of the brain from the body and the spirit becomes clear when people recount traumatic experiences, but express no emotional response as they speak. Often, people who have suffered from trauma use sex, drugs, alcohol, etc., to compensate for their inability to emotionally cope with their experiences. These stimulants engage the brain's "pleasure center" and cause the brain to remember the good feelings and relief that occur during the high (Henderson, 2000). For a traumatized individual, this can lead to a detrimental addiction.

The Body

A body's reaction to trauma directly relates to the brain's reaction. As mentioned above, disconnection and dissociation prevent the body from properly responding to an experience regardless of how pleasant or unpleasant the experience may have been. Victims of abuse or neglect are often disconnected from their bodies, because feelings of pleasure may bring back horrific memories, no matter how far removed from the experience they may be (Servan-Schreiber, 2003, p. 25). A common symptom of trauma is called dissociation, an unconscious strategy for "leaving" a place psychologically. Trauma survivors with this symptom sometimes cannot physically feel their bodies and are occasionally unaware of potentially dangerous situations (Cori, 2007, p. 32). For the trauma survivor, this can make one feel as though he or she has no "center, anchor, or root" (2007, p. 32). Internal continuity feels like it is non-existent, creating a sense of chaos and preventing a firm sense of self and identity from existing. This is why it is of the utmost importance that trauma care involves active physical grounding and centering exercises. These exercises help the victim gain control of their bodies and their surroundings. Jasmin Lee Cori (2007) says, "You may only become aware of how disconnected you are from your body when you have a contrasting experience of truly being present in it" (p. 33).

Because the body is so vulnerable after it suffers trauma, therapeutic movement may seem a challenging alternative to other therapies. However, a body must experience release of what it carries in order to heal (Goodill, 2005). Bessel Van der Kolk (2014) says, "Trauma victims cannot recover until they become familiar with and befriend the sensations in their bodies" (p. 100). Stressed out people live in stressed out bodies, which results in physical health issues such as heart disease, obesity, eating disorders, migraines, bowel disorders, liver failure (due to alcoholism and drug addiction), and even autoimmune disorders (Van der Kolk, 2014). These stem from a survivor's inability to cope or properly care for themselves (Banitt, 2012, p. 91). If they cannot cope in healthy ways, they cannot recover.

The Spirit

Finally, there is a spiritual component to trauma. The spirit is crushed by trauma. Though often ignored by many healthcare providers today, spirituality is the "understanding of ourselves beyond the level of our ego and is what gives depth to our experience" (Van Lith, 2014, p. 26). Trauma affects a person's character, personality, motivations, emotional well-being, and hope for something better. One of the major symptoms of PTSD and trauma is withdrawal and isolation (Delaney & Scheiber, 2011, p. 111). People tend to lose their sense of purpose and identity because they cannot cope with their experiences. Creative experiences have the ability to help survivors rebuild their sense of self, develop deeper meaning in their work (Van Lith, 2014), and reclaim hope and purpose for their lives.

The sense of self can be "understood in terms of interpersonal aspects such as roles, relationships and who we might become" (Van Lith, 2014, p. 20). According to Dr. Edith Grotberg (1995), a strong sense of self (I Am) is one of three main sources of post traumatic growth. Because trauma causes physical, mental, and emotional disconnection, trauma survivors are likely to feel as though they cannot control their environments, themselves, or their relationships, "resulting in a chaotic sense of self" (Van Lith, p. 20). Theresa Van Lith (2014) and Jasmin Lee Cori (2007) agree that finding self-congruence for trauma survivors is often a long process, and must be addressed with deliberate steps and experiences that promote healing. Van Lith states: "This is a task of great complexity, as it involves affirming the characteristics of self that were once of value and strength while simultaneously recognizing the need for change in other aspects" (2014, p. 20).

Mindfulness and intentionality in art making are also spiritual matters for trauma survivors. Having purpose, finding meaning, and being able to communicate through movement allow a trauma survivor to engage and connect with the world in ways that words cannot. It offers opportunity for people to express what cannot be spoken verbally, and still have others understand. Art making is communication and movement is language (Moore & Yamamoto, 2012). Metaphor becomes the method to finding meaning in life. Carol-Lynne Moore and Kaoru Yamamoto say:

Indeed, this physiognomic approach holds that not only are we biologically programmed to encode and decode feelings in universally fixed ways, but movements themselves, through their inherent qualities, carry intrinsic, expressive meanings that are immediately and viscerally apprehended. Sad movements sink, while happy movements rise with buoyancy. The defiant stand with arms akimbo, and the meek shrink with elbows held in. The vital, the ecstatic and the passionate are physically expansive, while the frightened, the intellectual, and the sickly are contained (2012, p. 70).

Movement identifies meaning and meaning identifies movement. Movements are metaphors for what one feels inside.

The development of empathy reflects another deep spiritual aspect of healing from trauma. The ability to tolerate, understand, and work with others in reality is important to a trauma survivor's success in the workplace, at home, or in any other social situation. Psychologist Dr. Diana Fischman (2009) says, "To understand other human beings sometimes implies overcoming distance through mechanisms such as:

simulation, imitation, echoing or using our imagination whereby we build theories matching our own and somebody else's experiences" (p. 45). A dance teacher can act as a "witness" for the subject by mirroring and reflecting the movements that she sees. This develops a greater sense of empathy between them. Fischman says, "...empathy happens in the bodies of witnesses when watching the dance of the dancer while focused on their own corporeal experience" (2009, p. 46). Time and weight of movements reflected from one body to another help subjects feel the emotion of those they mirror. This begins to re-establish safe emotional and social connections, removing focus from self, and helping people become more aware of those around them.

Necessities for Trauma-Informed Care

For anyone working with trauma survivors, it is necessary to be informed and aware of signs and triggers that may cause retraumatization. Babette Rothschild (2000) says, "The risk of a client's becoming overwhelmed, decompensating, having anxiety and panic attacks, flashbacks, or worse, retraumatization, always lingers" (p. 77). It is not, however, required that caregivers, teachers, and others working with trauma survivors have clinical degrees in order to be trauma-informed, and be able to provide trauma-sensitive care to their clients and students. Howard Bath's *Three Pillars of Trauma Informed Care* (2008) lays out a foundation for trauma-informed care within a non-clinical setting. He states: "One does not need to be a therapist to address these three crucial elements of healing: the development of safety, the promotion of healing relationships, and the teaching of self-management and coping skills" (2008, p. 18).

Safety

The first pillar of trauma-informed care is the development of safety. According to Bob Delaney and David Scheiber (2011), "...if major change is going to happen, it's going to come from within. So it's important to give people a sense that there is something *they* can do" (p. 107). Identifying fears, joys, desires, and things that make one feel safe all play a role in healing and regaining control of one's environment (Alcorn, 2008).

In Abraham Maslow's *Hierarchy of Needs: A Theory of Human Motivation* (2011), safety is the second most important need to be fulfilled, just after physiological needs (sleep, food, shelter, etc.). Bessel Van der Kolk (2014) says, "...traumatized people chronically feel unsafe inside their bodies: the past is alive in the form of gnawing interior discomfort" (p. 96). They are afraid of their own bodies, and sensory feelings that accompany distressing experiences. "People who cannot comfortably notice what is going on inside become vulnerable to respond to any sensory shift either by shutting down or by going into a panic - they develop a fear of fear itself" (Van der Kolk, 2014, p. 97). The development of a safe environment begins with "consistency, reliability, availability, predictability, honesty, and transparency," along with allowing subjects to make choices, attentive listening on the part of the facilitator, and mutual respect among the participants (Bath, p. 19).

Babette Rothschild suggests a "braking and accelerating" method for safety in trauma treatment (2000, p. 78). A facilitator must understand what kinds of trauma subjects have experienced and meet them where they are, not forcing them to recollect memories and experiences that may cause retraumatization. Knowing when to address the trauma, knowing when to take a "brake", and understanding the needs of the person are key to building a safe atmosphere.

Healing Relationships

The second pillar is promoting healing relationships. Howard Bath says, "Safety itself depends on the development of...comfortable connections between [subjects] and [the facilitator]" (2008, p. 19). This is one area where emotional and physical responses become entwined. Abuse in all forms causes relational trauma that is held in the body, usually unconsciously, causing one to feel distressed around certain types of people (Dayton, 2007). Daniel A. Hughes (2013) confirms that healthy relationships begin with safety. Much like an infant needs her parents to be present when she is frightened or distressed, adults need other people who they trust to help protect and comfort them. Hughes states: "...when we are secure in a relationship, knowing that it will persist even in the face of problems and that we are able to turn to the other when we are in distress, we are more open to learning about all sorts of things when we are in the presence of the other" (2013, p. 6).

Because of previous trauma and lack of relational stability, people may be distrustful of others - particularly adults - to the point that it is difficult to feel anything other than anger, suspicion, or avoidance when it comes to sharing information (Bath, 2008). Dr. Tian Dayton, author of *Emotional Sobriety: from Relationship Trauma to Resilience and Balance* (2007), writes that because a person's traumatized brain is trying to protect itself, "distorted thinking, hyperactivity, mistrust, and ambivalence can be some of the issues that become part of being in close relationships" (p. 73). It is not uncommon for anti-social and mental disorders to develop, causing dysfunction and interference with a person's ability to develop healthy relationships (Henderson, 2000). With the establishment of trust within a group, people begin to develop new patterns of relational health that benefit them going forward as they care for their families and friends.

Self-Regulation and Coping Skills

The third pillar is teaching skills for coping and self-regulation. While it is true that trauma creates disconnections and disruptions in the brain that can be incapacitating to some, Howard Bath believes that the brain can still be retrained "to learn new skills of emotion management" (2008, p. 20). Emotions naturally affect the body, whether one is conscious or unconscious of accompanying muscular tensions and somatic sensations. Accelerated heart rate, shallow breathing, and tension in various body parts all coincide with a person's emotional state. Dr. Tian Dayton says, "...one of the skills of self-regulation lies in the ability to balance and regulate our own behavior and adapt it to our environment" (2007, p. 77). Through various breath and body awareness experiences, greater levels of self-awareness and regulation can be achieved over time.

In congruence with Bath and Dayton, Jasmin Lee Cori (2007) also offers several "tasks of healing" that fall within the Three Pillars theory. Cori says one must learn to reset the nervous system and free the body of impacts and holding patterns derived from trauma by expanding the ability to stay present and regain mastery of trauma symptoms and emotions (2007). Lastly, Cori says giving back in small ways will aid in healing the whole person (2007). She says the healing process is lifelong, but there are several indicators of growing wholeness in a person:

Wholeness includes the presence of certain qualities, such as a sense of well-being; joy; humor; the heart qualities of kindness, compassion, and gratitude; effective life skills; a sense of empowerment; a capacity to love; a feeling of purpose; an ability to take care of yourself; and a sense of who you are on a very deep level (2007, p. 220).

Dance and Movement's Place in Healing

Movement and dance help reconnect the body, mind, and spirit. According to the American Dance Therapy Association, dance helps to "further the emotional, cognitive, physical, and social integration of the individual" (2014, http://adta.org/). Eric Jensen writes in his book *Arts with the Brain in Mind* (2001) that most of the brain is activated by the body's activity. Be it dance, woodworking, playing and instrument, or playing sports, the brain remembers kinesthetic and implicit (hands-on) activities. Many cognitive skills are learned through movement and play. For people who are unable to talk about their trauma, self-expression through movement offers a unique, less formal outlet for working out complicated and suppressed thoughts and emotions (Crenshaw, 2006). Movement also allows catharsis, or completion, to occur. The inability to react in the moment of abuse that has been stuck in the body is finally allowed to be released. This therapeutic catharsis allows the mind, body, and spirit to return to a state of homeostasis.

According to Babette Rothschild (2010), there are three potential benefits to physical movement and fitness. First, it provides "an antidote to a persistent freeze response" (2010, p. 117). This means that when natural reactions to stress and trauma are suppressed, that energy remains in the body, prohibiting easy, natural, day-to-day functioning. According to Susan Pease Banitt, LCSW (2012), when animals experience negative or traumatic situations, they often shake, spasm, or run in order to dispel the adrenaline that is released during the experience (p. 130). Their bodies are then able to move past the experience, without holding onto the freeze response. Judith Lynne Hanna, M.D. (1988) writes, "...when a person neither fights nor flees because physical action in the immediate situation is inappropriate, biochemical elements of energy may remain in the body" (p. 11). Because of this, Banitt states that "[one] could develop tension in the shoulders and upper back from the incomplete swing [one's] body wanted to take, tension whose origins are forgotten or unknown" (2012, p. 129). Jasmin Lee Cori agrees when she states:

...in somatic trauma therapies, there is a recognition that often there were defensive responses that were cut off during an overwhelming threat (e.g., an attempt to protect one's head, the urge to run, the impulse to strike out with a fist) and that allowing the body to spontaneously come back to these and play them out helps release such responses from the system (2007, p. 97).

Babette Rothschild's (2010) second benefit of physical activity is "to increase containment and self-control via increased muscle tone" (p. 119). When the body is well, so is the spirit and vice versa. Dr. Tian Dayton (2007) states, "...our emotional life is physical. It imprints itself on our bodies and on our neural systems" (p. 21). Sometimes people struggling with chronic tension and anxiety become more anxious when they try to relax. Exercise and building muscle tone relieves stress, releases endorphins, and according to Rothschild, results in emotional strength (2010). Exercises such as boxing, dancing, and running dispel pent up energy and provide feelings of freedom. With dance, meaning and symbolism begin manifesting in a person's movement, taking the individual to deeper, more meaningful, levels of healing. Exercise helps the body reset itself, and gives people opportunities to organize their thoughts and emotions if necessary. It helps them feel in control of their lives.

The third benefit dance and movement hold for trauma survivors is "to dissipate buildup of stress hormones and help regulate ongoing stress levels" (Rothschild, 2010, p. 117). Exercise releases endorphins in the brain that make people happy, and it also reduces adrenaline levels in the body. According to Dr. Tian Dayton (2007), "One of the developmental tasks of recovery is to learn new healthy skills of self-soothing and self-regulating and to make them part of our daily lives" (p. 202). This is especially important when working with people who struggle with addictions. Drugs, sex, alcohol, shopping, gambling, etc. are things people use to make themselves feel good; they provide a high. Dayton says, "We need to develop user-friendly ways to activate our body/mind's natural feel-good chemicals and our brain's pleasure centers so we can gradually become less dependent on unhealthy ways of getting that high or calm feeling" (2007, p. 202).

Dance also improves mindfulness. Dr. Bruce Kodish (2001) places an emphasis on exercises that not only increase strength, but improve body mechanics and awareness. Awareness of the body fosters a person's ability to remain in the moment and promotes mindfulness. Mindfulness lays the foundation for the development of decision-making skills and self-efficacy.

According to David Emerson and Elizabeth Hopper (2011), when teaching classes that involve the integration of mind, body and spirit, it is important to remember that survivors of trauma often have difficulty remaining in the present moment. Offering as many opportunities to make choices and build resilience is done through exercises that increase breathing awareness, grounding, promote feelings of self-efficacy and allow for choice-making. Emerson and Hopper state, "[The] profound lack of choice is a common denominator among trauma survivors" (2011, p. 44). Allowing the subjects to make decisions about how, when, and where they move their bodies helps them reclaim parts of themselves they thought were lost or forgotten. Subjects should have control in the classroom about how much or little they move, and if a movement makes them feel unsafe, they must be allowed the choice to stop and rest, or modify it in a way that makes it doable for them (2011). This provides the safety that Howard Bath deems necessary for therapeutic care.

Finally, dance can help to re-establish creativity and engage the brain in new ways, creating new neural pathways that help the brain re-learn healthy coping patterns. However, creating dances and encouraging creative movement with people who do not identify as "dancers" may present a few challenges. While "non-dancers" may find it easier to contribute creative, expressive ideas to a piece, their physical awareness of their bodies, time, and space are often disconnected from their mental and spiritual capacities, especially if they have suffered from trauma. If there is insecurity about one's body, or if a person has experienced physical trauma in her body, getting reconnected and feeling comfortable enough to literally reach out of her comfort zone poses a great challenge for the instructor. In many cases, however, a non-dancer's lack of experience in what movement "should" look like often allows for the greatest freedom from inhibition and opens the door for meaningful, expressive movements. Movement exercises for those with little movement experience must provide safe, beneficial, and practical instruction in order to be successful.

Dance educator Brenda Pugh McCutchen (2006) states, "Whether a [person] is working with a thematic structure, a narrative content, or abstract ideas, individuals create their own personal meaning as they make dances to communicate their perspectives" (p. 170). According to Pugh McCutchen, the creative process for choreography involves three basic steps: experimentation, composition and choreography, and polishing and sharing.

Experimentation begins with exploration. Facilitating the safe exploration of the body's capabilities (isolations, gestures, postures, stability, etc.) and its relation to the space is important for someone who is learning to reconnect with their body. Exploring levels in space such as high, medium, and low, as well as tempos and shapes are also key ingredients in the creative process. Someone who wants to express a feeling of despair or hopelessness may find an action such as falling to the floor helpful in expressing how their experience feels, while another may use high, reach movements that seem to lift them from the floor to express hope or joy.

Improvisation is the second key to experimentation (Pugh McCutchen, 2006). Dr. Hilda Wengrower (2009) states, "Improvisation encourages the mover to detach from typical or stereotyped reactions and connotations, so that new psychophysical forms may emerge and be explored" (p. 16). It allows a breaking from "norm" and the "shoulds" of everyday life and frees a person to authentically express how his body wishes to respond in a situation. Improvisational exercises must be done with care - always being guided and structured - for the highest benefit to the subject. Pugh McCutchen says, "Always define the parameters of an improvisation in the classroom to focus student's efforts in a way that makes room for their creativity and invites it within a structure" (2006, p. 175). If people are simply asked to move however they want, it can cause the environment to feel unsafe. Instead, every improvisation exercise done in a classroom should be themed or structured, allowing for *more* freedom and comfort, and resulting in a more productive class.

Next, composition and choreography take shape. This step contains the basics of composing a dance, building forms and structures, aesthetic principles of design, and choreographing (Pugh McCutchen, 2006). Brenda Pugh McCutchen states, "Composing involves using the body in space, designing timing and dynamic contrasts, and building relationships that convey the message of the dance…[it] is about organizing movement" (2006, p. 176). This process of organizing movement and allowing a group of dancers to make choices about their choreography opens the door for deeper levels of trust to be built among the group members. Subjects begin to take greater ownership of their work, and may begin to feel a sense of pride in what they are creating. It also develops problem solving skills and builds self-efficacy. Subjects make decisions about their pieces: What movements will they keep? What movements should change to make the piece flow? In what other ways can a movement be performed? In a group setting, subjects are also asked to work together to figure out how their individual pieces can fit together to make a larger piece of choreography. Not only does it empower group members to build their problem solving skills, it gives them opportunities to work through a potentially frustrating experience and come out on the other end of it with a deeper respect and empathy for their peers.

Sharing the compositions is the final step in Brenda Pugh McCutchen's creative process. She writes, "Compositions are often works in progress. But for students to improve at composing, their works need to be performed for qualitative feedback…" (2006, p. 176). Perhaps the most uncomfortable part of the process is the performance. It is an opportunity for someone who has been silenced for so long to now publicly share their story, and it may feel overwhelming or frightening for subjects. Because performing personal work can leave a person feeling vulnerable, it is important that this also be done in an environment that is safe for the group members. The group facilitator should make it clear from the beginning that a final performance is part of the group's collective goal, giving them purpose and something to work toward. Group members should invite people whom they trust and have a voice about who may come to witness their stories. While they may be nervous before and during the performance, feedback from a receptive audience has the potential to build their confidence and encourage subjects to continue in their post-traumatic growth.

Each of these elements - experimentation, composition and choreography, and polishing and sharing - builds the subject's ability to think critically about their work, solve problems, work closely with others, and push the boundaries of their creativity to discover new and exciting ways to communicate with the world.

THE METHODOLOGY

In 2015, five adults between ages nineteen and forty were selected to participate in a seven week study that implemented an arts-based movement curriculum as a method for storytelling. The participants were chosen based on experiences with past trauma and drug and alcohol addiction. Two males and three females, all Caucasian, with various backgrounds were asked to join the group. Their names have been changed for confidentiality purposes. One woman, Bridget, had been sexually assaulted. The second, Lydia, recently had a miscarriage. The third woman, Jessica, worked with women who were victims of sex trafficking in the United States. One of the men, Chad, struggled with bipolar disorder and alcoholism. The other man, Robert, had a family history of mental illness, abuse, and drug and alcohol addiction, and had been in recovery for nearly twenty years. All participants practiced some form of Christianity, which informed much of their content for drawings, movement, and writings. Subjects were asked to sign a consent form that gave the author permission to use quotations and original artwork from the group sessions.

The author was also well acquainted with four out of five participants preceding the curriculum, which was not originally intended. However, the established trust already existing between the author and participants allowed for openness and deeper vulnerability during sessions.

To keep from being biased, however, the author approached each participant as a new student. She taught each session with the same professionalism as she would in a dance studio or at a school, caring for and inviting the participants to engage with her, but also gently challenging them each week to literally take one or two steps out of their comfort zones. The author's role as instructor within the classroom clearly set the boundary for participants, and they allowed themselves to be guided through the curriculum as students, not as the author's acquaintances. This aided in a more unbiased assessment of each participant, however, the author was aware that this may also have created some limitations in assessing the curriculum, which will be discussed in a later section.

Structure and Overview of the Curriculum

This therapeutic movement curriculum was modeled after a structure designed by BuildaBridge, a nonprofit arts-intervention organization in Philadelphia. The curriculum was developed using the BuildaBridge Classroom sm model[1], and designed to be trauma-informed, hope-infused and person-centered. There are six elements that characterize the model:

- Ritual
- Art as metaphor
- Boundaries of space and behavior to promote safety
- Spoken blessings
- Holistic development that includes academic, social, artistic, and spiritual aspects
- Creative artist fulfills the roles of mentor, sage, shaman, and priest(ess)

The curriculum developed by this author contains four of the six elements: ritual, art as metaphor, boundaries of space and behavior to promote safety, and spoken blessings.

These elements assisted in making the curriculum trauma-informed. Ritual and safe spaces provided consistency and safety for the participants (Bath, 2008). Participants knew what to expect each week, and they were given choices about their levels of participation, putting control of the environment in their hands (Emerson & Hopper, 2011). The author developed and acquired experiences that promoted grounding and mindfulness with the hope of teaching participants new ways to manage their emotions and triggers. Careful instruction was also provided which offered choices, autonomy, and self-discovery, while keeping exploration structured enough to feel safe and anchored (Bartenieff, 2002).

Artistic experiences to develop metaphors for life were used to promote a deeper spiritual experience for the participants. The curriculum experiences were created to help the subjects see their world as it is, but also to envision the world as it could be in an effort to foster hope and future-orientation (Corbitt & Nix-Early, 2003). Allowing choice and building a sense of "I Can" (Grotberg, 1995) for trauma survivors was hoped to provide the participants with greater confidence and re-establish resilience. Edith Grotberg (1995) says, "The 'I Can' factors are [one's] interpersonal and social skills. The resilient [person] says I can communicate, problem solve, manage feelings and impulses, gauge the temperament of myself and others, and seek trusting relationships". All of these factors were addressed in this curriculum.

The curriculum consisted of seven 90-minute lessons, and the group met once per week for seven weeks. In the seventh week the group met for a celebration, inviting their friends and family to view a showcase of their work. Every session opened with a beginning ritual and ended with a closing ritual. They happened consistently every week, promoting safety and predictability, and set the classes up so participants knew what to expect, which also helped them acclimate to the space and to each others' presence before they started moving.

Every class opened with a ritual warm-up, followed by two other exercises that stemmed from the author's own experience. The lessons then proceeded to drawing symbols and maps about the participants' life experiences. From these drawings, participants were asked to find movements that told the story of what was drawn on their paper. Individuals shared their movements with the group, then they all worked together to further develop each other's movement phrases.

When every group finished sharing, a debrief or talk back was facilitated by the author. Subjects were given the opportunity to explain what they drew on their paper, and what their process was for developing their final choreography. The rest of the group was then given time to tell the choreographer(s) what they saw and how they related to the piece. Many blessings were spoken by the participants to each other, and by the author to the participants during this time.

The group closed every session by speaking the statement of affirmation. This was their own creation, stating what they thought should be affirmed about themselves personally, and also about the group as a whole:

Everything I do is worth watching.

Everything I say is worth listening to.

I was an idea that God thought was great!

I am a twinkle in God's eye.

Everything I am cannot be contained.

I will find the path, run the race, and finish well.

I am fully equipped. I am strong. I am fierce and safe.

I am a child of God.

Descriptions of the Curriculum Experiences

Grounding Experiences

One exercise that improves groundedness and body awareness is intentionally noticing one's feet on the floor (Emerson & Hopper, 2011). If they are comfortable with it, participants remove their shoes, and stand or sit in a way that allows the bottoms of their feet to make full contact with the floor. If they wish, subjects may close their eyes to help them draw their focus to their feet. They can experiment by tapping their heels or wiggling their toes to feel the floor (2011).

The curriculum also begins every session with a breath awareness exercise, intended to bring calm to the room and help participants relax and become comfortable in the space. Deep breathing resets the nervous system and frees muscles from tension, and deep inhalations and exhalations allow the body to expel toxins that are held up in the bloodstream. Intentional breaths help participants focus on the present state of their minds and bodies (Dayton, 2007).

The BrainDance

Anne Green Gilbert's BrainDance[2] promotes body control and body awareness. According to The Creative Dance Center, the BrainDance has several benefits. Enhancement of core support, building connectivity, and strengthening alignment of the body are just a few of the ways the BrainDance benefits the whole person (www.creativedance.org). The exercise begins with the tactile, gentle pats and brushes upon all parts of the body, paying attention to the areas that might be ignored such as the bottoms of the feet, top of the head, and back of the neck. Next is the core-distal warm up. Subjects reach out with legs, arms, heads, etc. to explore the space around them, searching for new shapes, different tempos, miniscule movement, and big movements. Following the core-distal exploration is the head-tail connection. Participants move their heads first, keeping their tailbones aligned with the rest of their body. Then, they explore with their tailbone and hips while keeping the head still. This progresses into the connection between the two, moving them simultaneously in the same directions as if the top of the head were reaching for the pelvis, hips, and tailbone, and vice versa. Next is the Upper/Lower Body experience. Participants explore the space with their upper bodies (torso, arms, head, etc.), while keeping their lower body still. Then, the lower body is explored while the upper body remains still. This progresses to the Side of the Body warm up, where participants explore the space using one side of their body while keeping the other side still. This also includes moving or isolating the facial muscles. It is repeated on the other side. Cross Lateral movement is next. Subjects move opposite arms and legs around, and then switch. Finally, there is the Vestibular movement: turning in circles, regaining balance, and then spinning the other direction, and regaining balance.

As participants grow more comfortable with the BrainDance, the facilitator can offer more specific ways to explore the space. Instead of saying "explore the space with your upper body", say: "With your upper body use small movements to explore the space near your center". Other stipulations could be given, such as only using quick, sharp movements, or smooth, large movements during the warm-up. The next week a facilitator could ask participants to explore the space far away from themselves. This brings closer attention to the body and its capabilities as well as increases the participant's body, space, and tempo awareness. It also teaches choreographic elements little by little allowing participants to grasp each concept fully before moving to the next element (McCutchen, 2006).

Circle Choreography

One exercise meant to help establish empathy in the group is the Circle Choreography experience. The group stands in a circle. Participants are asked how they are feeling in that moment. They then develop a motion or movement that expresses that emotion. Each individual presents their movement and the group repeats it. After each person presents, they begin again with the first presenter's movement and then the others' in order, adding each new movement to create a string of expressive movements.

Flocking

Another exercise intended for developing empathy is Flocking. Participants stand in a diamond or pyramid formation, and the person at the point of the shape begins to move. Everyone follows the leader's movements until leadership is passed to the next person. Leadership is passed when the current leader chooses to move in a given direction until he or she can no longer be seen by the person standing at the farthest point of vision. The person at the next point of vision then becomes the leader.

Drawing Symbols and Writing Haiku

Drawing and writing are two arts-based elements of the curriculum. These mediums are meant to provide safety for expressing arising emotions and thoughts before sharing them with the group. One of the first experiences of the curriculum involves drawing symbols to represent three categories: Things I Fear, Things I Love, and Things I am Hopeful For.

Next, participants create movement that conveys their symbols. Each participant develops a movement for each category, creating a short phrase to share with the others. One participant demonstrates the movement, the others repeat it and so forth, moving along so each person has an opportunity to share. This experience is meant to prompt new outlets for expressing stress, fear, hope, and love when words are overwhelming. It offers an opportunity for participants to tell their story without having to speak.

Teaching and Learning Choreography

The subject's main objective over the seven week time period is to develop his or her personal story through movement. There are three thematic options: Things I Fear, Things I Love, and Things I am Hopeful For. Participants create meaningful movement, expressing their ideas, feelings, and perspectives for each theme. Some may choose to focus on only one theme; some may decide to combine them to create a larger piece. Whatever their choice, "Creativity tends to bring with it a feeling of aliveness" (Cori, p. 189), which was essential for this process.

After they have created a short movement phrase, they divide into partners and teach their partner the choreography they have created. Each partner learns the other's choreography, and at the end of the experience they perform for the other groups, and talk about what it was like to both teach and learn. This is intended to provide the subjects with opportunities to "try on" another's movement, and open up opportunity for shared emotional experiences.

Talk Backs

Every session includes a debrief or "talk back", where the participants have an opportunity to talk about their pieces, and the other subjects give feedback on what they saw and felt as they watched or participated in the movement and choreographic process. Articulation of feedback regarding shapes, emotions, levels, metaphors, themes, etc. of the pieces they saw involves sharing what they perceive about the piece, what qualities and efforts create different metaphoric statements, and what things might be improved to create an even more expressive phrase.

Writing and Speaking the Statement of Affirmation

Developing the statement of affirmation provides another opportunity for problem solving and choice-making. Deciding what things as a whole are important to the participant, and what values they wish to affirm about themselves and each other aids in creating and taking ownership of the statement. Participant ownership of the statement makes it powerful, and every week at the end of class they say it together.

Emotion/Somatics Experience

Emotions such as fear, joy, love, hate, hope, etc. are presented to the group. Members take a moment to feel that emotion in their body and present their movement to the group. The group repeats each movement, empathizing with the presenter. These movements may become choreography material for future pieces. The group takes time to develop a mini dance from the movement they demonstrate, thinking of other synonyms for the words they are feeling to develop deeper meaning for their choreography. By moving as the other participants move, it is hoped that subjects will get a sense of how others are feeling in the moment, and develop the ability to relate by putting the same actions and physical tensions into their own bodies.

Life Map

The final exercise in this curriculum to promote empathy and develop communication skills is the Life Map. On a sheet of paper, individuals draw a map of their life - highs, lows, significant experiences, etc. - and begin moving through it at first by walking. Gradually, they begin using variating movement qualities (press, flick, thrust, glide, wring, dab, slash and float), levels, and tempos to move through the map again, expressing different feelings they experience as they share their story. One by one participants walk the group through their map; together the group follows the pattern and mirrors the given movements, in an effort to build empathy and connections among group members (Moyers & Grubin, 1997). Examples of Life Maps can be seen later in this chapter.

The Showcase

After subjects make editing decisions and polish their choreography, it is time to share their creations (McCutchen, 2006). Participants are encouraged to invite their friends and family to come and witness their creative work and stories. This celebration confirms the work that was done, and encourages the continuation of using the skills taught throughout the seven-week period. The pieces are intended to raise awareness of the inner plights of trauma survivors and present the hopes and dreams that were rediscovered during the process.

Goals and Objectives of the Curriculum

The goals of this curriculum are to teach coping skills and tools to help subjects manage stress and the side-effects of their trauma, and to teach participants to develop their stories through expressive movement. These goals were accomplished through several objectives, which can be seen in Table 1. This chart lists the objective, the method by which the objective was accomplished, the lesson in which it was taught, and upon which theoretical concept it was based.

Assessment Tools

There are several assessment tools used for this study to see if the curriculum met the goals set beforehand. The Circle Choreography assessment, a Movement Assessment Checklist, focus group interviews, and a participant evaluation survey were used to gather data and feedback about the curriculum. Formative and authentic assessments were made during class sessions and video recordings were used for further observation and data collection.

Circle Choreography Assessment

At the beginning of every class, the group was asked to think about how they felt in that moment, and then come up with a simple movement to express that feeling. At the end of every class they were asked to do it again. Change in movement qualities, mood of the movement, and attitude toward the exercise indicated that the lesson's experiences helped the subjects relax and feel more emotionally and physically free.

Focus Group Interviews

Every session finished with a group discussion (a.k.a. talk back) about the experiences in that week's lesson. Questions were asked about what worked in the experiences, what did not work, how the experiences affected the participants spiritually, mentally, and physically, and how the experiences applied to life metaphorically. The author acted as the moderator for the discussion, facilitating questions, but also participating in the discussion when appropriate. These focus groups helped "to explore the respondent group's views and experiences" as they worked through the sessions together (Savin-Baden & Major, 2013, p. 377). The author used this assessment to better understand the participants and their perspectives on therapeutic movement.

Table 1. Goals and Objectives of Curriculum

The Purpose of This Curriculum Is:	Method	Lesson #	Concept Idea[3]
To develop subjects' mindfulness in movement and increase their grounding in the present.	Grounding Experiences	All lessons	Mindfulness Groundedness Intentional breathing Self-management and coping skills
	BrainDance	All lessons	Body control and awareness
To teach basic stress and emotion management tools.	Grounding Experiences	All lessons	Mindfulness Groundedness Intentional breathing Self-management and coping skills
	Emotion/Somatics Experience	5, 6	Body awareness and release of emotional tension Self-management and coping skills
To teach methods and tools for communicating emotions and stories.	Circle Choreography	All lessons	Mirroring and reflecting movement to understand another's experience
	Life Map	3, 4	Non-verbal telling of one's story
	Drawing Symbols	1	Art making as communication
	Writing Haiku	2	Art making as communication
To encourage the development of subjects' self- efficacy.	Creating Choreography and Teaching Others	2, 3, 4	Decision-making and critical thinking about choreographic pieces
	Talk-Backs	All lessons	Sharing, critiquing, and polishing
To develop a greater sense of empathy among subjects in the group.	Circle Choreography	All lessons	Mirroring and reflecting movement to understand another's experience
	Learning Others' Choreography	2	Development of healing relationships
	Life Map	3, 4	Connecting with others' stories
	Emotion/Somatics Experience	5, 6	Mirroring and reflecting movement to understand another's experience
To promote the re-establishment of creativity.	Writing the Statement of Affirmation	1	Affirmation of characteristics of self that have value and strength
	Drawing Symbols	1	Thematic structure
	Writing Haiku	2	Thematic structure
	Flocking	4, 6	Improvisation and exploration free from inhibitions
To guide subjects as they create pieces of choreography and perform them at the end of the seven-week time period.	The Showcase	7	Celebration

Participant Evaluations

An anonymous evaluation for the participants to complete was created in Google Forms as a final assessment of how the curriculum benefited the subjects. The survey rendered important data regarding how the participants felt they had improved in the areas of mindfulness and body awareness, communication, self-efficacy, empathy, and creativity, and it provided feedback about what they found helpful in the curriculum and where they thought improvements could be made. Participants rated themselves on a scale of one to ten in each category before and after the completion of the sessions, and their ratings increased over the seven-week period.

Limitations

Several obstacles prevented the group from beginning on the scheduled date, putting the start date of the sessions more than a month behind schedule. Needs for space, funding, and liability insurance hindered the start of the class. In the beginning, the author had a space reserved for eight weeks at a church, but learned later, however, that the owners of the building decided to charge the group rent, costing between $400 and $500. This necessitated a move to a Plan B. In finding a new space to work, the need for liability insurance coverage prevented the group from having the first movement session on the newly designated start date. With the help of Eastern University, the details were worked out and the sessions were ready to commence. Once sessions commenced, they went very well, but the delays in getting started left very little time for assessments and writing before the deadline for the final study results.

Accessing the desired participants was also challenging. It was difficult to get people recovering from recent addictions to commit to the sessions. Many had to work during the class' designated times, some did not have the means of getting to the sessions, and others avoided communication altogether. Five participants were recruited. They made it to most sessions, and enthusiastically engaged in the experiences and exercises presented to them.

The study was also limited by the lack of diversity among the participants, and the fact that the curriculum was only tested with one focus group. Due to time and accessibility limitations, only one group was used, limiting further data possibilities.

The author's preceding relationships with many of the participants may have also caused limitations in the assessment of the curriculum. Honesty was constantly encouraged, but if any participant withheld constructive comments for the sake of his or her relationship with the author, that may have prevented important data findings in the research. While the author felt she had remained unbiased throughout the study, it is possible that the participants were not as unbiased. Had the group been comprised completely of people unacquainted with the author, the final results may have been very different due to lack of previously established trust.

FINDINGS

The curriculum was successful in teaching coping and stress management skills and in teaching participants how to develop their stories through expressive movement. This section outlines the indicators that demonstrated how the author knew which objectives had been achieved.

The first objective was *to develop subjects' mindfulness in movement and increase their grounding in the present.* Subjects reported that closing their eyes during the breath awareness and BrainDance experiences helped them feel more in-the-moment.

Metaphor and meaning were key for building mindfulness in the curriculum experiences. Every week during the talk back, the author asked participants how the experiences were metaphorical for life in an effort to help them find deeper meaning in their work. By lesson four, participants were making their own connections without being prompted by the author. This was an important indication of subjects' growing thoughtfulness and awareness of the applicability of the experiences in their everyday lives.

The Emotions/Somatics experience was also effective in building mindfulness. Robert spoke on more than one occasion about how disconnected he felt from his body. Having the opportunity to be guided safely into deeper connection gave him freedom to experience emotion and know how to handle it in the future. After completing the Emotions/Somatics Awareness experience, he said, "I feel like you collect stuff, and you don't even know it's there until someone guides you through the process of recognizing and managing it" (Session 5, April 14, 2015). The Emotions/Somatics experience also seemed to heighten awareness of which body parts held memories of previous trauma, enabling group members to better use the skills provided in the curriculum.

The second objective was *to teach basic stress and emotion management tools.* Drawing symbols for the three categories and Life Maps proved therapeutic for 100 percent of the participants. Drawing gave the subjects time to think and imagine without having to use words to communicate. The process also provided opportunities for participants to be honest and vulnerable with themselves before they began moving. Things the participants did not normally take time to think about were able to be processed.

The third objective was *to teach methods and tools for communicating emotions and stories.* Prior to this study, the participants were all well-spoken, thoughtful people, but the new means through which they discovered communication was exciting for them. To communicate with their bodies opened new possibilities for them. Finding ways to use movement, rather than words, to tell a story was empowering and non-threatening to the subjects. Jessica, in particular, held back and expressed discomfort with talking about her drawings and movement choices. However, when presented with the option to remain silent while showing her Life Map to the others, she became very animated and enthusiastic about the experience. She also later expressed gratitude for the opportunities to process and participate at her own pace and she said she never felt unsafe because of that.

The fourth objective was *to encourage the development of subjects' self-efficacy.* Most of the participants expressed feelings of awkwardness when they first started attending the movement sessions and timidity was expected during the first few lessons of the curriculum. They all agreed that movement made them feel exposed and vulnerable. As the sessions continued, however, each participant seemed to make a very conscious effort to participate fully.

Another indicator of self-efficacy was the participants' increasing confidence in their work. In the beginning, participants often looked to the author for cues about how to move and what to express. Bridget asked several times in the beginning lessons if she was doing an exercise correctly or what the author would do for a certain emotion. The author worked with her to help her connect with her body, and in lessons four, five, and six, a noticeable difference began to occur. Bridget seemed to be discovering new movement on her own without looking for approval from the author. In another instance, Jessica tended to place herself against a wall or as close to a corner of the room as possible. By the end of the sixth session, however, Jessica's use of eye contact with the author and others in the group had increased, she began to speak more boldly during the talk back time, and she offered ideas to the group and the author regarding future classes, indicating greater confidence in her own voice and greater trust in the other participants. When asked if she thought her confidence levels had changed, she responded, "I think doing these sessions has increased my confidence. I would have been reluctant to dance in front of others or share my movements before."

In the week preceding the showcase, Bridget also asked for the recordings of some of her previous choreography. She wanted to practice at home and continued refining her work for the celebration, an indication of deeper investment in and care about her work. This also demonstrated increased ownership in her choreography. Every week she worked to improve her movements and make them more genuine and true to the emotions she felt.

As the participants became better acquainted and more comfortable in the class, they also grew bolder in their improvisation and exploration, another indication of increased confidence and trust. For example, in the beginning sessions, most participants kept their movements relatively small and contained near the center of their bodies. In the last few sessions, however, an expansion of their movements and an opening of their bodies was noticed. They started using movements that reached farther away from their centers during the improvisational Flocking and Circle Choreography experiences.

The fifth objective was *to develop a greater sense of empathy among subjects in the group.* Discussions and feedback given during the talk backs indicated the achievement of this objective. Although most of the participants demonstrated empathy from the beginning, there was a consistent consensus that the experiences each week helped subjects gain a better sense of how those around them were feeling. Positive comments were made frequently by every participant about working with others and feeling what they felt as they "put on" each others' choreography.

The Emotions/Somatics experience rendered even greater results. Not only did the group members notice changes in their own bodies when an emotion was presented, but their awareness of others' body language was also heightened, helping them feel more connected to each other. Several participants noted how they saw other group members' posture, facial expressions, and movement quality change during the exercise, and how that affected their own attitudes and decision-making in the moment.

The sixth objective was *to promote the re-establishment of creativity.* From the first session to the sixth, participants seemed to grow increasingly confident in their abilities to create new movement. The Life Map experience provided the most opportunities for re-establishing the subjects' creativity. During the experience, participants were asked to feel their bodies' reactions at certain points on their maps and then create that sensation as a movement. This helped the participants dig deeper into the meaning and symbolism that informed their floor patterns. For example, Bridget, a survivor of sexual assault, used that experience on her map to fall and get up, but then stumble and fall in the other direction, repeating the movement to make a zig zag pattern on the floor. The others responded positively to experiencing that movement with her. Chad commented, "That was really tiring. I can only imagine how that must have felt trying to move on normally with your life, but feeling like you can't." Bridget finished her life map by spiraling in toward the center of the room, signifying her efforts to keep God at the center of her life and circumstances.

Another example of discovering deeper meaning during the Life Map experience was Lydia's decision to mark the path she had taken thus far in red over the other colors she used to signify various pieces of her journey. She said the red represented God's presence with her throughout the map. In her movements, Lydia moved from smaller to bigger steps to signify growing up, and low and high levels to represent struggle and victories. Every Life Map included some form of spiritual belief and intentional steps toward God for direction or healing.

The final objective was *to guide subjects as they create pieces of choreography and perform them at the end of the seven-week time period.* This objective was fulfilled in the seventh week of the curriculum. Participants enthusiastically polished and edited their pieces, and they invited their friends and families to share in their celebration. The pride and excitement they showed as they prepared for the showcase were not only indicators of subjects' confidence and self-efficacy, but also a sign that they felt they had something of importance to share with the people in their lives. Bridget remarked in the fifth week that she wanted her parents to be there so they could finally see how the assault from her past truly affected her. Jessica said performing for an audience, particularly her family, made the telling of her experience possible without risking their traumatization.

Group members also demonstrated their abilities to alter their movements in order to create a more harmonious piece together. Their movement grew more connected and smooth each week as they refined their pieces and explored with improvisation. In the Flocking and BrainDance experiences it became evident that subjects were not only finding new ways to move, but becoming more confident in their explorations. Rather than standing in one spot, they would take a few steps forward or to the side. Rather than remaining upright, many of them would kneel, hop, or bend at the hips for a moment.

Figure 1. Bridget's Life Map

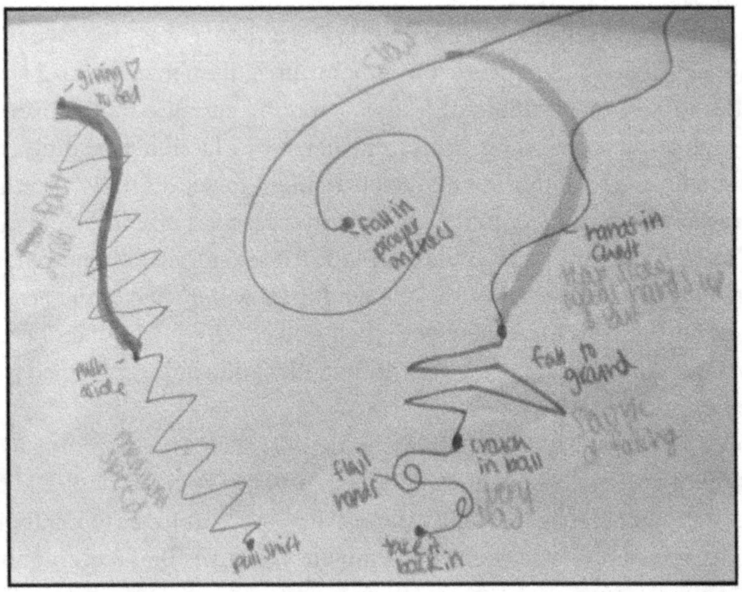

Figure 2. Lydia's Life Map

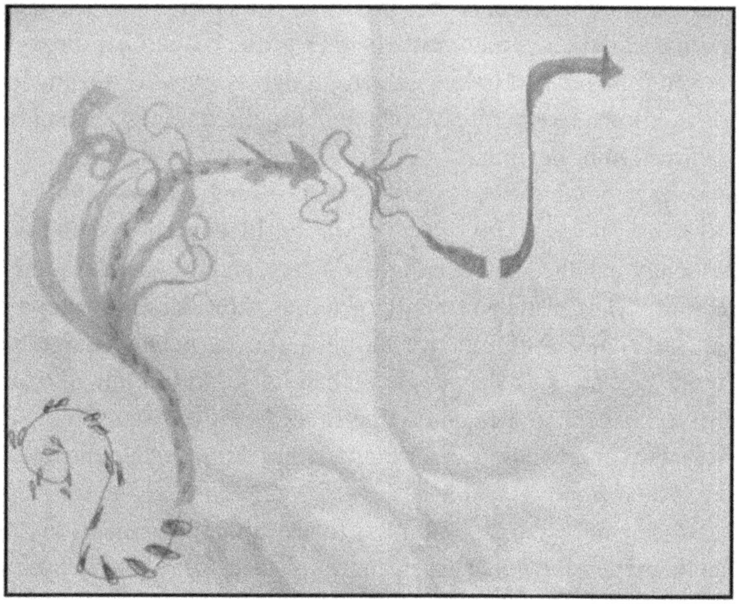

CONCLUSION

In conclusion, trauma affects mind, body, and spirit. This results in disconnection and imbalance that prevent a trauma survivor from maintaining healthy patterns in their thoughts, habits, and emotional care. Holistic, trauma-informed, hope-infused care can provide a way for the trauma survivor to safely work toward wholeness.

In an effort to become more informed about trauma and effective ways to serve those who have experienced it, the author developed a therapeutic movement curriculum to test with a small group of adults. Using Howard Bath's (2008) three pillars of trauma care, the author adopted exercises that promoted safety, taught self-regulation and coping skills, and helped to facilitate healing relationships. While there were some limitations, the author found the curriculum to successfully meet its goals and objectives. Participants responded positively to the guided arts-based experiences, and 100 percent reported increased levels of self-efficacy, body awareness, emotional self-regulation, communication, creativity, and empathy toward others. The success of this curriculum is widely due to the artistic experiences and the willingness of the participants to connect with their bodies, along with their comfort level with new forms of moving. While movement was awkward at first, the group quickly formed trust enough to begin reaching out of their comfort zones.

This curriculum can be replicated with other populations such as prison inmates, people who have suffered abuse, victims of trafficking, juvenile offenders, and those going through addiction rehabilitation. In fact, it is the hope of the author that eventually she will have opportunities to implement this curriculum in all of these areas as an effort to offer hope and wholeness in lives that feel forgotten and abandoned.

REFERENCES

Alcorn, N. (2008). *Violated: Mercy for sexual abuse*. Enumclaw, WA: Winepress Publishing.

American Dance Therapy Association. (2014). *About Dance/Movement Therapy*. Retrieved from: http://adta.org/About_DMT

American Psychological Association. (2014). *Trauma*. Retrieved from: http://www.apa.org/topics/trauma/index.aspx

Baer, R. A., Smith, G. T., & Allen, K. B. (2004). Assessment of mindfulness by self-report: The Kentucky inventory of mindfulness skills. *Assessment*, *11*(3), 191–206. doi:10.1177/1073191104268029 PMID:15358875

Bandura, A. (1994). Self-efficacy. In V. S. Ramachaudran (Ed.), *Encyclopedia of human behavior, 4* (pp. 71–81). New York: Academic Press.

Banitt, S. P. (2012). *The trauma tool kit: Healing PTSD from the inside out*. Wheaton, IL: Quest Books.

Bartenieff, I. (2002). Body movement: Coping with the environment. New York, NY: Routledge.

Bath, H. (2008). The three pillars of trauma-informed care. *Reclaiming Children and Youth*, *17*(3), 17–21. Retrieved from https://reclaimingjournal.com/sites/default/files/journal-article-pdfs/17_3_Bath.pdf

Behrens, G. A. (2014). *Arts in healing panel: Neurobiology of trauma and the arts* (PowerPoint slides). Retrieved from https://plus.google.com/u/1/communities

BuildaBridge. (2015). *Our Core Philosophy*. Retrieved from http://buildabridge.org/about-us/our-core-philosophy/

Camilleri, V. A. (Ed.). (2007). *Healing the inner city child: Creative arts therapies with at-risk youth*. London: Jessica Kingsley Publishers.

Corbitt, J. N., & Nix-Early, V. (2003). *Taking it to the streets: Using the arts to transform your community*. Grand Rapids, MI: Baker Books.

Cori, J. L. (2007). *Healing from trauma: A survivor's guide to understanding your symptoms and reclaiming your life*. New York, NY: Marlowe & Co.

Dayton, T. (2007). *Emotional sobriety: From relationship trauma to resilience and balance*. Deerfield Beach, FL: Health Communications, Inc.

Delaney, B. & Scheiber, D. (n.d.). *Surviving the shadows: A journey of hope into post-traumatic stress*. Naperville, IL: Sourcebooks, Inc.

Dell, C. (1970). *A primer for movement description: Using effort-shape and supplementary concepts*. New York, NY: Dance Notation Bureau Press.

Emerson, D., & Hopper, E. (2011). *Overcoming trauma through yoga: Reclaiming your body*. Berkeley, CA: North Atlantic Books.

Feder, B., & Feder, E. (1998). *The art and science of evaluation in the arts therapies: How do you know what's working?* Springfield, IL: Charles C. Thomas Publishers, LTD.

Fischman, D. (2009). Therapeutic relationship and kinesthetic empathy. In S. Chaiklin & H. Wengrower (Eds.), *The art and science of dance/movement therapy: Life is dance* (pp. 33–53). New York, NY: Routledge.

Goetz, T. (n.d.). *Movement matters - Brain dance workshop*. Retrieved from http://www.artstime.org/infors/documents/braindance_handoutgoetz.pdf

Goodill, S. W. (2005). *An introduction to medical dance/movement therapy*. London: Jessica Kingsley Publishers.

Grotberg, E. H. (1995). *A guide to promoting resilience in children: Strengthening the human spirit*. Retrieved from http://resilnet.uiuc.edu/library/grotb95b.html

Grotberg, E. H. (1996). *The international resilience project: Research and application*. Retrieved from http://resilnet.uiuc.edu/library/grotb96a.html

Grotberg, E. H. (2006). *Implications of the shift from diagnosis and treatment to recovery and resilience for research and practice*. Retrieved from http://resilnet.uiuc.edu/library/grotberg2006_implications-diagnosis-recovery-georgeton.pdf

Hanna, J. L. (1988). *Dance and stress: Resistance, reduction and euphoria*. New York, NY: AMS Press, Inc.

Hanna, T. (1988). *Somatics: Reawakening the mind's control of movement, flexibility, and health*. Cambridge, MA: Da Capo Press.

Hari, J. (2015, January 20). *The likely cause of addiction has been discovered, and it is not what you think*. Retrieved from: http://www.huffingtonpost.com/johann-hari/the-real-cause-of-addicti_b_6506936.html

Harris, D. A. (2007). Pathways to embodied empathy and reconciliation after atrocity: Former boy soldiers in a dance/movement therapy group in Sierra Leone. *Intervention (Amstelveen, Netherlands)*, *5*(3), 203–231. doi:10.1097/WTF.0b013e3282f211c8

Henderson, E. C. (2000). *Understanding addiction*. Jackson, MS: University Press of Mississippi.

Hughes, D. A. (2013). *8 keys to building your best relationships*. New York, NY: W.W. Norton.

Jensen, E. (2001). *Arts with the brain in mind*. Alexandria, VA: Association for Supervision and Curriculum Development.

Kodish, B. I. (2001). *Back pain solutions: How to help yourself with posture-movement therapy and education*. Pasadena, CA: Extensional Publishing.

Kreitler, H., & Kreitler, S. (1972). *The psychology of the arts*. Durham, NC: Duke University Press.

Loman, S. T. (2005). Dance/movement therapy. In Expressive therapies (pp. 68-89). The Guildford Press.

Malchiodi, C. (2009, February 19). *Be here now: Mindfulness and the creative spirit*. Retrieved from https://www.psychologytoday.com/blog/arts-and-health/200902/be-here-now-mindfulness-and-the-creative-spirit

Maslow, A. H. (2011). *Hierarchy of needs: A theory of human motivation* [Kindle Edition]. Retrieved from Amazon.com.

Moore, C. L., & Yamamoto, K. (2012). *Beyond words: Movement observation and analysis*. New York, NY: Routledge.

Moyers, B. (Producer), & Grubin, D. (Director). (1997). *The Moyers Collection - Bill T. Jones: Still Here with Bill Moyers* [Motion Picture]. United States: Films for the Humanities and Sciences.

Pugh McCutchen, B. (2006). *Teaching dance as art in education*. Champaign, IL: Human Kinetics.

Rothschild, B. (2000). *The body remembers: The psychophysiology of trauma and trauma treatment*. New York, NY: W.W. Norton.

Rothschild, B. (2010). *8 keys to safe trauma recovery: Take-charge strategies to empower your healing*. New York, NY: W. W. Norton.

Savin-Baden, M., & Major, C. H. (2013). *Qualitative research: The essential guide to theory and practice*. New York, NY: Routledge.

Servan-Schreiber, D. (2003). *The instinct to heal: Curing depression, anxiety, and stress without drugs and without talk therapy*. Paris, France: Rodale.

Substance Abuse and Mental Health Services Administration. (2014). *SAMHSA's Concept of Trauma and Guidance for a Trauma-Informed Approach. HHS Publication No. (SMA) 14-4884*. Rockville, MD: Substance Abuse and Mental Health Services Administration.

Tan, C. (2008). Manifestations of Hope Chart. In *Manifestations of Hope in Music Therapy with Hospitalized Pediatric Patients*. Philadelphia, PA: Drexel University.

The Center for Somatic Studies. (2014). *Developmental somatic psychotherapy*. Retrieved from somaticstudies.com/

The Merriam-Webster Dictionary. (2015, April 13). *Trauma*. Retrieved from: http://www.merriam-webster.com/dictionary/

Tortora, S. (2006). *The dancing dialogue: Using the communicative power of movement with young children*. Baltimore, MD: Paul H. Brookes Publishing Co.

Van der Kolk, B. (2014). *The body keeps score: Brain, mind and body in the healing of trauma*. New York, NY: Penguin Group.

Van Lith, T. (2014). Painting to find my spirit: Art making as the vehicle to find meaning and connection in the mental health recovery process. *Journal of Spirituality in Mental Health, 16*(1), 19–36. doi:10.1080/19349637.2013.864542

Wengrower, H. (2009). The creative-artistic process in dance/movement therapy. In S. Chaiklin & H. Wengrower (Eds.), *The art and science of dance/movement therapy: Life is dance* (pp. 13–32). New York, NY: Routledge.

ENDNOTES

1 For a more detailed explanation of the BuildaBridge Classroom sm model, visit http://buildabridge.org/about-us/our-core-philosophy/

2 For a more detailed explanation of the BrainDance, visit http://creativedance.org/about/braindance/

3 Bath, 2008; Corbitt & Nix-Early, 2003; Cori, 2007; Dayton, 2007; Emmerson & Hopper, 2011; Fischman, 2009; Green Gilbert, 2014; McCutchen, 2006; Moore & Yamamoto, 2012; Moyers & Grubin, 1997; Van Lith, 2014; Wengrower, 2009

APPENDIX

Table 2. Curriculum Lesson 1

Curriculum Project Title: Movement and Storytelling Curriculum
Lesson No.: 1
Lesson Overview: This is the introductory lesson to the storytelling and movement curriculum. It begins the storytelling process by getting subjects to start thinking about expression of their thoughts and feelings.
Goals: 1. To create a safe environment and community that allows for freedom for self-expression and honesty. 2. To teach choreographic and movement skills.
Questions: What does fear feel like in our bodies? What kind of movements look like fear? What does love feel like? What kinds of movements express love? Do you notice any similarities among all of our movements depending on the category?
Lesson Objectives: 1. Develop body and breath awareness 2. Work together in groups to create meaningful movement 3. Understand purposefulness in movement and life
Lesson Breakdown: 1. Warm up - Begin with Breath Awareness exercise and Brain Dance movement. (10 mins) 2. Circle choreography - Each person says their name and presents a movement that expresses something about themselves. The group repeats it together and then move to the next person, adding each movement onto the first, until the circle is complete (15 mins). 3. Experience 1 - Pass out paper and pens. Ask each person to make three columns on one side of the paper and label them Fears, Love, and Desires. In the columns each person draws symbols pertaining to each category and how they apply to their personal lives. Ask: "What are your fears?" "What things do you love?" and "What do you desire in life? Today? Tomorrow? For your children? etc." (15 mins) 4. Experience 2 - In their own space, each subject will develop one simple movement for each category they just wrote about. Divided into small groups, they will present their movements to each other and together develop and record (on paper) a short phrase that incorporates each movement. (20 mins) 5. Presentations - each group will demonstrate their movement phrase. (15 mins) 6. Talk-back - Subjects will give feedback about what they saw - emotions, movements, expressions - to each group, and allow groups to explain their piece. (5 mins per group) 7. Assessment - Subjects participate enthusiastically in activities, and will have a short piece of choreography to present with their group by the end of the class. 8. Experience 3 - Write the statement of affirmation. Ask: What things do we want to affirm about ourselves in this group? 9. Close by saying the statement of affirmation together. (2 mins) 10. Final assessment - Circle Choreography - Ask participants how they currently feel and to put that feeling into a simple movement. Take note of the differences between movement from the beginning and movement at the end of the class. *Note: This will usually be done before the statement, but because of the flow of this lesson, it should be done afterward.
Books, Materials, Supplies: Paper, pencils, pens, colored pencils, instrumental music
Assessment Method(s) Authentic Assessment, Circle Choreography before and after assessment

Table 3. Curriculum Lesson 2

Curriculum Project Title: Movement and Storytelling Curriculum
Lesson No.: 2
Lesson Overview: Participants begin to identify movements that signify their emotions, fears, hopes, and desires through writing haiku poems and choreographing small phrases to coincide with those poems. They will then teach and learn each other's choreography.
Goals: 1. To teach choreographic and movement skills. 2. To develop greater empathy among subjects in the group. 3. To encourage the development of subjects' self-efficacy.
Questions: • What did you see and feel as you watched & and performed each person's dance? • What emotions did you hear and see? • Do you notice any similarities among the movements depending on the choreographer? For the choreographers: • What was the process of creating a dance like for you? • What were you thinking about as you choreographed? • How was your experience working together? • What did you like/dislike about it? • What would make it better for next time? • How is life like this?
Lesson Objectives: 1. Develop time and tempo awareness - working on contrasting movements 2. Work together in groups to create a meaningful movement 3. Understand purposefulness in movement and life
Lesson Breakdown: 1. Warm-up - Begin with Breath Awareness exercise and Brain Dance movement. (10 mins) 2. Circle choreography - Each person demonstrates a movement that expresses how they are feeling at the moment. The group repeats it together and then move to the next person, adding each movement onto the first, until the circle is complete (15 mins). 3. Mini Lecture and Experience 1 - Hand out sheets from the last class. Subjects should review their symbols on the first side of their paper. On the back of the paper have subjects write a haiku for each category. (15 mins) a. 5 - 7 - 5 syllabic pattern b. Poignant Experience, environments, emotions, relationships, etc. c. Seasonal or nature references d. Contrast/subject change e. Details/sensory descriptions f. Example 1 - "Whitecaps on the bay/ A broken signboard banging/ In the April wind." g. Example 2 - "Finding life anew/ Out of twisted lies and storms/ Standing on The Rock." 4. Experience 2.a - Subjects pick one of their haikus and create a short movement phrase. (15 mins) 5. Experience 2.b - With a partner, subjects teach and learn their phrases to their partners. (15 mins) 6. Presentations - Each duet will demonstrate their movement phrases. If they are comfortable, the choreographer will read their haiku while their partner dances. (15 mins) 7. Talk-back - Subjects will give feedback to each duo, and allow duos to explain their pieces. (5 mins per group) 8. Assessment - Subjects participate enthusiastically in activities, and will have a short piece of choreography to present with their partners by the end of the class. 9. Circle Choreography - Ask: *Now* how do you feel? Put that feeling into a simple movement to share with the rest of the group. 10. Close by saying the statement of affirmation together. (2 mins)
Books, Materials, Supplies: Paper, pencils, pens, instrumental music
Assessment Method(s) Authentic Assessment, Circle Choreography before and after assessment

Table 4. Curriculum Lesson 3

Curriculum Project Title: Movement and Storytelling Curriculum
Lesson No.: 3
Lesson Overview: Participants will tell their stories by walking each other through their life maps. The goal of this exercise is to increase empathy among the group as they listen to and walk with the leader through their journey.
Goals: 1. To develop greater empathy among subjects in the group. 2. To develop subjects' awareness of time, space, their own bodies, and of others.
Questions: • What did you see and feel as you walked with each person? • What emotions did you hear and see? • How did your respond to the others' life maps? For the choreographer: • What was the process of creating a dance like for you? • Why was it easy/hard? • What were you thinking about as you choreographed? • How is life like this?
Lesson Objectives: 1. Develop space awareness 2. Work together in groups to create a meaningful movement 3. Understand purposefulness in movement and life
Lesson Breakdown: 1. Warm-up - Begin with Breath Awareness exercise and BrainDance movement. (10 mins) 2. Circle choreography - Each person demonstrates a movement that expresses how they are feeling at the moment. The group repeats it together and then move to the next person, adding each movement onto the first, until the circle is complete. (15 mins) Experience 1.a - Mapping exercise - on a large piece of paper, participants draw a map of their individual lives, from birth through present day. They draw the ups and downs, fears and joys, and anything else they desire to include on their map. Participants walk through and memorize their maps to teach to the other subjects. (20 mins) 3. Experience 1.b - Map walkthrough - one subject leads the group around the room in the pattern of their map, and *describes what is happening at each point. The group follows the participant copying any movement qualities, level changes exemplified. (20 mins) 4. Talk-back - Each participant is given time to debrief about their map and what feelings and thoughts arose for them as they were drawing and creating it. (10 mins each) 5. Circle Choreography - Ask: *Now* how do you feel? Put that feeling into a simple movement to share with the rest of the group. 6. Close by saying the statement of affirmation together. (2 mins) *Note: Descriptions should only be given if the participant is comfortable sharing their experiences with the group. It is better to do the first walk-through without using words.
Books, Materials, Supplies: Paper, pencils, pens, colored pencils, instrumental music
Assessment Method(s) Authentic Assessment, Circle Choreography before and after assessment

Table 5. Curriculum Lesson 4

Curriculum Project Title: Movement and Storytelling Curriculum
Lesson No.: 4
Lesson Overview: This lesson teaches flocking, another choreographic skill used for creating movement and developing connectedness among participants. Participants may use this skill as they continue to develop their life maps and mini haiku phrases.
Goals: 1. To teach choreographic and movement skills. 2. To create a safe environment and community that allows for freedom for self-expression and honesty. 3. To encourage the development of subjects' self-efficacy.
Questions: • What emotions are present in your map? • What does that feel like in your body? • How does it look when you move it around the floor? • What themes (in floor patterns and movement) do you see throughout these maps? • How is life like this?
Lesson Objectives: 1. Introduce Flocking as another choreographic skill 2. Develop space, body, and tempo awareness 3. Work together in groups to create a meaningful movement
Lesson Breakdown: 1. Warm-up - Begin with Breath Awareness exercise and Brain Dance movement. (10 mins) 2. Introduce Flocking - Like birds fly in a flock across the sky, we can move as a flock as well. Participants should stand in a pyramid, diamond, or square formation. Researcher explains that everyone will follow the person at the point of the pyramid until he/she feels like passing the lead off to someone else. Passing requires turning in either direction. When the person at the next point can no longer see anyone that makes them the lead. This continues around the formation. Participants may move in any direction in the room, but keeping the movement simple enough so everyone else may follow. No spinning allowed! As soon as the person at a point loses sight of the leader, it's their turn to lead. (15 mins). 3. Experience 1.a - Map walkthroughs continued (go through any maps that did not get shared last week) - one subject leads the group around the room in the pattern of their map, and describes what is happening at each point. The group follows the participant copying any movement qualities, level changes exemplified. (20 mins) 4. Experience 1.b - Locomotion study - Ask participants to travel through their maps again, this time thinking about *how* they want to travel. Ask them to be mindful about the levels (high, medium, low) and tempos (quick, moderate, slow) with which they move. 5. Talk-back - Each participant is given time to debrief about their map and what feelings and thoughts arose for them as they were drawing and creating it. (10 mins each) 6. Circle Choreography - Ask: *Now* how do you feel? Put that feeling into a simple movement to share with the rest of the group. 7. Close by saying the statement of affirmation together. (2 mins)
Books, Materials, Supplies: Paper, pencils, pens, instrumental music
Assessment Method(s) Authentic Assessment, Circle Choreography before and after assessment

Table 6. Curriculum Lesson 5

Curriculum Project Title: Movement and Storytelling Curriculum

Lesson No.: 5

Lesson Overview: This lesson is a review and solidification of which pieces will be shown at the showcase. Participants will need to decide what they feel ready for, and how they will present their work. This decision-making process may be guided by the author as to maintain a feeling of safety and structure without taking control away from the participants.

Goals:

1. Decide on which pieces to present at the showcase

Questions:

- How is life like this?

Lesson Objectives:

1. Work together in groups to create a meaningful movement
2. Understand purposefulness in movement and everyday life

Lesson Breakdown:

1. Warm-up - Begin with Breathing exercise and Brain Dance and Circle Choreography movement on the floor today. (10 mins)
2. Flocking exercise. (15 mins)
3. Experience 1 - Somatics/Emotion study - Participants are asked to provide emotions they would like to explore (relevant to their maps). Each person takes time to feel those emotions in their body, and then creates a movement expressing that feeling. Like in the Circle Choreography, one person presents and the other mirror the presenter's movement.
4. Experience 2 - Mapping - Using movements from the Somatics/Emotion study, they begin to add those into their map dances where they deem appropriate. Participants should feel free to change and expand or shrink movements, and are encouraged to add contrast in quality/effort, time, and level. (30 mins)
5. Discussion of the final celebration: What parts of what we are working on do we want to continue to expand and then share with our community? Do we want to make one big piece that includes our maps and haikus, or a bunch of little pieces with just parts of maps and haikus?

   Suggestions:

   a. Pick one map and have members break off into little pieces of their maps here and there.

   b. Haiku pieces - add all three haikus together and create a couple big pieces, do a bunch of small pieces, and/or ask for their ideas
6. Circle Choreography - Ask: *Now* how do you feel? Put that feeling into a simple movement to share with the rest of the group.
7. Close by saying the statement of affirmation together. (2 mins)

Books, Materials, Supplies: Paper, pencils, pens, instrumental music

Assessment Method(s)

Authentic Assessment, Circle Choreography before and after assessment

Table 7. Curriculum Lesson 6

Curriculum Project Title: Movement and Storytelling Curriculum
Lesson No.: 6
Lesson Overview: Participants will begin to polish the pieces they have agreed to work on for the showcase.
Goals: 1. Develop a plan for the celebration. 2. Presentation pieces completed. 3. To guide subjects as they create pieces of choreography and perform them at the end of the 7-week time period.
Questions: • How is life like this?
Lesson Objectives: 1. Work together in groups to create a meaningful movement and a rehearse celebration pieces 2. Solidify and polish the pieces being prepared for the showcase 3. Solidify an order for the pieces being shown
Lesson Breakdown: 1. Warm-up - Begin with Breath Awareness exercise and Brain Dance movement. (5 mins) 2. Circle choreography or Flocking. (15 mins) 3. Work on presentation pieces: a. Brief review of haiku dances. Share them with the group followed by a brief discussion of each piece. (20 mins) i. Combine groups. ii. Participants choose two poems and teach the movements to each other. iii. Now there will be one person reading the haiku, and four people dancing each piece. iv. If there's time, have them try out different levels and tempos. b. Combine mapping pieces together to make one big piece (40 mins): i. Ask the most confident participant to begin with their moving through their map followed by everyone else. ii. Every person picks a part of their map to perform - they pick a moment to break away and do their part. iii. Every participant should have a part of their piece in it, and leader must also have a chance to break away for a moment as well. iv. The map dance could involve some of the haiku readings. c. Work on flocking, levels, and tempos 4. Presentation and talk back of pieces and their progress. (10 mins) 5. Circle Choreography - Ask: *Now* how do you feel? Put that feeling into a simple movement to share with the rest of the group. 6. Close by saying the statement of affirmation together. (2 mins)
Books, Materials, Supplies: Paper, pencils, pens, colored pencils, instrumental music
Assessment Method(s) Authentic Assessment, Circle Choreography before and after assessment

Table 8. Curriculum Lesson 7

Curriculum Project Title: Movement and Storytelling Curriculum
Lesson No.: 7
Lesson Overview: Showcase/Celebration
Goals: 1. Participants will perform for their friends and family at an informal showcase.
Questions:
Lesson Objectives: 1. Work together in groups to create a meaningful movement 2. Understand purposefulness in movement and life
Lesson Breakdown: 1. Welcome 2. Presentation of pieces: a. Flocking b. Map Dance c. Haiku Dances 3. Close by saying the statement of affirmation together. (2 mins)
Books, Materials, Supplies: Music picked by the participants
Assessment Method(s) Authentic Assessment, Observation

Section 4

Mastery and Self-Regulation

Too often a traumatic experience can hinder a person's ability to self-regulate and gain mastery over their emotional responses. Unfortunately, the absence of mastery and self-regulation can result in the development of mental illness, feelings of hopelessness, depression, etc. These can be crippling and prevent people from leading full and healthy lives. The following chapters offer strategies for non-clinicians to help their constituents develop mastery of life skills and self-regulation in their everyday lives.

Chapter 10
Healing Together:
The Lid Project

Kristine Vuocolo
Human Services Inc., USA

ABSTRACT

This chapter emphasizes several key concepts concerning mental illness in today's society. The author strongly believes that mental health recovery is possible and that it is an individualized journey. People struggling with mental health issues can find hope and healing through the use of artistic expression. This chapter is designed to encourage and inspire others to use everyday items and turn them into art. The author describes how collaboration can be a key ingredient to the success of the healing that takes place while doing art together.

INTRODUCTION

While trauma disorders are currently receiving significant attention, countless other mental health disorders often remain undiagnosed, ignored, and stigmatized. Statistically, 1 in 4 adults struggle with a mental illness in a year (Johns Hopkins Medicine). That is 1 out of every 4 people in a family, 1 out of every 4 coworkers, students, friends and neighbors. In other words, a quarter of the population is struggling with a mental illness at any given moment. Mental illness is non-discriminatory and crosses all cultural lines, age brackets, and economical statuses. So while communities and schools rush to become trauma-informed, it may be more poignant to acknowledge, educate, and respond to the extremely high percentage of people living with mental illnesses beyond those associated with trauma.

Fortunately, the benefits of art making do not discriminate either. Regardless of diagnosis, the arts have repeatedly demonstrated an ability to heal. Engaging in music correlated to a form of relaxation, a decrease of tension and anxiety, and control of chronic pain. Making art led to a reduction of the stress producing hormone cortisol, and also gave participants a sense of identity. The findings of movement expression and expressive writing are similar, but added findings of a boost in immune functioning, significant improvement in physical health, and an overall improvement in quality of life (Stuckey and Nobel, 2010).

DOI: 10.4018/978-1-5225-5981-8.ch010

Collaborative art projects seek to intertwine people traveling similar paths; building trust and connections in an effort to simultaneously decrease feelings of isolation while providing movement towards coping and healing. This chapter shares the story of The Lid Project, a collaborative art project set at Transitions, a psychiatric rehabilitation program. While the story may offer the reader a project to replicate, the more substantial takeaway is the richness of metaphor for the healing journey found within the story and the process of creating art together.

Collaborative Art Making

Strategically planned arts based experiences can play a very valuable role in healing for those living with mental illness. The arts have been shown to improve focus, mood, brain function, communication, and social skills, all of which are necessary for working toward healthy living and thinking (Nurrie-Stearns, 2013). The arts offer choice and opportunities to take control. For those who have experienced trauma or live with a mental health diagnosis, art making can promote skills to help regulate emotions, build confidence and self-esteem, and foster therapeutic communities and relationships through collaboration.

The shared experience of group art making in particular has many benefits. First it provides safety, which aids in building trust and stronger relationships among members of a group. The art maker is able to be vulnerable and understood by the group, without having to verbalize his experience, making it a safe form of communication and expression (Moon, 2010). Secondly, collaborative work lessens the pressure for one person to achieve an end goal successfully on their own. Both the individual and the community around him are empowered as they work together to achieve their goals (Moon, 2010). Finally, according to art therapist Dr. Bruce L. Moon (2010), "Making art in the presence of others is an expression of hope" (p. 8). When an individual is free to express and be understood by others through his artwork, he can begin to trust in something outside of, or greater than, himself. Ultimately, working collaboratively can move the participant away from feelings of isolation towards being part of a community (Rossetto, 2012).

Feelings of isolation are common among people who are in the midst of mental illness, addiction, grief and other traumatic experiences. These experiences may be difficult to talk about, which is why art making can be a valuable and effective method of therapy for many. Moon says, "In art-based group therapy we often witness creative expressions of feelings that are beyond the communicative abilities of conventional speech" (2010, p. 29). Making art within a group context allows people to share their stories without having to verbally articulate their experiences. This helps to establish an atmosphere of safety and trust, which is key to successful group therapies.

Artwork in any form (dance, music, painting, writing, etc.) can be considered a "partial self-portrait that metaphorically represents that artist's life" (Moon, 2010, p. 67). This makes one very vulnerable to the group when they share their work. However, when other group members are able to see and relate to the experience of the art maker, organic relationships begin to form, and the power of understanding that one is not alone in the world begins to establish feelings of hope. Moon says, "Acts of creating are invitations to relate. By making things, artists take images from within and give them visible form in the world" (2010, p. 4). Art making offers an alternative way for one to reconnect not only with himself, but with the world beyond.

When in a group, an individual is part of a collective whole working to achieve a common goal. This can set a participant at ease because he/she is not solely responsible for a final outcome of a project. The potential for creativity magnifies as ideas from one participant are able to expand off of ideas of the other group members. Working through ideas with others changes isolation into connection (Moon, 2010), and gives group members choices about how they work together, and what they want to achieve as a collective whole. After that achievement is met, a sense of pride and ownership becomes evident, and group members find the confidence to continue trying new things and working together.

Description of Facility Program and Population

Psychiatric Rehabilitation (Psych Rehab) programs are designed to promote recovery, community integration, and an overall improvement in life for those diagnosed with a mental illness (Psychiatric Rehabilitation Association, n.d.). Transitions, located in Chester County, Pennsylvania, is a group-based model that utilizes evidence-based practices within a rotating twelve-week schedule. These groups vary based on the needs of the current membership and the goals they have set for themselves. Transitions serves adults who live with severe and persistent mental illness.

Upon arrival, new members are assigned a Primary Coach. These Psych Rehab workers are not therapists, but are there to support the client and assist them in achieving goals they set for themselves in areas such as living, learning, working, and socialization. The Primary Coach also helps to navigate the mental health system, which is vast and can be intimidating.

Participants

According to the Mayo Clinic's website, the definition of mental illness is, "disorders that affect your mood, thinking and behavior." Among the different diagnoses, the symptoms of mental illness are vast. Those who are accepted into the Transitions program exhibit characteristics associated with mental illness that can be nuanced or overt. Symptoms of schizophrenia, bipolar disorder and major depression disorder tend to be more widely recognized. However, symptoms associated with personality disorders, anxiety disorders, and trauma related disorders may not be so obvious.

Any and all mental health symptoms may cause those experiencing the symptoms to feel disconnected to friends and family or just as likely, have friends and family reject or turn away from them. Symptoms demonstrated by individuals with schizophrenia and bipolar disorder include depression and anxiety, hopelessness and thoughts of suicide, lack of social skills, and cognitive impairment. Those with bipolar disorder may also experience rapid mood swings, mania, or insomnia (Rodseth, 2011). Individuals diagnosed with major depressive disorders may demonstrate a lack of interest in activities, lack of energy and appetite, have trouble sleeping and may have suicidal thoughts or behaviors. Symptoms of anxiety disorders manifest as excessive worry, restlessness, irritability, and sleep disturbance (Smith, 2018). Trauma symptoms are similar to those of anxiety and depression and may include fear and anxiety, sleep disturbance, hypervigilance, difficulty concentrating, and problems controlling anger. Trauma survivors also struggle with feelings of safety and the ability to trust others (Setti & Argentero, 2014).

Many people facing mental illness find it very challenging to make friends, obtain jobs, and even complete simple tasks if these symptoms are not managed (NIMH, 2016). There are many reasons why adults struggling with mental health issues would come to Transitions: some are looking for people to whom they can relate; some need support going back to school, getting their driver's license and/or finding a job; others are there to learn a new skill set based on the impact of their mental illness symptoms.

From the inception of the Transitions program, there are a handful of groups that remain consistent in the different twelve-week schedules. Within these groups, participants develop coping skills for mental health issues, relationship skills, job development skills, and artistic expression. The groups themselves have several goals including but not limited to building on skills, increasing natural supports, connection to community services, and building self-esteem. Through the use of art, it is possible to accomplish all of these.

Primary Coaches and Specialists

Psych Rehab workers or Primary Coaches along with Psych Rehab Specialists believe in the philosophy of mental health recovery. The term recovery has been historically linked to drugs and alcohol rehabilitation. However, the term recovery is also associated with mental illness. In 2005, the Pennsylvania Department of Mental Health and Substance Abuse Services released a publication titled, *A Call For Change: Toward A Recovery-Oriented Mental Health Service System for Adults.* This document was a proclamation of the Department's dedication to the Recovery Movement.

Certified Psychiatric Rehabilitation Specialists (CPRP) are professionals who have worked at least two years in the mental health field and have completed a minimum of 45 hours of training specific to "the treatment and/or rehabilitation of adults with serious mental illness" (PRA & PRF). After that time they are eligible to take the exam to become certified. CPRPs believe that people living with mental illness are first and foremost individuals. They believe that they have skills and talents unique to them, and recovery pulls on these strengths. Recovery is an individualized journey and different for everyone. They also work through the belief that recovery means people living with mental illness can find meaningful employment, stable housing, a supportive network and live a fulfilling life (PRA & PRF). It is this philosophical stance that guided the Lid Project.

The Creation of the Lid Project

The Transitions program is part of Human Services. Inc., which is a non-profit agency. As many staff of non-profits would attest, money for art can be tight or non-existent. When approaching this project the staff at Transitions began by working with the supplies they already had available to them: paints, paint brushes, and a large canvas they found tucked away in a closet. They also reached out to people in their network. During the daily morning meetings the Primary Coaches asked all of the Transitions' members to bring in lids of various shapes and sizes. They then approached other staff in the agency and local stakeholders to ask them to save lids as well. Rather quickly bags of lids started showing up. Peanut butter jar lids, soda lids, pickle jar lids, jam lids and so forth. No lid was too big or too small!

After the lids were gathered the project was officially started. Members were told that this was a group project and asked to decorate the lids. Staff presented the theme of mental health recovery and expressed that the lids were to represent what that means to them. Members asked about what the finished project would look like and the facilitator at the time was honest in saying that she wasn't sure what the end result would be. This actually excited the members! There was anticipation about what the lids would turn into.

During that first art group, some of the lids were painted. Members and staff worked side-by-side, each painting a lid or two. Some members were nervous because they hadn't really painted before. Yet, the staff watched as other members encouraged them, saying things like, "That's ok, just put some dots on them, or squiggly lines." This set the members who were nervous at ease and they joined in.

A few weeks went by and more people became involved in the lid project. There were times when the art room was buzzing with laughter and chatter. Other times music was heard up the halls. On some lids words started to appear: hope, discovery, journey, etc. Other lids were painted in solid colors with a few accents. The colors ranged from loud primary colors to pastel tones. Each one was unique and symbolized a different artist.

As weeks passed something magical started to happen. The first was that as the members and staff painted, conversations unfolded about past experiences, the realities of mental illness, past traumas as well as fears mixed in with conversations of everyday life. Bonds started to form that didn't previously exist. Relationships between both staff and members became stronger. The members who participated were set at ease and went more in depth with sharing their stories. Around the program there was a genuine camaraderie that developed. Through spending time painting together the members found other members who had gone through similar experiences. They realized that others dealt with comparable mental health symptoms, and they began to share coping skills that had worked for them.

The second was that members started to become even more creative. The art room was a place that had a wall of storage closets. In these storage closets were unused art supplies of projects past. Members and staff alike started rummaging for items that could be glued to the lids. This was a surprising yet welcomed development!

At this point lids started taking on personalities all their own. Some had faces others had entire scenes painted on them, birds flying over grass and fish swimming in the ocean just to name a few. Then there were the more abstract pieces that were left to interpretation. Suddenly lids started appearing with feathers and beads on them and even mini dream catchers were attached for decoration. The creativity was contagious and this brought even more participation.

Approximately 100 lids later, the staff and members of Transitions thought it was time to look at the canvas and try to envision the final outcome.

What to do with the lids? At first the staff thought that they would just glue all of the lids on the canvas until the canvas was full. The canvas turned out to be bigger than they thought, and it was decided by the group that there might be too many lids. This is where members and staff started discussing some alternative options.

To get started they took some of the lids and arranged them on the canvas to see what it would look like with lid next to lid. It looked good, but it was observed during this process that pressing the lids up next to each other left gaps due to the different sizes of the lids. What to do with the gaps?

Again as a team they went back to the storage closets and, as luck would have it, found a bag of clear decorative glass gems. They fit perfectly in between the caps. This was the inspiration needed and a group went for exploration purposes to the dollar store. There they picked up more glass gems and some small round mirrors, which seemed like great options to glue onto the canvas as well.

It took a bit of dreaming, some more conversation between members and staff, and the vision finally emerged: "Journey of Recovery, River of Hope." Over the next few weeks staff and members jointly painted the canvas, and glued finished lids as well as glass gems and mirrors onto the canvas. The lids and gems became the bank of a river. Then a river was painted with lids lazily floating down it. Above that was a night sky with an artistic moon leaving a shadow reflecting off the river. Finally the mirrors were artistically positioned within the sky to reflect the onlooker. After a few months, good conversations, much laughter and some tears, the masterpiece was complete!

Healing Effects Observed

In the mental health field of today, employees at every level are being trained in trauma informed care. It is more commonly accepted that mental health issues can be connected with past traumas and vice versa. As facilitators, when approaching a group art project, it is important to remember that we do not know what traumatic experiences have impacted our participants, and it is impossible to know what might trigger the individuals we are working with. With that in mind, the Transitions Psych Rehab staff found that providing an activity with no specific end goal was more welcoming and safe than a more specific project. This allowed the project to focus on working collaboratively, providing choice and helping to set the participants at ease with making art. Even though no formal therapy was done during these sessions, healing effects were noticeable.

Members who participated felt pride in the finished project, and their confidence seemed to rise when they saw their painted cap(s) put into a collective project. When individuals who did not think that they could make art became involved, their self-esteem improved by being included.

Working on the same project as a group encouraged the development of meaningful relationships and natural supports within the group. New friendships developed through conversations that took place during the art groups. The Psych Rehab workers developed bonds with the participating members, leading to deeper therapeutic conversations that helped with breakthroughs and healing. Many of those participating in the project shared that the process was very therapeutic for them, and they began making art at home with everyday items. The shared experience helped build a sense of camaraderie among community members, and the continued openness with which they shared their experiences after the project was completed demonstrated the establishment of hope.

As the project progressed, more and more members took part in the art sessions. After The Lid Project was completed, more individuals participated in future art projects, and the walls of the Psych Rehab center are now covered with artistic expression. When visitors and new members arrive at Transitions, they stop at the mural and read the words associated with the journey of recovery. This has created an atmosphere of hope.

Metaphors Discovered in the Process

The destination is not always known at the onset of a journey

The Lid Project began as a way for the Primary Coaches to make art with their members as inexpensively as possible, but ended up being a very valuable journey. Through this process, participants learned to focus not on working towards something, but to trust in the process and be present in the moment. In recovery, this is a valuable lesson to learn. By focusing on neither the past or the future, participants can truly engage in the present moment, the present treatment method, and the present environment and community.

We can always reach deeper within to find new tools and resources.

As confidence and trust in the creative process and the project grew, participants began searching for more materials to use. They had become comfortable using the tools already on hand and were both prepared and excited to try new things. The supply closet became a treasure trove; providing creative

Figure 1. The completed lid mural

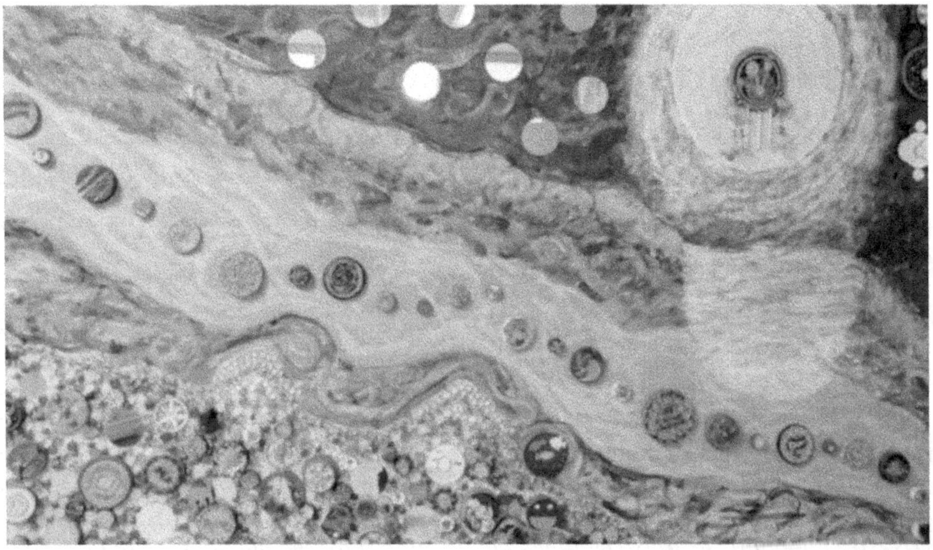

materials once passed over or discarded as being useless. It was not until later in the process that the participants were able to recognize the value of what was on hand and how it could be incorporated into the artwork. In a similar fashion, as the healing process unfolds, with guidance and support participants are able to reach deeper into themselves to find more tools, untapped strength and energy, and deepened commitment to support further healing.

The small steps we take at the beginning still move us down the path.

The first few lids created were simple and unadorned. Yet, each simple, first lid moved the project forward towards the final 100 lids decorated and collected. The beginning of a treatment method or the beginning of a new program or even the beginning of a new relationship can feel overwhelming. It may seem at the start that every step must be completed simultaneously or that the first steps are so insignificant that they can not possibly be going anywhere. Those first lids helped to demonstrate the very opposite. Every small step, in any direction, is part of the journey and a valuable step towards healing.

CONCLUSION

Admittedly, at the start of this project, the Psych Rehab workers did not recognize the value of the journey they were about to embark on with their clients. They simply sought to build relationships using art in its most therapeutic form; to work through past traumas, build self-worth, and bring hope. A collaborative art project seemed like the best way to bridge the gap between someone who struggles with a mental illness and someone who wants to connect with him/her. The Lid Project accomplished all of these things and more.

REFERENCES

American Psychological Association. (n.d.). *Recovering Emotionally from Disaster.* Retrieved from http://www.apa.org/topics/trauma/index.aspx

Bell, C. E., & Robbins, S. J. (2007). Effect of Art Production on Negative Mood: A Randomized, Controlled Trial. *Art Therapy: Journal of the American Art Therapy Association, 24*(2), 71-75.

Bussing-Birks, M. (n.d.). *Mental Illness and Substance Abuse.* Retrieved from https://www.nber.org/digest/apr02/w8699.html

Foundations Recovery Network. (n.d.). *The Connection Between Mental Illness and Substance Abuse.* Retrieved from https://www.dualdiagnosis.org/mental-health-and-addiction/the-connection/

Geist, J. H. (2014). *Overview of Trauma and Stress Related Disorders.* Retrieved from https://www.merckmanuals.com/professional/psychiatric-disorders/anxiety-and-st ressor-related-disorders/overview-of-trauma-and-stressor-related-disorders

Godman, H. (2018). *Regular exercise changes the brain to improve memory, thinking skills.* Retrieved from http://www.dhs.pa.gov/cs/groups/webcontent/documents/document/s_002537.pdf

Guggenheim Museum, R. (n.d.). *Visitor Studies, Evaluation & Audience Research.* Retrieved from http://www.artsedsearch.org/summaries/educational-research-the-art-of-problem-solving

Johns Hopkins Medicine. (n.d.). *Mental Health Disorder Statistics.* Retrieved from https://www.hopkinsmedicine.org/healthlibrary/conditions/mental_health_disorders/ment

Korn, R. (2010). *Educational research: The art of problem solving*. New York: Solomon.

Mayo Clinic. (n.d.). *Mental Illness.* Retrieved from https://www.mayoclinic.org/diseases-conditions/mental-illness/symptoms-causes/syc-20374968

Moon, B. L. (2010). *Art-based group therapy: Theory and practice*. Springfield, IL: Charles C. Thomas Publisher, Ltd.

National Institute of Mental Illness (NIMH). (2016a). *Bipolar Disorder.* Retrieved from https://www.nimh.nih.gov/health/topics/bipolar-disorder/index.shtml

National Institute of Mental Illness (NIMH). (2016b). *Schizophrenia.* Retrieved from https://www.nimh.nih.gov/health/topics/schizophrenia/index.shtml

Nurrie-Stearns, M., & Nurrie-Stearns, R. (2013). *Yoga for emotional trauma: Meditations and practices for healing pain and suffering*. Oakland, CA: New Harbinger Publishing, Inc.

Pennsylvania Office of Mental Health and Substance Abuse Services. (2005). *A Call to Change: Towards A Recovery-Oriented Mental Health Service System For Adults.* Retrieved from http://www.dhs.pa.gov/cs/groups/webcontent/documents/document/s_002537.pdf

Psychiatric Rehabilitation Association (PRA) and Psychiatric Rehabilitation Foundation (PRF). (n.d.). Retrieved from https://www.psychrehabassociation.org/who-we-are/core-principles-and-values

Rodseth, D. (2011). Dealing with bipolar disorder in general practice. *South African Family Practice, 53*(6), 549–553. doi:10.1080/20786204.2011.10874150

Rossetto, E. (2012). A hermeneutic phenomenological study of community mural making and social action art therapy. *Art Therapy: Journal of the American Art Therapy Association, 29*(1), 19–26. doi:10.1080/07421656.2012.648105

Setti, I., & Argentero, P. (2014). The role of mindfulness in protecting firefighters from psychosomatic malaise. *Traumatology, 20*(2), 134–141. doi:10.1037/h0099398

Smith, K. (2018, February 13). *Anxiety vs depression: Tips to help understand the difference.* Retrieved from https://www.psycom.net/anxiety-depression-difference

Stuckey, H. L., & Nobel, J. (2010). The Connection Between Art, Healing, and Public Health: A Review of Current Literature. *Am J. Public Health, 100*(2), 254-263. Retrieved from https://www.ncbi.nlm.nih.gov/pmc/articles/PMC2804629/

Substance Abuse and Mental Health Services Administration (SAMHSA). (2015). *Trauma-Informed Approach and Trauma-Specific Interventions.* Retrieved from https://www.samhsa.gov/nctic/trauma-interventions

U.S. Department of Health and Human Services. (2017). *What is Mental Health.* Retrieved from https://www.mentalhealth.gov/basics/what-is-mental-health

Chapter 11
Story Dances:
Identity and Power in the Dance Classroom

Julia Ann Crawford
J. Crawford Dance, USA

ABSTRACT

The motivation of this chapter is to add to the literature about the practice of teaching dance with a critical and somatic approach and to contribute to illuminating the reality of negotiating power in the dance classroom and the complexity of the influence of cultural values on this dynamic. This chapter reflects on the process of teaching a dance curriculum that explores identity to three different cultural groups in order to gain knowledge of best practices for nurturing somatic authority and providing meaningful choice opportunities while developing dance skills.

INTRODUCTION

Dance has always been a vessel for healing and transformation. People and communities have engaged in dance as part of rituals for healing, war, and celebration throughout all of time. As the more performative traditions of dance from the European world developed, forms such as Classical Ballet and Modern Dance, which is steeped in the appropriation of the aesthetics and costuming of other culture's dance rituals, so did an authoritarian teaching tradition. In this tradition dancer's strive to perfectly mimic the command of the teacher rather than experience catharsis through movement. When dance is taught and engaged with in this way, it is stripped of its healing attributes and the dance classroom perpetuates oppression and manifests disorders with social, psychological, physical, and spiritual ramifications.

This chapter offers an approach to invite healing possibilities into the dance classroom and spaces where dance is utilized through nurturing the whole person, cultivating artistic voice, promoting ownership of story, and nurturing people to reconnect to their body as they develop and explore dance skills. The author's primary goal is social justice in dance through teaching approach, class content, inclusion of bodies, and access to excellence in dance. The author strives towards a critical and somatic teaching approach in order to promote healing, wholeness, transformation, and holistic development (Shapiro, 1999; Friere, 2000; Green, 1998).

DOI: 10.4018/978-1-5225-5981-8.ch011

Western dance education has a long-standing custom of authoritarianism in the dance classroom. A common outcome of authoritarian teaching in dance is the systematic breaking down of dancers to be built up in the image of the teacher (Smith, 1998). As dancers submerge their unique identities and surrender their authority in the dance classroom, 'docile bodies' are created (Green, 1998). The dancers become objects that the teacher or choreographer uses for their personal artistic creation, shaping and molding them into their own image and vision (Smith, 1998). Dancers as objects build their skill from the outside in without attaching the depth of their experience, story, and expertise of their own body and self.

In the authoritarian tradition, dance teachers often hold absolute power over dance students in deeply harmful ways. Smith (1998) writes, "I understood the dance classroom to be an ideal climate for authoritarian behavior. The student has already consented to being in a situation in which he or she is usually attempting to replicate as perfectly as possible the example and the demands of the teacher" (p. 128). The definitive power exerted over dancers often includes a predesigned mold the dancer is expected to make him or her self fit. This mold often includes very specific body types and the perfection of skills that are not necessarily anatomically possible for all bodies.

However, in order to continue participating, dancers must obey and adhere to the rules determined by those in power (Kelso, 2003). Smith (1998) offers, "Because dancers are generally scantily clad, evenly distributed in space, and eager to please, they are easily observed and controlled. A dancer who will not or cannot participate at the general group level is easily picked out" (p. 128). This predetermined perfection limits those that may participate to only the elite few that are able to fulfill the requirements. Clement (2007) writes, "The body is under constant scrutiny and within the dance discipline, failing to acquire the ideal body shape and mannerisms is grounds for exclusion" (p. 51).

There is an ever-present comparison to perfection that is perpetuated by constant surveillance and correction from the teacher and the obligation to observe oneself in the mirror and consistently "fix" one's self throughout dance class. The experience of constant surveillance leads to self-surveillance (Smith, 1998). Smith (1998) writes, "The dance classroom, with its mirrors, watchful teachers, and self-critical students, is a key site for both the external and internal surveillance of dancing bodies…" (p. 131).

These norms in dance education provide that dance students are often not given the opportunity to think critically or truly engage their creativity. The teacher decides the values of the classroom culture, requiring dancers to submerge their own values and life stories upon entering the dance classroom. Through this paradigm dependence on the dance teacher is created; "Dancers rely on their teachers for support and guidance, but also for approval and selection of parts in ballets. This leads to a generalized fear instilled in the dancers" (Kelso, 2003).

The depth of this control is alarming as dancers begin to interpret attention that tears them down as positive, "…a criticism, even a hurtful one, can be taken as a compliment because at least the management is not ignoring her" (Kelso, 2003). Smith (1998) also offers, "In addition, because dancers are typically dependent on the teacher's feedback, any comments or lack of comments take on exaggerated import… Unfortunately the line between what we as dancers term a correction and what others might call an insult can be quite thin" (p. 128). Largely, dancers have come to accept abusive treatment as normal.

While this describes the worst of authoritarianism in the dance classroom it is important to note that it is present, albeit at varying degrees, in many dance classrooms even those that aim to implement holistic development teaching practices. Clement (2007) writes, "Even in dance classes where collaborative learning is encouraged, students ultimately do not question their teachers or the information they are supposed to unequivocally accept" (p. 41). This is in part because there is great importance placed on specific bodily positions and standardized movement sequences (Smith, 1998). This creates an empty ritual that is performed with little to no awareness of why, but with an unattainable ideal of perfection in mind.

Further, the damage this can cause to dancers is not limited to their experience inside the dance classroom; it overflows into their whole being and existence (Stinson, 1998). Clement (2007) adds, "I came to realize that while dance classes are expressly designed to regulate human bodies (at least the bodies that have access to these courses), during the time spent in class or onstage, these regulations also influence a dancer's actions outside of the studio" (p. 51). The repetitive experience of submitting to the authority of the teacher by sacrificing one's own authority creates a split between the mind and body (Johnson, 1983).

The split between mind and body and sole reliance on outside experts rather than developing one's own expertise causes doubt in one's own knowledge and perception and habituates people to look outside themselves for direction. In turn, this split between mind and body perpetuates authoritarianism (Johnson, 1983). Johnson (1983) writes, "...with our physical training to adopt rigid stances, a 'habit of performance.' The muscular rigidities that come from holding those stances for years dull perception and make it difficult for people to adapt to each other and to new situations" (p. 171).

In the field of dance, application of critical pedagogy and somatics has begun to sway the traditionally hierarchal or authoritarian way that teachers approach teaching dance (Medina, n.d.). Fortin (1998) even suggests that a somatic approach provides people of non-dominant cultures the possibility of resisting dominant culture. Critical Pedagogy offers a theoretical basis for moving towards holistic development and the balance of power in the dance classroom, but in practice it is complex (Ellsworth, 1989; Anttila, 2003). Anttila (2003) states that the process of critical pedagogy is complicated and is limited in bringing about equality and justice. However, she maintains that hearing student voices and helping to bring about awareness of their life situation is still a crucial part of making learning meaningful (Anttila, 2003).

Shue and Beck (2001) contribute that some dance teachers who claim to be teaching with a critical philosophy are not; their actions are communicating the opposite. The teachers were unaware that they were not living their philosophy (Shue & Beck, 2001). Green (1998) writes,

Particularly in modern dance, educators and artists often believe that dance is a liberating experience and teachers often focus on offering students access to an ability to free themselves through movement. Yet, dance teachers do not always attempt to be self-reflexive regarding the ways the student dance body may be mechanized or habituated into an ideal form that represents the teacher's learned belief system and presumed ideas about what the body should be and do (p. 4).

It is important to continue to construct and reconstruct knowledge about the practice of using a critical and somatic teaching approach in order to uncover best practices that do not feed the cycle of oppression in order to make space for and invite healing and transformation through dance.

BACKGROUND

The way we perceive and understand the world is rooted in our lived experience, which is directly determined by our cultural background and identity. Our identity informs the way we fulfill roles and group membership. Therefore, the way a teacher carries out a critical and somatic approach to teaching dance is informed and guided by their identity and has the potential to nurture power in people or to oppress. Identity also informs the way people participate in the learning experience.

Identity

Identity theory maintains that the self consists of a collection of identities based on the roles a person has and fills. Role identity, such as identifying one's self as a mother or a dancer, influences behavior based on the interpretation of the role and the social expectations of the role. Since the self has many role identities, a hierarchy of roles is developed, which influences the effort put into fulfilling each role (Stets and Burke, 2000).

Social identity theory illuminates the influence of group membership on self-perception (Stets and Burke, 2000). A person has several identities that correlate to memberships in different groups. Different social contexts draw out different identities. This is different from a personal level of identity, which is comprised of unique personal attributes. Social Identity theory is primarily concerned with the identities created due to differentiating between belonging to groups and not belonging to others (Tajfel and Turner, 1986).

Stets and Burke (2000) propose a theory of Self that combines identity theory and social identity theory to form a more integrated view of the micro, meso, and macro levels of identity. This theory considers role and group membership influences on identity, as well as, unique personal attributes. Group membership takes place at the macro level, role identity takes place at the meso level, and personal attributes of self-esteem, self-efficacy, and authenticity take place at the micro level (Stets and Burke, 2000). In an effort towards an inclusive definition of identity, embodied identity or the lived body experience must be included.

Embodied Identity

One's body contains and shapes their identity, it is the vessel in which one develops, experiences, and fulfills their roles and group memberships. Johnson (1983) writes, "Your whole body transmits data and organizes meaning" (p. 50). The experience of living in the body is a process of doing and being. The study of Somatics addresses this by seeking to access the wisdom of the body by exploring and reflecting on the lived body experience (Hanna, 1985). Including the lived body in the definition of identity calls attention to the constant evolving, adapting, and negotiating that is characteristic of identity formation.

Thomas Hanna poses that somatic awareness allows a person to find wisdom from within the body and to perceive the self from the inside out (Eddy, 2002; Hanna, 1985). Hanna proposed a biological view of somatics, viewing the body's wisdom or internal sensing as secluded from the social settings that the body exists within (Hanna, 1985). A much later developed view of somatics, encompassed in social somatic theory, shifts from Hanna's micro view of the lived body experience to a macro socio-political view by widening the scope to approach lived body experience as taking place within social and cultural context (Green, 2008).

Social somatic theory views lived body experiences as bearing the imprint of culture. This approach to somatics values the social experience within which the inner body experience takes place (Green, 2008). Eddy (2002) adds that the body's wisdom forms and adapts to its social environment and cannot be viewed separately from its social, cultural, and relational context. Further, when exploring lived body experience, even if intending to only explore the body in isolation from social experience, discoveries will be influenced by social and cultural values and experiences (Eddy, 2002). In other words, the lived body experience is not separate from the social context in which it exists, or the multiple group memberships, roles, and personal attributes that combine to create and influence it.

The lived body experience or awareness of the body is not separate from identity formation or awareness. In a qualitative study of participants in somatic movement work, the theme of "embodied identity" developed as a result of participant experience. Subcategories of "living in the body" and "living in relation to others in society" also developed. Living in the body was defined as becoming more aware of the body from the inside in order to strengthen awareness of identity. Living in relation to others and in society was defined as acknowledging one's embodied identity and the need for support from others (Gyllensten et al., 2010).

Becoming aware of soma, or somatic awareness, uncovers intuitive meaning of lived experiences, which through critical reflection can reveal how they affect and influence our lives (Medina, n.d.). Medina poses that our understanding of the world is, "...deeply embedded in our bodies in the form of embodied memories" (Medina, n.d.). Stinson (2004) writes, "...I have found that my body is, in a sense, a microcosm of the world, and thus a laboratory for understanding its meaning" (p. 160). She poses that feeling on a body level or exploring lived body experience requires critical reflection in order to interpret and make meaning of it (Stinson, 2004). The body holds memories of lived experiences, which must be interpreted. However, Stinson warns, "Because our bodily experiences are constructed within cultural context, there are no universal truths which derive from them" (Stinson, p. 163).

Green (1998) defines "somatic authority" as affirmation and awareness of the intuitive knowing that is felt inside the body. This is different from viewing the body based only on appearance or how the body should conduct itself, which is typical of cultures that consider the mind and body to be separate from one another (Green, 1998). In a study Green (1998) conducted, dance students explained that they experienced somatic authority in action to mean personal engagement in learning and ownership of their own body. Johnson (1983) uses the term "sensual wisdom" to describe this same sense of somatic authority and describes that people relinquish somatic authority when there is a split between the mind and body because they question their own intuitive knowing. Dominant cultures maintain this split in order that non-dominant cultures will not know their sensual wisdom or somatic authority and power (Johnson, 1983). Taking a somatic approach to teaching dance offers an alternative to perpetuating the mind-body split in the dance classroom.

Somatic Approach to Dance

Supporting and fostering the somatic authority of students, particularly of non-dominant cultures, in dance education is taking a somatic approach. Green (1998) clarifies that taking a somatic approach means to move beyond treating students' bodies as objects based on external appearance and towards facilitating possibilities for inner sensory awareness. Dance educators intending to foster somatic authority and not damage it must teach students to value and trust their bodies as valid sources of knowledge (Shue and Beck, 2001; Shapiro, 1998).

Anna Halprin began working with dance as a healing and transformative art in the 1950's. She has since developed the Life/Art Process with her daughter Daria Halprin. The Life/Art Process integrates dance, other art forms, and therapeutic practices to explore the wisdom of the body. Halprin's approach maintains that movement reveals themes from our lives. Daria Halprin writes, "The body holds our entire life experience. We understand movement as the body's primary language" (Halprin, n.d.). She further describes the wisdom of the body as revealing our social context and identity, "Body sensations, postures, and gestures reflect our history, our culture and our current ways of being" (Halprin, n.d.).

Similarly, Arkin (1994) views the body and unique experience as sources for choreography in dance. She further contends that a lifetime of transformations exist in the body. Movement and meanings can be generated and derived from the body (Arkin, 1994). Somatics is a tool and an approach to the work of understanding the lived body experience (Green, 2008). Using inner sensing to produce meaningful movements, which can be recreated repeatedly and formed into choreography, allows for critical reflection on the meaning of movement. Combining a somatic approach with a critical approach further strengthens the possibilities for critical awareness in the dance classroom.

Critical Pedagogy in Dance

The most common and accepted way of teaching dance is hierarchical and gives the teacher absolute power to treat the dancers' bodies as objects. Not only does the teacher treat bodies as objects, but also the dancers themselves are taught to objectify their own bodies and give up their somatic authority (Shapiro, 1999). Shapiro (1999) states that this does not let the dancer as subject engage in the class or develop through dance. When the body is treated as an object, a person's identity and power is fragmented and undermined. However, when the body is viewed as subject or a source of knowledge the pedagogy begins to have the undertones of social justice and liberation. Blume (2003) contributes that critical dance pedagogy can limit the oppressive split between mind and body and help to reinstate somatic authority.

Shapiro writes, "Dance must be connected to the world in order to re-create and re-shape the world" (Shapiro, 1999, p. 136). In this effort, Shapiro (1999) pioneered a critical pedagogy of the body in dance that places the body as subject, values the voice and lived experience of participants, and is for the purpose of empowerment and critical understanding. Shapiro (1998) developed the practice of the pedagogy by weaving movement vocabulary based on the framework of Laban Movement Analysis with student experiences and context (Dell, 1977).

The critical understanding or awareness sought in this approach is of the self in relation to the larger context of society (Shapiro, 1999). Shapiro (1998) writes, "It is through the critical process of reflecting upon 'lived experiences' that students can interpret the individual and social relationships in which they interact and can begin to understand their own power to reshape and recreate those relationships, hence, their own lived world" (p. 8). Critical pedagogy in dance incorporates attention to issues of power and identity, and views the body as a map that contributes to our understanding of oppression and liberation by revealing how we have been shaped by the dominant society (Shapiro, 1998). Shapiro (1998) writes, "Arts education, then, becomes revolutionary as it shows us reality – the 'what is' of our lives – in ways that heighten our perception of reality and present images to us of 'what should be'" (p. 18). However, even in this approach, the complexity of power and negotiating authority exists.

Power and Negotiating Authority

One of the complexities of implementing critical pedagogy is negotiating authority in the classroom. Establishing the dancer as subject and creating an authentic democratic way of forming content is complicated in practice. Ellsworth (1989) contends that critical approaches give the illusion of equality between teacher and students while leaving the teacher with absolute power. Further, teachers often assume that they are more critically aware or know how to "free" students from oppression and ultimately intensify the oppression they intend to work against by reproducing domination (Ellsworth, 1989).

While critical pedagogy makes direct attempts to negotiate the typical hierarchical structure of authority it is difficult to foster student autonomy without directing them in some form (Brubaker, 2009; Ellsworth, 1989). Stinson (2004) describes the tension between directing and wanting to move students towards making their own choices. She presented options for students to choose from, which resulted in students telling themselves to do what they knew the teacher wanted them to do. To this end Stinson (2004) writes, "I wanted to empower them – but did I really? Or was I just using more seductive means to produce docility?" (p. 158). Anttila writes, "A teacher can maintain external authority and control over students in many ways, even respectfully. That is why distinguishing the difference between fear of authority and genuine respect is so difficult" (2003).

Ellsworth (1989) describes that the disparity of power present in society due to culture, ethnicity, gender, and socioeconomic background is also present in the classroom. This difference in power warps our ability to engage in real dialogue in the larger society, and thus it is also warps the ability for real dialogue in the classroom. The imbalance of power cannot be transformed in a classroom regardless of the intention and effort made. Our ways of knowing, perceiving, and understanding the world are rooted in our lived experience, which is directly determined by our cultural background and identity. Teachers must seek to be critically self-aware of how they approach fostering awareness (Ellsworth, 1989). Dyer (2010) expresses the process of moving between acknowledging her own identity and facilitating empowering opportunities for students, "I came to comprehend how the line could easily be blurred between facilitating emancipatory opportunities for students, and teaching from the perspective of a cultural tourist. Further, was my realization that this perspective could easily lead to the pedagogical implementation of my own form of social indoctrination – from the perspective of how I believed the world should be" (p. 16).

Brubaker (2009) observed a teacher educator that proclaimed to be practicing critical pedagogy and arrived at the conclusion that democracy was never established but that authority was exhibited in extremes. The students were either in full control with teacher abdicating all authority or the teacher was dictating content with no student input (Brubaker, 2009). Dyer (2010) discusses how she orchestrated the components of a dance performance experience to include diverse students that created predictable and positive outcomes, "…that although an important outcome ensued that appeared to be empowering to these students, the same results may not have been achieved or topics addressed, given different social dynamics and without my acts to craft contextual factors of the experience" (p. 17). She brings another necessary dynamic to the surface by acknowledging the power she asserted to begin the project. This project moved students towards empowerment but it required that she prescribe the context to make the positive outcome a possibility.

Despite the limitations, critical pedagogy has led teachers who practice the pedagogy to understand that the "other" can never be understood (Anttila, 2003; Ellsworth, 1989). It is impossible for a teacher to be aware and inclusive of every student's reality at once, but it is possible for the teacher to be aware that they can never understand the other completely (Anttila, 2003). Ellsworth writes, "If you can talk to me in ways that show you understand that your knowledge of me, the world, and 'the Right thing to do' will always be partial, interested, and potentially oppressive to others, and if I can do the same, then we can work together on shaping and reshaping alliances for constructing circumstances in which students of difference can thrive" (Ellsworth, 1989). Uncovering the complexity of identity is a starting point for revealing that "otherness" is not finite (Ellsworth, 1989).

Stinson (2004) suggests the use of "kinesthetic empathy" as a tool to be used to seek to feel what others are feeling. However, she warns that what we sense about others may not be their reality. She discusses that verbal dialogue might be used in an effort to gain understanding, but that words have different meanings to different people. She concludes that, "...words cannot directly and completely represent our lived experiences" (p. 155). This reiterates the necessity of seeking to become aware of the lived body experience. We must unlock our identities, shedding light on our blind spots, to become aware of how our identity influences or impedes the identity formation of others. Stinson (2004) writes, "Oppression comes from outside as well as inside the self, and we must address both if we are to live in the kind of world in which freedom of expression exists for everyone" (p. 159 – 160). Teachers must seek to unlock their own identities in an effort to be self-aware of how they fill the role of teacher.

Identity Role of Teacher

The specific identity role of teacher is influenced by the previous lived body experience and the context and social group in which one teaches, which in turn creates new lived body experiences. The identity that teachers use in the context of their teaching is shaped by the culture or cultures from which it was obtained (Nevin, et al., 2009). Danielewicz (2001) contends that teachers must engage with their identity as a necessary means to "be" a teacher and not just behave as a teacher, deeming methodology and approach secondary to this engagement with identity. This illuminates why it is imperative to acknowledge and seek to become continually self-aware of the social, historical, and cultural contextual influences that develop teacher identity (Nevin et al., 2009).

Every teacher occupies the role of teaching differently and this difference is informed by skin color and gender, as well as the aforementioned personal attributes and cultural and social norms and values. Each teacher must develop strategies for negotiating how they respond to embodying the role of teacher (Ford, 2011). Teacher identity begins with a collection of values that depend on an ever-developing construction of context, experiences, and relationships (Andrzejewski, 2008). As such, a teacher's identity continues to be shaped, informed, and changed through their engagement in teaching. Hoffman-Kipp (2008) similarly discusses that teacher identity forms within classroom engagement. Identity is therefore not set, but shifting or evolving and adapting based upon social interaction and cultural influence.

The effects of dominant culture teachers on learning outcomes of non-dominant culture students is of great concern in the discussion of teacher educators seeking to better prepare teachers for multicultural teaching (Haviland et al., 2009; Ladson-Billings, 2001). Andrzejewski (2008) states that teachers' identities play a crucial role in their classroom behavior and teaching. Hoffman-Kipp (2008) provides an ample definition of teacher identity, "Given the active process of identity construction, I see teacher identity as a mix of values, beliefs, attitudes, approaches to interaction, and language that has been developed in personal realms (life history, family, community of origin) combined with understandings, pedagogical commitments and approaches, and routines of professional practice developed in teacher education programs and on the job" (Hoffman-Kipp, 2008). Teacher identity is also constructed in the body and communicated through the body, both verbally and non-verbally, as it is constantly evolving and becoming through lived body experiences. Teachers communicate their values both explicitly and implicitly in every interaction with students, which informs the structure of the teacher student relationship.

Teacher Student Relationship

The teacher student relationship is based in the tension between students needing modeling and guiding wisdom to grow and needing to be respected as experts in their own lives and experiences. There is a delicate balance between students as experts of themselves and students as non-experts of content in need of wisdom. Cultural differences add to the complexity of this, particularly when the teacher is of dominant culture. Wisdom is a result of our lived experience, which develops as a result of experiences shaped by social interactions that are shaped by cultural identity. Teachers must move toward becoming critically aware of their own cultural identity and values in order to realize the power and influence this has on their actions in the classroom and their interactions with students (Anttila, 2003).

Hoffman-Kipp (2008) states that when dominant culture identities of teachers are uninspected, engagement of students is impeded. Teachers must be aware of the reality of the various social roles and group memberships their students exist within and are influenced by. Translating the identities of students, as they are adapting and evolving, is a skill that informs the teacher's own identity (Hoffman-Kipp, 2008). Teachers, in relating with students, must be aware that self-concept and ethnic identity is influenced by relationships with others. Pena offers, "There is a variety of ways individuals practice different aspects of their social identity therefore, it is imperative for teachers to consider multiple perspectives in their teaching" (Pena, p. 19). Providing space for multiple perspectives allows students to practice and form themselves within identity roles and group memberships that are relevant to their cultural identities.

This is of great importance as students who are able to navigate learning without losing their identity are better prepared for life. Thus, students must be provided the opportunity to grow in their knowledge of their own culture in order to develop their own identity. Teachers who are self-aware of their own culture and identities are better able to facilitate students becoming aware of their own culture and identity (Ladson-Billings, 2001). In a study done with primarily dominant culture teachers who teach non-dominant culture students, it was found that being able to see the self through the eyes of others is important. Not only must teachers be able to critically evaluate their own cultural identity, but they must also acquire the skill of viewing themselves from the perspective of their students. A necessary objective in teaching cross-culturally is to move the relationship between teacher and student beyond surface level, to acknowledge cultural differences and break stereotypes (Haviland et al., 2009).

Ottey (1996) describes that it is through the teacher student relationship that dance can be a transformative power in society. Dance teachers and students must engage in the process of critical awareness and understanding together by fusing artistic content material and lived experiences to guide their exploration. The relationship is complex because students often struggle with viewing the teacher as a resource and guide as opposed to the absolute power and source of information due to previous educational experiences. However, dialogue must be established if students are to be subjects in their own learning (Ottey, 1996). The call for dialogue and dancers as subjects illuminates the need to continue discovering the possibilities for holistic development in a critical and somatic approach to dance.

Possibilities for Critical and Somatic Approach

Using a dialogical method or critical pedagogy provides the possibility of students as creators of the content explored (Freire, 2000; Nevin et al., 2009). A critical pedagogy approach can help students understand how experiences are manipulated by culture, and how the body can be used to interpret these experiences (Medina, n.d.). Similarly, somatic work participants are experts of their own bodies. Fortin writes, "Students are empowered, in turn, by being able to give input, where normally they wouldn't. Furthermore, there is a shift from alienation to authenticity. By giving the authority to the individual rather than to the experts, empowerment is achieved through personal control over one's body" (Fortin, 1998). A critical and somatic approach provides the framework and possibility of nurturing dancers towards power and agency.

REDEFINING CLASSROOM CULTURE

Co-Created Classroom Culture

Creating a "co-created" classroom culture requires input and influence from the students and teacher. Smith writes, "We must recognize the ultimate autonomy of each participant as well as the relative wisdom of teacher and student" (Smith, p. 144). This challenges the model of authoritarian teaching where the teacher is the sole creator of the classroom culture. Teachers should prepare curriculum and lesson plans that give opportunity for participant contribution and choice integrated with specific dance skills that impart experienced wisdom of content. Curriculum and lesson plans, while created by the teacher, serve as a means to hem in the teacher's influence and hold them accountable to making space for the voices and influence of the participants.

Participant Influence: Cultural Imprint

The dancers' stories or identities directly and indirectly influence the culture of the class in many ways. Each unique person participating has a story that is brought into the classroom and influences the collective experience. Each group of people establishes norms for the way they go about sharing and dancing with one another resulting in the creation of a new culture within each class.

Groups of people may have something that connected them prior to participating in a class together. Themes develop around these initial cultural connectors that influence the newly created culture of the class. Specifically, movement languages, themes in narrative, and approaches to learning movement skills and material reveal the cultural imprints of the participants and the formation of new classroom cultures.

Dance skills are interpreted through cultural lenses and therefore appear in dancers' bodies in different ways according to their life experience and stories. The difference in approach to learning a movement phrase with familiar or unfamiliar movement characteristics for various groups of people illuminates the need for space for dancers to sort out the dance skills being explored. This allows dancers to explore the skills on their own terms and in ways that are most meaningful to them as a part of the group.

Teacher Influence: Class Emphasis

Teachers should purposefully set out to get to know the people in a class with experiences to establish safety, trust, and an invitation to share one's story on their own terms. As teachers come to know students, they can then begin to emphasize specific exploration and learning that might be most meaningful. Based upon the knowledge of the participants and their development stage or phase of life, how a teacher nurtures somatic authority, provides opportunity for meaningful choice, and engages participants in dance skill will be different. The process of guiding a class over time requires constant inviting, co-creating, listening, and adapting. It is the teacher's role and responsibility to ensure that somatic authority is being nurtured, meaningful choice is being offered, and dancers are developing dance skill.

Somatic Authority

Somatic Authority. Being the expert of one's self in relation to others and environment by accepting and being aware of the inner sensing of the body as a resource of intuitive knowing and sensual wisdom (Green, 1998; Johnson, 1983)

Somatic authority is nurtured through expanding awareness of the body, self, and others. Discoveries of self and the body's capability and wisdom are accomplished in relation to others and one's social context. It is through interaction with others that we can become more aware of ourselves. To be aware of others requires understanding one's role in relation to others and perceiving others as complex beings that cannot be fully understood (Ellsworth, 1989). The more critical understanding and awareness one has, the more possible it is to exist in sensual wisdom or somatic authority.

Body Awareness

Body awareness is a necessary component of Somatic Authority. It includes how one experiences their moving body with a realistic sense of what one's body is doing, can do, and what one can challenge it to do. To be conscious or aware of movement patterns allows us to become critically aware of how we conform or resist the norms of movement and behavior (Johnson, 1983). Johnson (1983) writes, "Developing a clear awareness of how we relate to various molds is the key to recovering our authority" (p. 67). Perceiving the sensations of the body as a valid source of knowledge opens up the possibility of existing in somatic authority.

As one develops their awareness of their physical experience they can begin to become attuned to how body-shaping patterns occur in the dance classroom and everyday life (Johnson, 1983). This is beneficial to the dancer because it assists them in being the expert of self by listening to the body's cues about discomfort and new possibilities in range. The teacher can provide opportunities that encourage students to exist in their somatic authority by asking questions that help students become more aware of their bodily experience, providing exposure to new ways of moving, affirming students in trusting their own bodies, and providing pauses that allow students to listen to the sensations of the body.

Self-Awareness

Critical awareness of self is a necessary component of somatic authority. To be the expert of one's self requires knowing one's self. The embodied self, with unique attributes, is ever developing, adapting, and negotiating in response to identity roles and group membership (Stets and Burke, 2000). A dance classroom that provides space for the dancers' unique story creates opportunity for critical awareness and understanding of self. What can be discovered about self in the dance classroom is not limited to knowing one's self in this context alone, rather what can be illuminated and uncovered is beneficial to the dancer in many contexts.

Other Awareness

Connecting to others is a necessary and highly important component of somatic authority.

Johnson (1983) writes, "The more isolated a person is, the more impoverished will be the amount of sensual experience he or she has available for making decisions" (p. 175). It is through connecting and interacting with others that our sensual wisdom or somatic authority is developed. Johnson (1983) continues, "Truly reliable judgments are based on experiences that we have shared with others, honed by feedback, contrasts, and comparisons" (p. 175).

In order for awareness of others to occur in the dance classroom teachers must provide space for dancers' stories. This creates the possibility of becoming aware of the complexity and depth of others. This can occur explicitly through verbal or movement interaction, but it may also take place implicitly. The teacher's own self-awareness is imperative in ensuring that competition and comparison between dancers is not fostered, but that critical awareness of the complexity, depth, and value of others is. In providing space for unique stories, the contribution of each dancer will shape the collective story of the group.

Inside-Out Dancing

Nurturing dancers towards the experience of inside-out dancing is the primary purpose and goal of teaching with a critical and somatic approach. It is the experience of inside-out dancing that can illuminate one's somatic authority. Johnson (1983) writes, "Pressures to shape ourselves according to external images disconnect us from our own experience. Preoccupation with these images – the 'proper' way to sit, the 'correct' way to move our feet while dancing or playing a sport, the ideal alignment of the spine, the sexiest shape – distracts us from information our own bodies give us about how to do any activity most efficiently" (p. 85). Inside-out dancing is the act of bringing to life through dance the information your body is giving. It is being deeply connected in the body, with full integration of mind-body-spirit, and in relationship with the outside world as one moves. It involves listening or sensing, doing, giving, and receiving simultaneously. Dancing from the inside-out is an act of transformational art. Transformational art externalizes the internal experience and brings forth or commemorates experiences that can often not be described by words alone (Corbitt and Nix-Early, 2003).

Inside-out dancing is not limited to improvisation or self-created choreography. It can take place in repeated movement phrases when there is whole integration in each moment of movement and not just a mimicking of shapes or a sole focus on the technique needed to do the next planned movement. As a movement phrase is repeated, inside-out dancing can take place when the dancer engages in the ever-unfolding discovery of new and deeper meaning in the movement. Dancing from the inside-out is to be fully present in a moment of movement, so much so, that every cell of the body is breathing out the meaning of what is being performed and is reaching out to connect to the world; the dancer is in it, immersed, present, and connected.

The dance teacher can actively participate in facilitating the experience of inside-out dancing by intentionally calling upon dancers to connect cognitive, emotional, and physical experiences. Inquiry-based questions that engage imagination and challenge dancers to connect classroom experiences to their life experiences help to illuminate what students do know about themselves, their bodies, and others and also what there is to discover. Asking questions such as, "What does this feel like in your body?" "Does this remind you of something in life?" "How does this make you feel?" and "What did you notice about others during this experience?" assist in integrating experiences. This line of questioning activates imagination and creativity pours out. Connecting dancers to their imagination engages inner sensing and deepens the embodiment of the dance.

Meaningful Choice

Meaningful Choice. Practicing somatic authority by making decisions to steer one's learning and experience with awareness of self and others.

Providing opportunity for meaningful choice in the dance classroom nurtures somatic authority. Meaningful choice requires inner sensing and perception of others in the social context as well as an interaction with the knowledge conveyed by the teacher. However, a truly meaningful choice does not include dancers making choices based upon what they believe the teacher wants them to choose (Clement, 2007; Stinson, 2004). The development of dance skills also contributes to the dancer's ability to make meaningful choices in the dance classroom. The more developed a dancer's skills the more there is available to choose from to convey the lived body experience through movement. A dancer existing in somatic authority and equipped with dance skills is able to make meaningful choices that influence and steer growth and critical awareness.

Safety in Parameters

Providing opportunity for meaningful choices begins with teachers contributing to a sense of safety. Parameters or contained experiences with specific objectives or limitations can create a sense of safety that allows students to explore. Limits and structure give way to discovery and the formation of opinions and ideas, as well as critical awareness of self and others.

Parameters also serve as a means to facilitate student interaction with new skills. However, parameters should not be created with one fixed outcome in mind; rather they are a way to provide an entrance point to interacting with skills. For instance, the Story Dances curriculum included in this chapter results in a cumulative dance. Participants are not asked to create a dance together on the first day of class, rather the teacher facilitates contained experiences in each lesson that assist participants in developing content and movement material to be woven together to build a dance on the last day of class. Participants make choices throughout each experience, but as they develop through the course of the classes their choices become more meaningful or more influential over the whole group and the overall direction of learning. Parameters need to be created in accordance with students' dance skill awareness, comfort with creativity, and developmental stage or phase of life. Parameters for art experiences will be different for every group of students.

Listening and Adapting

As a sense of self-efficacy blossoms in students, teachers must develop with them by adapting parameters or removing them all together. This growth is a part of the dialogical exchange in the dance classroom. It occurs both verbally and non-verbally and the teacher must be attentive to both. This exchange alerts the teacher to when too many parameters are limiting creativity and discovery and when too few parameters have limited students' sense of safety to explore.

Cutler and Huntsberry (2007) discovered through their work with Sonomama Improvisation Dance Theater, "Listening implies an openness of mind, a state free of prejudice and fully alert to the present. It connotes willingness rather than willfulness and includes qualities such as receptivity, vigilance, expectancy, flexibility, vitality, trust, poise, patience, empathy, and compassion. This is the creative state" (p. 43). Students and teachers must engage in a creative state together in order for choice opportunities to be meaningful. Teachers must create an atmosphere in which the creative state can occur by listening to both verbal and non-verbal cues in order to adapt to what students are exploring, discovering, and experiencing. Parameters provide safety to explore, but as exploration begins and as students develop teachers must adapt to what unfolds.

Dialogical Exchange Indicators

As a classroom culture develops, every group will approach communicating about parameters differently. This requires the teacher to listen and adapt in different ways for each group they teach and occasionally for specific participants.

- Students will let the teacher know when they are ready to make more choices. Either with or without prompting they will begin to make more choices, expressing them verbally or physically, indicating their comfort with new skills. When this occurs it is time for the teacher to give more ongoing responsibility.
- The teacher should let students know when they are making choices and do not realize it. When students are comfortable and feel connected they will intuitively begin to make choices as a group and individually, teachers should acknowledge what is taking place so that they can be aware of their authority and excellence.
- Students will let the teacher know when the parameters are not enough. If students appear too overwhelmed to begin a task or are just not getting started it may be that there is not a clear entrance point or the uncertainty of outcomes feels unsafe. Teachers should model an example, incorporate more limitations, or work through the task once with the whole group before requiring students to be independent.
- Students will let the teacher know when the parameters are wrong all together. Students may refuse to engage, protest verbally or physically, negotiate new parameters, or the group may show relief when a new idea is presented. Teachers should gather ideas from students first, but if they do not have alternatives, teachers should create an alternate option that does not sacrifice excellence.
- Students may not engage with new skills unless there are parameters. Specific directions and limitations provide more predictability with a limited outcome. Engaging in something new this way first can then lead to experimentation and eventually greater choice in the use of the skill.
- Students will let the teacher know when to redirect an experience to follow their lead. When teachers facilitate open-ended experiences, things can unfold differently than planned and sometimes for the better. When something unfolds spontaneously that is meaningful and useful to students, teachers should quickly direct the experience to continue in the most meaningful direction.
- Students will lead if the teacher will follow. Spontaneous moments of student leadership can be profoundly meaningful. The teacher should participate and ensure safety and inclusion of all participants, being ready to shift back to leading when appropriate.

- Students will let the teacher know when to step out. As students master something they will begin to respond to one another's questions or challenges. There is no need for a teacher to interject themselves if good assistance is taking place.

Dance Skill

Dance Skill. Tools used in the art of dance in the domains of movement (how one moves the body), choreography (how one creates dance), critical analysis (how one interprets dance), and performance (how one relates to an audience).

Developing dance skill has the possibility of supporting somatic authority and broadening opportunities for meaningful choice when they are presented as tools for the dancer as subject to utilize. Thus, learning and developing dance skills involves becoming aware of the self in the experience of dance; how one moves, performs, creates, and perceives the movement of others.

Dance skills in turn become embodied knowledge as they help to articulate embodied experience. The teacher's role is to contribute their knowledge of dance skill while facilitating dancers' exploration and discovery of the use of the skills in their bodies. Modeling might be used to convey new skill information, but the teacher must be careful to prompt the focus back to what the dancer is experiencing from the inside-out.

Skill Integration

It can occur that dance skills are cognitively understood but not bodily, while others are bodily understood but not cognitively. Some dancers can define or identify a skill in another dancer's movement and practice it in contained moments, but can not apply the skill or integrate it into their own movement. Others innately or from past training have dance skills integrated into their movement but are unaware that they are skills that can be utilized intentionally. Skills that dancers are aware of only cognitively are not available for use and skills that are understood only bodily cannot be used to their fullest potential because they are not cognitively available to choose from.

When creating curriculum and lesson plans, teachers should plan dance skills appropriate to teach the group they are teaching. Teachers should also be prepared to identify and teach skills spontaneously. The spontaneous skills come about in learning based upon participant requests for more information or due to the teacher taking the opportunity to identify a skill that was being used unknowingly. It is the teacher's role to provide experiences that allow for contained and creative practice with the intended dance skills in many different contexts within the class and to creatively listen or perceive the dance skills that introduce themselves as participants explore (Cutler & Huntsberry, 2007). Teachers should ask themselves:

1. Did participants cognitively understand the skill? Could they describe it or identify it?
2. Were participants able to practice the skill in a contained moment?
3. Were participants able to integrate the skill in their dancing? Is the integration long-term?

CONCLUSION AND IMPLICATIONS

The possibility of nurturing somatic authority exponentially expands as dancers develop integrated awareness of dance skills and engage in the act of making meaningful choices. As meaningful choices increasingly result in positive outcomes affirmed by others and the teacher, trust in perception and sensing grows. This more readily enables the dancer to exist in their somatic authority. Somatic authority without meaningful choice is dormant authority. Somatic authority without skill is less critically informed.

Ability to make meaningful choice grows exponentially with a dancer's ability to exist in somatic authority and integrate dance skills. Meaningful choice is an act of somatic authority and thus the more one exists in somatic authority the more meaningful choices become. Dance skills are best utilized and most effective when they are like tools in a toolbox for the dancer to choose from. The dance classroom can provide a safe space to make meaningful choices with immediate feedback or affirmation from the group and teacher. Choice without somatic authority results in choosing what the expert would do. Choice without skill is less expansive because there are fewer options to choose from.

The development of dance skill is enhanced by the ownership that comes with somatic authority and by the choice to use skills intentionally. The dance classroom can provide a safe space to explore and discover the use of dance skills when the creativity of the dancer is engaged. Engaging creativity ushers the dancer towards steering learning and away from sole reliance on the teacher as expert. Dance skills without somatic authority are empty rituals without meaning. Bodies that can only replicate and perform the rituals of movement have not discovered the full range of possibility in the use of dance skills. Without meaningful choice, the dance skills acquired can only be used with someone else's direction.

In order to truly shift the paradigm of dance education from training dancers with the goal of perfection towards fostering dancers capable of inside-out dancing, we must begin to assess dancers based upon the values strived for in teaching with a critical and somatic approach. To teach with a holistic approach but not change the way we practice evaluation in dance education is contradictory. What one evaluates determines what is important. If only dance skill is assessed then we cannot begin to hope that somatic authority and meaningful choice are being nurtured. It is palpable that an imbalance in somatic authority and choice can exist. Perceiving when student sensing is occurring predominantly inward or outward informs how the teacher might facilitate experiences that foster critical awareness and growth.

There is still much to be discovered about what it means to holistically develop dancers in different dance classroom contexts. However, in the medium of dance that begins with the body the antithesis of using the body as a resource has been perpetuated. Treating the dancer as an object by forcing the submergence of identity and story is oppression. Acknowledging the dancer as subject with authority and power is agency. Dance educators must continue to actively seek ways to foster holistic development in practice. This gives way to healing, wholeness, and transformation.

The whole dancer must be nurtured. The focus must move from perfection to person. Nurturing the whole person allows for development without the baggage of pre-determined perfection that is culturally and body-type exclusive. Facilitating the growth of dancers who are self and other aware is beneficial not only to the dancer, but also to the art of dance. Dancers have life experience, embodied knowledge, and the capability of critical thinking to contribute to the dance classroom.

In order to practice a truly transformative critical and somatic approach, teachers must nurture dancers to explore, discover, and challenge the growth of their own range. Dancers must also be guided in enjoying the complexity of the beings that surround them in the dance classroom. Dance has the potential to intentionally nurture dancers to live in the authority and power they have been intended to live. This can nurture self-aware dancers who are able to connect to their sensual wisdom as they dance from the inside-out.

Teachers have the responsibility to nurture body, self, and other awareness in the dancers they teach. They have the responsibility to provide opportunities for meaningful choice that ebbs and flows with the growth of the dancer. Teachers have the responsibility of conveying their wisdom of the body and dance in ways that advocate for the critical use of skills. Teachers have the responsibility to engage student creativity in order that the dancers themselves will explore and discover in ways that do not make them solely dependent on the teacher as master. The greatest resources in the dance classroom are the dancers themselves.

REFERENCES

Andrzejewski, C. E. (2008). *A Holistic Investigation of Teacher Identity, Knowledge, and Practice* (Doctoral Dissertation). Ohio State University. Retrieved October 5, 2011, from http://etd.ohiolink.edu/send-pdf.cgi/Andrzejewski%20Carey%20Ellen.pdf?osu1217014454

Annual. (n.d.). *BuildaBridge*. Retrieved May 1, 2012, from http://www.buildabridge.org/programs/institute-programs/annual

Anttila, E. (2003). *A Dream Journey to the Unknown: Searching for Dialogue in Dance Education* (Doctoral dissertation). Theatre Academy, Department of Dance and Theatre Pedagogy.

Arkin, L. C. (1994). Dancing the Body: Women and Dance Performance. *Journal of Physical Education, Recreation & Dance*, 65.

Bell, J. S. (2002). Narrative Inquiry: More Than Just Telling Stories. *TESOL Quarterly*, *36*(2), 207. doi:10.2307/3588331

Blume, L. B. (2003). Embodied (by) Dance: Adolescent De/constructions of body, sex and gender in Physical Education. *Sex Education*, *3*(2), 95–103. doi:10.1080/14681810309035

Brubaker, N. D. (2009). Negotiating Authority in an Undergraduate Teacher Education Course: A Qualitative Investigation. *Teacher Education Quarterly*, 99–118.

Clement, J. (2007). *Reforming Dance Pedagogy: A Feminist Perspective on the Art of Performance and Dance Education.* University of South Florida Scholar Commons, Paper 673.

Coe, D., & Strachan, J. (2002). Writing Dance: Tensions in Researching Movement or Aesthetic Experiences. *International Journal of Qualitative Studies in Education: QSE*, *15*(5), 497–511. doi:10.1080/0951839022000019795

Corbitt, J. N., & Nix-Early, V. (2003). *Taking it to the Streets: Using the Arts to Transform your Community*. Grand Rapids, MI: Baker Books.

Cutler, C. V., & Huntsberry, R. (2007). Creative Listening: Overcoming Fear in Life & Work. Lincoln, NE: iUniverse.

Danielewicz, J. (2001). *Teaching selves identity, pedagogy, and teacher education*. Albany, NY: State University Of New York Press.

Dell, C. (1977). *A primer for movement description using effort-shape and supplementary concepts* (Rev. ed.). New York: Dance Notation Bureau Press.

Dyer, B. (2010). Ruminations of a Road Traveled Towards Empowerment: Musing Narratives of Teaching, Learning, and Self-realization. *Research in Dance Education, 11*(1), 5–18. doi:10.1080/14647891003653393

Eddy, M. (2002). Somatic Practices and Dance: Global Influences. *Dance Research Journal, 34*(2), 46–62. doi:10.2307/1478459

Ellsworth, E. (1989). Why Doesn't This Feel Empowering? Working Through the Repressive Myths of Critical Pedagogy. *Harvard Educational Review, 59*(3), 297–325. doi:10.17763/haer.59.3.058342114k266250

Erikson, E. H. (1995). *Childhood and Society*. London: Vintage.

Fortin, S. (1998). *Somatics: A Tool for Empowering Modern Dance Teachers. In Dance, power, and difference: critical and feminist perspectives on dance education* (pp. 49–74). Champaign, IL: Human Kinetics.

Freire, P. (2000). Pedagogy of the oppressed (30th ann. ed.). New York: Continuum.

Green, J. (1998). *Engendering Bodies: Somatic Stories in Dance Education*. Annual Meeting of the American Educational Research Association. Retrieved November 3, 2011, from http://www.eric.ed.gov/PDFS/ED432552.pdf

Green, J. (2008). *American Body Pedagogies: Somatics and the Cultural Construction of Bodies in the Institution of Higher Education*. Retrieved October 5, 2011, from http://content3.bestthinking.com/s/1/thinkers/864/media/75cd883e-c887-4589-b101-5a0d3b901bdc.pdf

Gyllensten, A. L., Skar, L., Miller, L., & Gard, G. (2010). Embodied Identity: A Deeper Understanding of Body Awareness. *Physiotherapy Theory and Practice, 26*(7), 439–446. doi:10.3109/09593980903422956 PMID:20649495

Halprin, D. (n.d.). *Tamalpa Institute - Our Philosophy - Statement by Co-Founder Daria Halprin*. Tamalpa Institute. Retrieved October 20, 2011, from http://www.tamalpa.org/about/philosophy.html

Hanna, T. (1972). *Bodies in revolt: a primer in somatic thinking*. New York: Dell.

Haviland, V. S., Gere, A. R., Buehler, J., & Dallavis, C. (2009). Making the Journey Toward Cultural Competence With Poetry. *Multicultural Perspectives, 11*(1), 19–26. doi:10.1080/15210960902743870

Hoffman-Kipp, P. (2008, Summer). Actualizing Democracy: The Praxis of Teacher Identity Construction. *Teacher Education Quarterly.*

Johnson, D. H. (1983). *Body: Recovering Our Sensual Wisdom.* Berkeley, CA: North Atlantic Books.

Kelso, P. T. (2003). Behind the Curtain: The Body, Control, and Ballet. *Edwardsville Journal of Sociology, 3*(2). Retrieved April 2, 2012, from http://www.siue.edu/sociology/EJS/v32kelso.htm

Ladson-Billings, G. (2001). *Crossing over to Canaan: the journey of new teachers in diverse classrooms.* San Francisco: Jossey-Bass.

Medina, Y. (n.d.). *Critical Aesthetic Pedagogy: Toward a Theory of Self and Social Understanding.* Retrieved October 6, 2011, from http://qcpages.qc.cuny.edu/Education/AE%20Conference%20Proceedings/articles/Critical%20A esthetic%20Pedagogy.pdf

Nevin, A., Bradshaw, L., Cardelle-Elawar, M., & Diaz-Greenburg, M. (2009). *Becoming a Teacher: A Cross-Cultural Analysis of Motivation and Teacher Identity Formation.* Retrieved October 6, 2011, from the ERIC database.

Ottey, S. D. (1996). Critical Pedagogical Theory and the Dance Educator. *Arts Education Policy Review, 98*(2), 31–39. doi:10.1080/10632913.1996.9935096

Pena, D. C. (1998). *Three Teachers' Histories.* Retrieved October 11, 2011, from the ERIC database.

Shapiro, S. B. (1998). *Toward Transformative Teachers: Critical and Feminist Perspectives in Dance Education. Dance, Power, and Difference.* Champaign, IL: Human Kinetics.

Shapiro, S. B. (1999). *Pedagogy and the politics of the body: A critical praxis.* New York: Garland Pub.

Shue, L. L., & Beck, C. S. (2001). Stepping Out of Bounds: Performing Feminist Pedagogy within a Dance Education Community. *Communication Education, 50*(2), 125–143. doi:10.1080/03634520109379239

Smith, C. (1998). *On Authoritarianism in the Dance Classroom. Dance, Power, and Difference.* Champaign, IL: Human Kinetics.

Stets, J. E., & Burke, P. J. (2000). Identity Theory and Social Identity Theory. *Social Psychology Quarterly, 63*(3), 224–237. doi:10.2307/2695870

Stinson, S. W. (2004). *My Body/Myself: Lessons From Dance Education. In Knowing bodies, moving minds: towards embodied teaching and learning* (pp. 153–167). New York: Kluwer Academic Publishers.

Tajfel, H., & Turner, J. C. (1986). *The Social Identity Theory of Inter-group Behavior. Psychology of intergroup relations* (2nd ed.). Chicago: Nelson-Hall Publishers.

KEY TERMS AND DEFINITIONS

Dance Skill: Tools used in the art of dance in the domains of movement (how one moves the body), choreography (how one creates dance), critical analysis (how one interprets dance), and performance (how one relates to an audience).

Meaningful Choice: Practicing somatic authority by making decisions to steer one's learning and experience with awareness of self and others.

APPENDIX: STORY DANCES CURRICULUM

Story Dances

Lesson No. 1

Lesson Title: I Am From: Part I

Lesson Overview: Students will write self-reflective poems about where they are from and create symbolic movements to be combined into a movement phrase.

Goal: Increase students' ability to create symbolic movement, to work with others, and to identify influences on identity formation. Increase student awareness of inner sensing and somatic authority.

Lesson Objectives:

1. Engage students' creativity (artistic)
2. Increase students' ability to work together (social/spiritual)
3. Increase students' experience with writing self-reflective poetry (artistic/academic)
4. Increase students' experience with choreographing symbolic movement (artistic)

Measurable Outcomes: By the end of this lesson,

1. 100% of students will perform a movement phrase.
2. 100% of students will be able to create symbolic movement.
3. 100% of students will be able to write a self-reflective poem as demonstrated by the poem written.

Lesson Breakdown:

1. **Name Game With Movement And Adjective:** Standing in a circle each student chooses a word that describes them and makes a movement that expresses their chosen word. Going around the circle, each student says their word coupled with their name while doing their movement. The group then responds by repeating it back to them. As each new name and movement is added, the group repeats all that have been done. To close the game, the movements will be performed as a movement phrase without speaking the words. *Speak the blessing that students have now choreographed their first dance.
2. **Call and Response Affirmation:** "I am beautifully and wonderfully name. I am more precious than all that is valuable in this world. I will surround myself with people who want the best for me. I will surround myself with people who see me. Everything I do is worth watching. Everything I say is worth listening to" Debrief the affirmation by asking students what they think each line means.
3. **Movement Phrase:** Discuss style values and meaning of movement.
   a. Decide collectively what each movement in the sequence could mean creating a narrative and/or symbolism.
   b. Hope circle symbolic movement:

c. Standing in a circle teacher asks students to create a movement that represents "hope." Movements will be linked together to create one movement phrase.

4. **"I am From" Poems:** Using the prompts (derived from Trapeta B. Mayson's "I Am From" poem prompts, BuildaBridge Institute 2011) participants will write their own "I am From" poem. Participants may use as many or as few of the prompts as they choose.

I am from (list your favorite place in your home) ____________________
I am from (list two of your favorite relatives by name or nickname) __________ and __________
From (list a smell that reminds you of home) ____________________
From (list two favorite foods that don't come from the corner store, like "fried plantains") ________ and ____________
I am from (list 2 family sayings that are said in your home like "a hard head makes a soft behind") ____________________ and __________________
From ____________________
I am from________________
I am from______________
From ______________

5. **Sharing:** After completing the poems, participants will choose one, two, or three lines from their "I am from" poems to share with one another.
6. **Closing Ritual Affirmation With Movement:** "My hands hold my purpose, my worth, my experience, my story. I cannot do all the things the world needs, but the world needs all that I can do."
7. **Journal Free Write:** Students will write about their experience in the class session.
   a. Materials & Supplies
   b. Writing utensils
   c. Music
   d. Student journals

Lesson No. 2

Lesson Title: I Am From: Part II

Lesson Overview: Students will create symbolic movement, both independently and collaboratively, based upon the content of their poetry.

Goal: Increase students' ability to recall memories and influences of identity formation. Increase students' ability to empathize with others, to create symbolic movement, and to work with others. Also, increase student awareness of inner sensing and somatic authority.

Lesson Objectives:

1. Engage students' inner sensing and somatic authority (spiritual)
2. Engage students' creativity (artistic)
3. Increase students' ability to work together (social/spiritual)
4. Increase students' experience with choreographing symbolic movement (artistic)

5. Increase students' ability to recall lived body experience (artistic/spiritual)

Measurable Outcomes: By the end of this lesson,

1. 100% of students will be able to create symbolic gestural movement and postural movement.
2. 100% of students will be able to collaboratively choreograph a movement phrase.

Lesson Breakdown:

1. **Name Game With Movement And Adjective:** Standing in a circle, students will share one word and a movement that represents how they feel.
2. Call and Response Affirmation
3. **Movement Phrase:** Explanation of gestural and postural movement as students try movement:
    a. **Gestural Movement:** Peripherally initiated, involving only part of the body.
    b. **Postural Movement:** Centrally initiated, involving full body.

Ask students what the other movements in the phrase are, gestural or postural?

4. **Hope Circle:** Students to come up with a new word to create to this week.
    a. "We need hope in life, what are some other things we need in life?"
    b. Each student creates a GESTURAL movement that represents the chosen word.
    c. Students develop their GESTURAL movement into a POSTURAL movement.
    d. Weave movements together to create a movement phrase.
5. **Choreographing Uniqueness:** "I am from" movement: Students will choose a space in the room and create two movements, one gestural and one postural, that represent one or two poem lines that are most meaningful to them.
6. **Weaving Uniqueness Together for a Collective Voice:** Students teach one another their movement and weave it together to create a movement phrase. Students to invite next person through Mutual Invitation.
7. Closing ritual affirmation
8. **Journal Free Write:**
    a. Materials & Supplies
    b. Music
    c. Writing utensils
    d. Student journals

Lesson No. 3

Lesson Title: I am Going

Lesson Overview: Students will write poems about where they are going in life and continue to choreograph, both independently and collaboratively, movement that represents this to them.

Goal: Increase students' ability to write self-reflective poetry, to imagine, to create symbolic movement, and to work with others. Also, increase student awareness of inner sensing and somatic authority.

Lesson Objectives:

1. Engage students' inner sensing and somatic authority (spiritual)
2. Engage students' creativity (artistic)
3. Increase students' ability to work together (social/spiritual)
4. Increase students' experience with writing self-reflective poetry (artistic/academic)
5. Increase students' experience with choreographing symbolic movement (artistic)

Measurable Outcomes: By the end of this lesson,

1. 100% of students will be able to choreograph movement intentionally using at least one LMA effort-shape concept.
2. 100% of students will be able to write a self-reflective poem as demonstrated by the poem written.

Lesson Breakdown:

1. Name game with movement and adjective.
2. Call and Response Affirmation.
3. Movement phrase.
4. **Improvisation:**
   a. Body part initiation and Effort-shape concept improvisation (Dell, 1977): Body part initiation.
   b. Call specific body parts to lead the rest of the body in movement pathways.
   c. Effort-shape.
   d. Time: Quick and sustained time.
   e. Weight: Strong and Light.
   f. Flow: Bound and Free.
   g. Space: Direct and Indirect.
   h. Free improvisation.
5. **"I am Going" Poems:** Students will write "I am Going" poems beginning with prompts provided, but not limited to the prompts.

I Am Going
I am going (a place) ______________________
I am going (how it smells, looks, feels, and tastes) __________, __________, __________, and ____________________
I am going (what is valued there) ________________________
I am going ____________________

6. **Sharing:** Standing in a circle. Participants choose two to three lines from their "I am Going" poems that are most meaningful to them to share. Mutual Invitation through dancing to another person.
7. **Choreographing Uniqueness:** Students to create movement using at least one effort-shape concept that represents one or two poem lines that are most meaningful to them.

8. **Weaving Uniqueness Together for a Collective Voice:** Students teach one another their movement and weave it together to create a movement phrase. Students to invite next person through Mutual Invitation.
    a. Closing ritual affirmation
    b. Journal free write
    c. Materials & Supplies
    d. Writing utensils
    e. Music
    f. Student journals

Lesson No. 4

Lesson Title: I Am

Lesson Overview: Students will draw self-portraits, create verbal and non-verbal self-affirming statements, and choreograph a cumulative dance.

Goal: Increase students' ability to self-affirm, to identify barriers and envision solutions, to create symbolic movement, and to work with others. Also, increase student awareness of inner sensing and somatic authority.

Lesson Objectives:

1. Engage students' inner sensing and somatic authority (spiritual)
2. Engage students' creativity (artistic)
3. Increase students' ability to work together (social/spiritual)
4. Increase students' experience with drawing a self-reflective visual art piece (artistic)
5. Increase students' experience with choreographing symbolic movement (artistic)

Measurable Outcomes: By the end of this lesson,

1. 100% of students will be able to draw a self-reflective visual art piece as demonstrated by the drawing completed.
2. 100% of students will be able to collaboratively choreograph a movement image using all participating people.
3. 100% of students will be able to choreograph movement and structure as demonstrated in the final dance made.

Lesson Breakdown:

1. Name game with movement and adjective.
2. Call and Response Affirmation.
3. **"I Am" Self Portraits:** Ask students again what the affirmation "I will surround myself with people who see me" means to them. (Possible teacher contributions: people who seek to see the inside of you and do not define you based on appearance alone, as well as, being a person that seeks to

"see" others). Then ask students to draw a self portrait of their inside self in order to be seen and see others. When portraits are complete, ask students to reflect on what they see about themselves in their portraits.

4. **Sharing:** Describe your portrait and what it says about you.
5. **Self Affirmation Statements:** "I am from ________, I am going ________, because I am ___________. Consider using imagery, metaphor, or symbolism.
6. **Movement Affirmation Statements:** Collectively choose a spot in the space that represents where we are "from" and create a still shape that represents or symbolizes this to you. All students will stand in their shape and say the"I am from _____" portion of their statement.
   a. Collectively choose a new spot in the space that represents where we are "going" and create a still shape that represents or symbolizes this to you. All students will stand in their shape and say the "I am going _______" portion of their statement.
   b. Students solidify a pathway to walk that is direct or indirect to move between "from" and "going" points in space.
   c. Ask students to then begin to talk out loud about what barriers they might or do experience to getting to where they are going as they walk between their "from" and "going" spots. Then repeat the walking pattern and have students talk out loud about what they have that will help them overcome the barriers
   d. Concept derived from Theatre of the Oppressed "walk and talk" experience.
   e. Students share barriers and ways to overcome barriers. What things do we need to get where we are going? What things will help us overcome the barriers? What things do we have uniquely and collectively?
7. **Collaborative Movement Image:** Collectively create one movement image that expresses a barrier being overcome.
8. Students create one shape that represents "because I am _____" portion of statement.
9. **Choreograph Cumulative Dance:** Collaboratively decide how to weave together all parts previously choreographed. OR

Teacher selects sequence.
"From" statue
Speak statements
"From" collective movement phrase in unison
Walk pathway
"Overcoming barriers" large group image
Walk pathway
"Going" statue
speak statements
"Going" solos
"I am" statue
speak "I am" statement

10. Closing ritual affirmation
11. Journal free write
12. **Celebration:**
    a. Materials & Supplies
    b. Colored pencils, crayons, markers, colored pens, pencils, and sketch paper
    c. Music
    d. Student journals

Chapter 12
Collaborative Art and Relationships

Tessa L. Hitz
Eastern University, USA

ABSTRACT

This study supports the value of collaborative visual artmaking in the pursuit of strong relationships, healthy bonding, and the development of the whole child. Based on educational, artistic, and child development theory, this mixed-methods study utilized arts-based collaborative experiences to measure potential growth in the areas of bonding, attachment, and relationship development between child and caregiver pairs (dyads). Through informal art-making sessions, caregivers and their child experienced collaborative artmaking and rated their own personal view of their relationship and bond with their dyad partner in pre and post-assessment surveys, through interviews and storytelling, and through observation using a bonding assessment chart. It was found that collaborative artmaking does indeed have a positive effect on the deepening of relationships and supports an increase in positive family behaviors and dynamics.

INTRODUCTION

Relationship is at the core of how we live and who we are as human beings. Our desire for human interaction comes from how we are wonderfully designed and factors into how we mature, grow, and survive. Our basic social structures, our happiness, even our all-encompassing health and whole development depend upon how we are influenced by relationship. We are designed as relational beings that crave connection and thrive when appropriate social supports are present and active in our lives. The relationships we have with people who care for us while we are young and who are an integral presence in our younger years influence and directly shape who we become as adults (Siegel, 2015).

In today's digital and fast-paced age, intimate and in-person connection and deep relationship is often glossed over or simply overlooked. Many people have lost the ability to enter into deep relationship with another individual or a group and truly connect on a personal level. Trust is difficult to find and attachment and close personal bonds are difficult to develop within a culture and society that screams

DOI: 10.4018/978-1-5225-5981-8.ch012

for individuality, independence, and making it "on your own." Social Capital, or value in relationships and in the reciprocal benefit of social relationship is not a priority or even something that individuals or communities consider. Sadly this is a trend that affects family structures as well. The availability of technology in the home has impacted how families communicate and how children learn to socialize. Increased screen time and decreased face-to-face time is slowly taking its toll on socialization skills and how children interact with and communicate with those around them. "Social capital matters for children's successful development in life" (Putnam, 2000, p. 299) and in turn affects our families and communities in which they live (2000).

Collaborative creativity fosters an instant connection to others through our five senses. We see artwork, watch a dance theatre production, hear music, and taste carefully prepared foods. These sensory experiences immediately connect us as both the creator and participant or as the observer, creating common thought processes and opening opportunities for communication and interaction. Music and movement have been utilized for years as educational, developmental, and social supports for young children and their families. This chapter further explores this creative realm and offers observations on how the visual arts may support and enhance family relationships through collaborative creativity and art making experiences.

Thankfully the arts have a natural ability to reach across borders and create connections. Music can speak across language barriers even if one cannot understand the lyrics. Dance, facial expressions and movement are universal, and visual art can communicate without words or sounds. This expressive ability has powerful potential within relationships and specifically within the realm of mental health and education when verbal and direct communication is not always possible or effective.

Relationship bonding and social attachment is essential from birth. Attachment is the mammalian capacity for an infant to depend on a parent for his or her survival. Determined by the limbic area of the brain, attachment is essential to bonding and full and holistic social development(Siegel, 2015, p. 141). Our social development is essentially "the way in which our brains remember the attachment relationship(s) we have had, or still have, and how we have adapted to these formative attachment experiences" (Siegel, 2015, p. 141).

Even "infants depend on their caregivers for healthy internal development" (Colle, 2013, p. 7), setting the foundation for a healthy internal development that has a lasting effect on our physical, mental, and emotional systems as we grow and mature. This long-term effect "makes it important for adults that did not have the chance to develop a healthy attachment to *learn* how to form a healthy stable attachment" (Colle, 2013, p. 7).

Sometimes physical touch and presence are not possible during the early critical development time of a child's life due to circumstance or trauma (Grigsby, 1994). The statistics of American children related to a possible lack of relationship and attachment is startling. According to the US Department of Health, of the American children "who experienced maltreatment or abuse, nearly 80% suffered neglect" in 2013 (2015). Non-traditional family dynamics, fostering and adoptive situations, parent's military deployment, incarceration or chronic illnesses sometimes prevent the development of long-term deepening relationships (Lowenstein, 2010). Words and verbal communication are not always available to support bonding, attachment, and the development of a relationship with young children or non-verbal individuals. Traditional methods of education and bonding can fall short and not effectively serve all members of a population. People's lives are busy and difficult and some days the simple truth is that devices and screens can be an easy choice on a hard day (Steiner-Adair & Barker, 2013).

In a constantly changing digital society that puts less and less importance on interpersonal skills and family connections, it is imperative to find the means to have quality time and create connections. Taking time away from the screen, off of devices, and making time to connect directly with one another creates lasting connections that will carry through to the later stages of life and may influence how individuals will interact with others on a societal level.

Brains and Bodies by Design

Our brains and bodies are designed in an amazing and intricate way when it comes to growth, development, and health. The intricacies of how the brain and body react and influence emotions, thoughts, and communication with other people is even more fascinating, and the most integral concept is that each of these realms are all connected. The neuroscience behind relationship and holistic health is complex and compelling. Daniel Seigel defines the term *relationship* as "the sharing of energy and information flow" (2015, p. 52), and he discusses this not only referring to other people but as the connections between the basic systems within our bodies. Our physical body, emotional state, and spirituality all share information in relationship to make up our identity and our personality. We learn, grow, and adapt through the transfer of energy and information shared with us through our surroundings and the people that we interact with on a daily basis.

Our ability as humans to take in information and not just instinctively react to it, but to process and intellectually choose our response is unique. Our ability to relate to others is essential to our ability to develop and hold relationships. One integral part of successful relationships is our ability to recognize the spiritual capital (value and abilities) in ourselves and recognize it in others (Zohar & Marshall, 2004). Once value is recognized in another individual, this sparks the transfer of energy that leads to relationship. The first and most valuable spiritual capitol we come into contact with is that of our own family members in childhood. If this bonding foundation is unable to happen, or a disruption causes this process to be stopped early on in a child's life it can cause a lasting affect. These long-term effects can impact adult relationships and holistic development (Stams, Juffer, & van IJzendoorn, 2002). A sense of empathy, ability to trust others, and an awareness of others needs can all be compromised.

The Whole Child

As we grow and mature, our most integral times of growth and development occur as young children. Once we are old enough to begin communicating and responding with those around us, our social interactions become a huge influence on our learning and growth in all development areas. According to Maslow's theory of the Whole Child this includes an awareness of and sensitivity to a child's physical health, safety, social engagement, emotional support system, and intellectual stimulation or challenge. When these areas are all met, a child is able to learn, grow, and thrive. Each of these development areas is essential and intertwined in the complete development of the whole child. Negative effects on physical health and development can impact emotional and social development, self-esteem, and even academic growth and ability (Maslow, 1943).

Relationships, Attachment, and Bonding

Relationships, attachment, and bonding are essential parts of natural human development. Attachment is a natural development within a healthy relationship and it "is generally accepted that children who are securely attached to a caregiver usually appear relaxed, happy, and enthusiastic while interacting with that person" (Alexander, 2015). Relationship and bonding is integral for holistic health at any age, but it is essential in the first year and even weeks of life. Research has already proven that physical contact can improve health from early on, but there seems to be an even deeper and intrinsic effect from healthy attachment. "When an internally stable caregiver provides sensorial contact, it promotes the development of a healthy central nervous system in infants. Research is revealing evidence for a link between maternal attachment and brain development" (Colle, 2013, p. 7). At such an early age, brain development is vital to the rest of an infant's physical, emotional, and mental development. In her book *Creative Arts and Play Therapy for Attachment Problems*, Cathy Malchiodi (2013) explains succinctly just how important the role of attachment is in our healthy development. She discusses the effect of age on brain development and attachment, stating that "brain plasticity is greater earlier in life - a fact underscoring the importance of appropriate intervention with young children in order not only to enhance attachment, but also to support the development of appropriate affect regulation, interpersonal skills, and cognition" (p. 7).

While attachment does have a physical aspect that provides comfort, it is much more than the simple physical need for contact. According to John Seigel, attachment is about being *seen*, being and feeling *safe*, and being *soothed* (2015). "Contact or gaze, which provides focus and an early form of communication is an event that gives the infant a sense of self" (Kerr & Hoshino, 2008, p. 66). Seigel's three "S's" of attachment formulate his comprehensive approach to bonding. Individuals who have formed healthy attachment can go to their caregiver and feel as if they are not just physically seen and acknowledged but fully understood. They feel safe and nurtured, and they feel calm, regulated, and cared for. If one of these "S" areas is not present, then there is likely a gap in the attachment bond.

The Power of the Dyad

Dyadic therapy allows for new venues of communication between individuals. In parent-child-dyad therapy there are two sets of pair relationships. The two relationships are between the therapist and the dyad, and between the parent and the child. This approach to therapy allows for a relationship to develop, and therefore more than observation is needed. The therapist and the parent become more than observers and listeners and are encouraged to be active participants alongside the child.

In arts-based dyad therapy, the communication lines are opened up in a whole new way, allowing for non-verbal cues and communication, as well as audible conversation and written words. Dyadic experiences are also valuable in the non-clinical setting, encouraging intentional relationship and collaborative communication. The aim of this type of intervention and experience is meant to increase bonding and work on the relationship between one caregiver at a time. Therefore, "a child cannot participate in this art therapy intervention without a primary adult to contain him and help him through the process" (Proulx, 2003, p. 36).

When working with preschool aged children and toddlers who cannot yet write or draw recognizable figures, a familiarity of "non-representative art" (Proulx, 2003) is encouraged to make sense of the mark making done by the youngest child participants. This difference in visual communication brings about a unique opportunity for the therapist to set the parent to work at the child's level, both challenging themselves to let go of the pressures of their age-appropriate abilities and to meet and support the child on their level. This encourages and advocates the child in his/her abilities and helps the parent to better understand where his/her child developmental level is. It also provides a method of non-verbal communication for children who are too young to speak fluently or who have a non-verbal condition or block. Giampaolo gives great insight into the challenges of children who are on the autistic spectrum and how art can benefit them. He discusses how difficult it can be for parents to build relationships with their children due to the social engagement and communication impairments that can manifest as a result of living with autism. He goes into detail explaining how children with autism do in fact show secure attachment patterns; the parent-child relationship is often strained because of the child's impairments in social interaction. These impairments include: the child's lack of motivation for relating, an inability to understand another person's thoughts and feelings, mentalization, and difficulty with joint attention. (2013)

Group dyad interventions can be useful as well. The primary goal of group dyad intervention also helps to reinforce the emotional ties between the caregiver and child and "transmits information about the emotional, social, and cognitive development of the child, and the age appropriate capabilities of the child" (Proulx, 2002, p. 42). In addition, group dyad interventions can create an atmosphere and environment that fosters commonality and solidarity between the caregivers as well. This support network and social interaction can be just as important of a development. This author's proposed study will most likely involve such groups that form a community working toward healthy attachment.

Collaboration and Play

Collaborative and play interventions could easily be applied to individuals who are experiencing long-term effects from trauma and stress and who may be working on healing and coping skills within a clinical setting. Thobaben (2013) discusses how "(these) activities can give children some of the emotional support they need to help them heal and provide an opportunity for children to maintain healthy cognitive and emotional developmental growth even while they are homebound." While the article is specifically discussing a physical healing, the connectedness of physical and mental health is widely known and an influence in how a whole persona is holistically healthy. "Whenever the child plays, there is some degree of transformation" (Levine, 1998, p. 260). Play is how we naturally experiment in various settings and in turn, learn. Successful playgroup experiences and "mommy and me" classes are based around the musical arts and its imperative role in development. *Mother Goose on the Loose,* for example, is a highly successful early literacy program based on music and rhythm and collaborative play between the parent/caregiver and the child (mgol.com, 2015). The design of this program provides a setting for playful interactions between a child and caregiver through the use of music and movement. The music, instruments and toys, and rhythmic movements provide opportunities for interactive sharing and collaboration. The give and take of play interactions encourages moments of non-verbal communication, even with children who are not yet literate or verbal.

Thobaben explains and delves into the importance of creative thought and play in a child's holistic development and states that neglecting those areas can hinder healing. She also discusses specifically how reading and writing should be included in these creative experiences, and how nurses and other home-caregivers can incorporate them into a child's routine. This author maintains that these same activities and experiences could be just as valuable within a dyad relationship and collaborative setting. Further research could be done with this concept in mind.

Play has an ability to create connection, allow expression and freedom, and create co-creators and participants of artists. Through the work of philosophers and psychologists, Katarzyna Zimna discusses the concept of "childsplay" and the transition from viewer and observer to participant (2010, p. 143). Writing from a high school and adult age focus, the discussed concepts of play, active participant, and creative expression and communication are very integral concepts to attachment and relationship. Her discussions correlate well with this potential study and will be of use in learning and defining concepts, terms, and defending the worthwhile need for collaborative art making and play in healthy relational development. A healthy environment for this to happen is one that is safe and one that allows for mess and chaos in a contained way so it is emotionally manageable for participants. (Hosea, 2006).

Zimna's primary focus is based on the concept of play theory and supports how it is a tangible and useful approach not only in clinical therapy but also in the healthy growth and development of an individual. Her discussions on the transition from observer to active participant in art making will translate well to parents and guardians growing from the position of observer to active and engaged participant with his/her child. Malchiodi (2013) mentions the model of *Theraplay,* developed in the 1970's, which focuses on healthy parent-child interactions and attachment. Theraplay allows for families to interact together in a fun, playful and natural way while fostering healthy communication and deepening attachment. This model has become particularly valuable with adoptive families (Weir et al, 2013).

Why the Arts?

Sometimes healing requires more than talking about the problem. Holistic healing and whole development considers the whole person and can provide various methods, activities, and options for wellness and growth within many different settings and for many different purposes. The arts and creative therapy provides a tangible outlet that goes beyond the normal realms of communication and experience. "Music has an important role as healer when it brings about a holistic wellness that includes the body, mind, soul, and community" (Corbitt, 1998. p. 145). Visual art at its core, is non-verbal, and provides a new way to communicate that does not require words. As an infant, obviously words are not an option, and even as a child, sometimes the words and vocabulary simply are not yet present. Emotional blocks may be present and communicating may become difficult, inaccurate or even impossible. The arts can provide a place of safety where thoughts and feelings can be expressed without words.

Even in adults, "for some individuals, conveying a memory or story through one or more expressive modalities is more easily tolerated than verbalization" (Malchiodi, 2014). A creative avenue can provide a new form of communication that will not only help an individual tell his/her story, but also process his/her memories and information. "Meaningful exchanges through art experiences for intergenerational partners are those shared events that have personal relevance" (Whiteland, 2012). Non-verbal communication traverses through generations.

Music has long been an artistic avenue that has sparked discussion about the arts and its benefit for health and social interaction. In the 1700's, the first documented article that discusses music therapy is found. In the 1950's, Alfred Schutz proposed that music making influenced social relationships (Schutz, 1951). Just a year earlier, the first organized music therapy group "the National Association for Music Therapy (NAMT) was founded at a meeting in New York City" (musictherapy.org, 2016).

At their foundation, growth and development are holistic. Creative development is also intertwined into this as well. If music has been successful in the development and support of social skills, bonding, and relationships, why not visual art? Artistic development can sometimes be a tangible indicator of emotional and intellectual development (Levick, 1998). Research has proven that "the visual arts are an important part of a brain-based education. They can enhance cognition, emotional expression, perception, cultural awareness, and aesthetics; they can play a significant role in the learning process" (Jensen, 2001). Art can be used as an experience to foster growth and can also be used as an indicator of growth and development.

The theories behind this designed intervention are based on various theories in education, child development, and the arts. A strong focus is on the needs of healthy development of the Whole Child as described by Maslow's (1943*) Hierarchy of Needs* and how Bonding and Attachment builds the basic layers of that hierarchy. When caregivers, who provide a child's basic physiological needs and provide a safe and healthy environment, emotional support and love are present, a child has the chance to grow and develop to his/her full potential. Eric Jensen proposes that the arts are essential to child development and absolutely must be part of a holistic education and intellectual development (2001). Together, the application of these theories can provide the healthy foundation and ideal environment for whole child development. The following described arts intervention was designed to support parenting skills and increase awareness of collaborative art making as a valuable tool in child development and relationship building.

METHODS AND APPROACH

In support of the development of the whole child and the deepening of family social relationships, the author developed an arts-focused intervention based on her exploration of the realm of visual art as a method of communication and creative outlet. Bonding skills, social-emotional connection, and relational ability are essential to an individual having a support network and to successfully develop social awareness skills. This is especially important for a developing child. Arts-based experiences are a meaningful and essential way to develop and build these skills. The results of this art intervention provide support for this under-researched facet of psychology and education, allowing for potential insight into helpful arts-based activities and experiences that could be used by caregivers at home and in the community and by educators in the classroom to support family bonding and healthy child development.

Participating in the arts activates different areas of the brain that can allow for alternate methods of communication and for increasingly open dialogue and interaction (Beiver, 2015). While this intervention certainly did not intend to provide therapy, the author recognizes that for families facing the effects of trauma or children dealing with difficulty in language acquisition or communicative issues, art making experiences could be incredibly helpful in providing an alternative experience to cope and communicate within the home setting. This new flexibility or alternate means of communication and interaction could assist in the growth and healing process of family relationships and of the individual. Parents wanting to better connect with their young child in a new way could experience deeper connections, better bonding, and a new form of communication. "Such a shared experience, weekly or periodically, may indeed help them to develop a new mode of communication" (Proulx, 2003, p. 25).

The following described intervention is built on the use of the visual arts in a safe, meaningful, and trauma-informed setting. There, children and their parents or guardians can collaborate and create together as they bond and communicate visually through their artwork experience. The collaborative art making intervention took place with community members who willingly volunteered to participate in art experiences with their child and who were willing to be open and possibly grow and experience change through the process. Arts Based Community Development (ABCD) utilizes "art-centered activities that contribute to the sustained advancement of human dignity, health and/or productivity within a community" (Corbitt & Nix-Early, 2003, p. 28). For the purposes of this intervention experience, the family unit was viewed as a small, intimate community. Therefore, this author's intent is to support the developing growth, relationship attachment and overall health of local families who participate in this study through the arts.

The experiences of the intervention were designed and executed from the perspective of an educator, artist, and one who desires to support and strengthen parenting and family relationships. The author has witnessed the ability of the arts to transform and enhance quality of life and build relational connection. When done collaboratively, art making becomes more than just creating and making, and becomes a form of communication. Caregiver relationships are essential to the development of a healthy and whole child. The author is confident in the ability of the arts to reinforce parent–child relationships and hopes to support the research and validity of the arts in child development and relationship.

Designing the Intervention

To test the efficacy of this intervention, the author conducted a study through a series of ten art making sessions that took place over the course of seven weeks. Child and caregiver pairs (dyads) were split and scheduled into groups based upon the age of the child to create communities that were developmentally appropriate to be taught and create art together effectively. Participants were voluntarily assessed prior to the first session and again after the last session using questionnaires and verbal surveys. Questionnaires and surveys assessed both the caregiver and child on how closely bonded they believed their relationship to be. Each session provided a visual arts based experience for the caregiver and child to share collaboratively. The arts based experiences intentionally fostered situations for the caregiver and child to practice both verbal and non-verbal communication and encourage moments of teamwork, sharing, leading, and receptive following. A focus was kept on process and teamwork and not on the final product. Observational data on bonding and interactions was collected using a Parent Child Observation Tool (Heffron, Children's Hospital and Research Center, 2006). Caregivers and older children were also interviewed at the close of the study for qualitative data and personal storytelling opportunities. The purpose of the study was to explore how regular collaborative art making would encourage deeper communication and foster bonding between caregivers and children. Information gleaned from this study will equip caregivers with art based activities and tools to increase creative bonding with their children in the comfort of their own home.

The study collected quantitative and qualitative assessment of nine families after their experiences of creating and exploring art making together. Calling on art teaching experience, the author designed and guided each art experience to foster an environment of collaboration, communication, and teamwork between each child and parent.

The study sought to address the following questions:

1. *How does the phenomenon of collaborative visual art making impact relational bonding and attachment between child and caregiver dyads?*
2. *Does collaborative art making increase communication between young pre-verbal/preschool children and their caregiver?*

Sampling

Convenience sampling was utilized to form the study population. The author's personal connections and professional networking within educational and holistic health fields provided a population with diverse family histories ranging from traditional nuclear families, adoptive and foster families, and non-traditional homes. Careful consideration of and sensitivity to past experiences and traumas were taken while selecting families to participate. This consideration aimed to ensure a mixed group that provides a realistic and well-rounded sample. Though the sampling represented the overall population trend of the geographic area, the sampling was not as diverse ethnically as would lend to a strengthened study. The participating group was made up of working middle-class Caucasian families with children between the ages of 2 to 10 years. The parents ranged between 30 to 50 years of age, and varied as to whether they were employed full-time, part-time or worked as a stay-at-home parent. There was also variation as to whether the participating child was the parent's first born child or not. Various family dynamics and structures were represented such as intact nuclear families, divorced or separated parents, adopted children, and children with learning disabilities.

The nine families that participated in this study were split into two groups by the ages of their children. Children under school age (ages 2-4 years) gather as one group while elementary aged children gather as a second group. This allowed for age-appropriate activities to be planned to cater to motor and cognitive skill levels as well as for children with similar social and language levels to be in sessions together. These consistencies allowed for more genuine social interactions between both child-to-child and parent-to-parent.

Data Collection and Analysis Procedure

Data was collected through a variety of methods. As a qualitative mixed-methods study, storytelling and interviews with both the parents and children were utilized as well as quantitative and qualitative pre and post-assessments completed with surveys. A Bonding Assessment Chart is utilized to collect quantitative data through observation during the art making sessions. This chart aids in focusing on specific behaviors and actions that give indicators into the depth and connection of a relationship. Video recordings of the sessions as well as photographs of the participant artwork were also taken into consideration for assessment.

Analysis involved looking for changes in knowledge, behavior and outlook through surveys, in-person discussion, and storytelling as well as increases in specific measurable behaviors and actions. A Bonding Assessment Chart was utilized to document and quantifiably measure behaviors and actions that display bonding and attachment qualities. Behaviors observed and documented on the chart included intentional and subconscious actions such as meaningful and safe touch, effective or ineffective communication, eye contact, displays of empathy and understanding, and appearing or not appearing to enjoy one another's company. It was intended to see if a growth in any of these behaviors or areas was seen from the first session to the last. A bonding chart was filled out for each dyad pair by a research assistant each art making session.

The bonding charts were then compared with the video recordings and instructor notes to catch any additional behaviors and interactions. Pre and Post Surveys and Final Survey comments and informal discussion interviews provided qualitative data on the opinions and thought processes of the participations during and after the sessions completed.

INTERVENTION ACTIVITIES AND RESPONSES

Artwork and Art Experiences

The artwork and art experiences were designed to create spaces and times for participants to engage in collaborative, communicative art making. A unique activity and art making experience was planned and organized for each weekly session. These experiences resulted in multiple finished works of art, but also some artwork that focused more on process than product. It was intentionally communicated to families that the experience of working together as a team was the priority of the exercise – not necessarily the creation of a beautiful piece of art. The art making process served as a vehicle for the partnering dyads to work cohesively and intentionally together toward a goal.

Various art materials and processes were used throughout the sessions. Drawing, painting, collage, sculpture and construction, basic printmaking, and non-traditional art tools were all explored. Each day's session focused on a different material and process to provide a variety of experiences and to speak to all abilities and interests. Participants were always highly encouraged to use a material in new ways an in a manner that facilitated teamwork between the child and parent.

Parents were often timid at first, and less likely to be playful than their child, but every parent eventually relaxed, loosened up, and allowed themselves to have fun and get messy by the end of a session. Multiple parents voiced specifically how the experiences altered their own personal view of art making. One parent even said that they now have an increased desire and ability to engage in art activities at home with their child.

Figure 1. Parents and child creating together

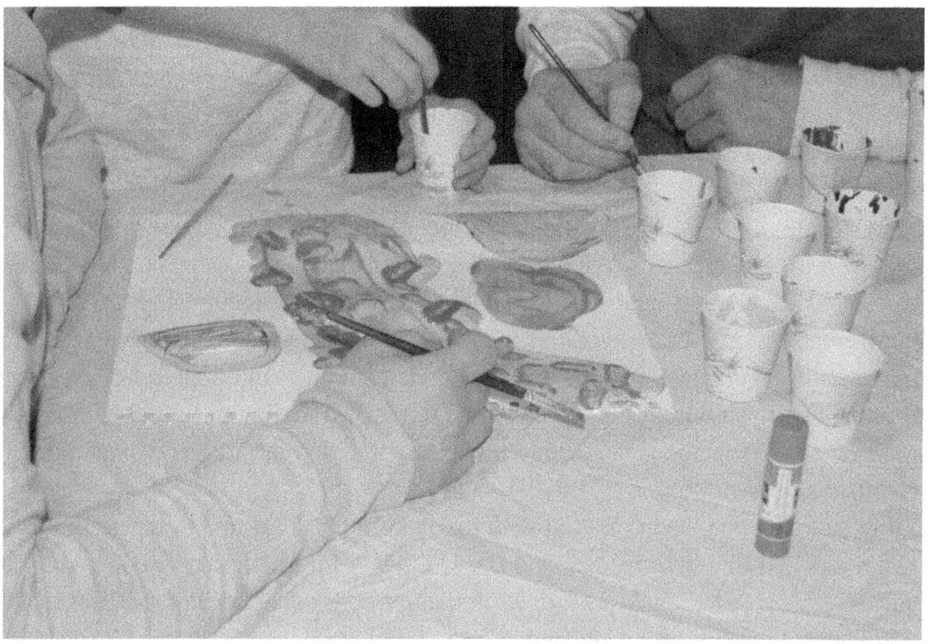

Figure 2. Mother and child together

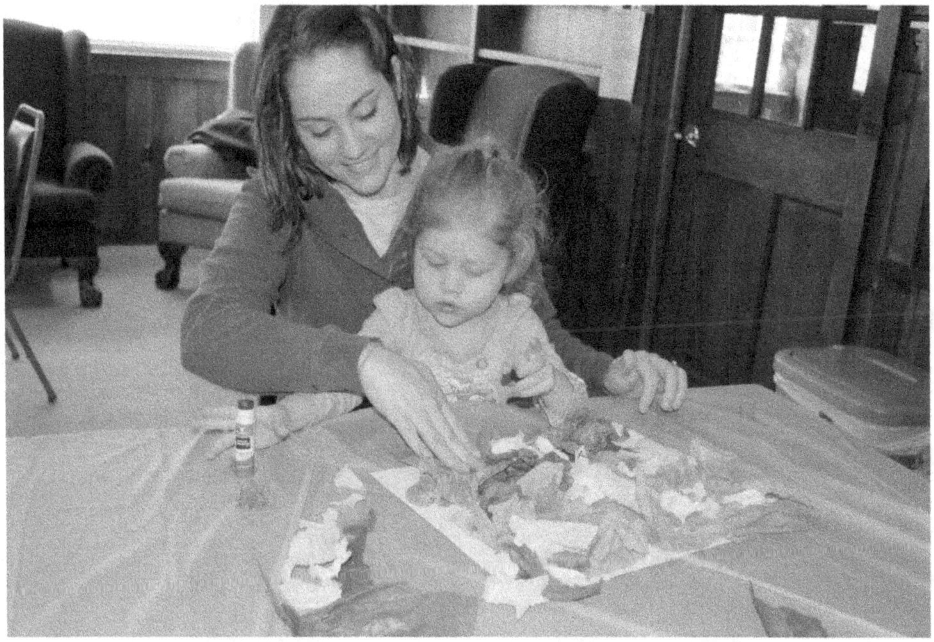

Pre-School Age Experience

The pre-school aged group activities and experiences were designed to encourage interaction between parent and child without the need for extensive verbal conversation. This consideration was necessary in a group with ages ranging from 2 years to 4 years. This covers a large range of developmental stages and also includes a child who is identified as highly functioning on the autism spectrum. Instead, activities were designed to foster situations that encouraged the dyadic pairs to participate in turn-taking, responding to one another's choices and actions, expressing their own ideas, and in partnering physically and mentally in the artistic tasks set before them.

Elementary Age Experience

The elementary aged group followed similarly to the pre-school group in the materials and types of finished art pieces they produced, but their journey to arrive at that goal was altered to fit the appropriate developmental and verbal levels (see Table 2). Dyadic pairs were certainly still encouraged and guided to participate in taking turns, responding to one another's choices and actions, and overall teamwork behaviors. However, the higher levels of communication skills and developmental abilities allowed for a different level of teamwork that required both child and parent to actively listen to their partners' requests, desires, thoughts, creative ideas, and dislikes.

Figure 3. Mother and child building

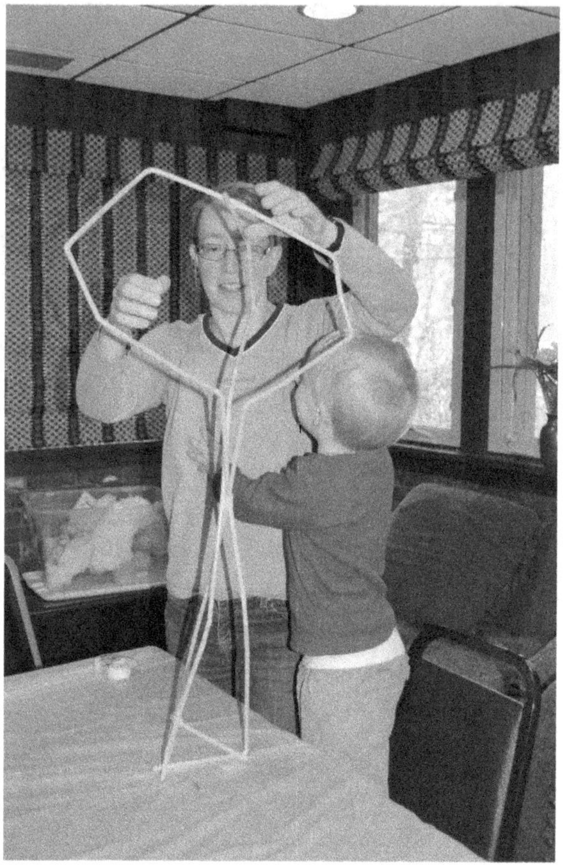

Video Recordings, Photographs and Personal Observations

Video recordings of each session were taken during instruction of art making processes, while participants were taking part in their art making experiences, and during any closing discussions and comments to aid in observation and recollection of specific interactions and happenings during each class session. Photographs of collaborative artworks were collected to document art making processes and final creations. Photographs were also taken to document moments of teamwork and collaboration between the parent and child while creating together.

Bonding Assessment Charts

Bonding assessment charts were utilized to rate dyadic behaviors and interactions during each class session. A chart was completed for each dyad pair for each weekly session. Allowing for such abnormalities and outliers such as illness, fatigue, and off-days, these assessment charts show minimal or no growth or change in attachment and bonding behaviors for any of the participants. It is the author's belief that growth in these areas happened but assessment over a longer time frame would produce more accurate and meaningful quantitative results.

Table 1. Pre-School Aged Art Making Experiences

	Activity/Theme	Positive Behavior/Interaction Encouraged
Session 1	*Masking Tape Painting:* Parent and child took turns placing pieces of tape on their paper to create designs and shapes. *Color Mixing Discovery/Finger Painting:* Dyads were given primary color pairs to allow child to discover color mixing by finger painting over their masking tape designs. Parents were highly encouraged to finger paint alongside their child. Tape was then removed at the end of the session to reveal designs and patterns.	Loosening up/Relaxation, Turn-taking, Exploration, Verbal Communication, Child-like discovery and play, Paying attention to and connecting with child. Creating ***with*** instead of just alongside one another.
Session 2	*Parent-See, Parent-Do* - Parents were instructed to follow along and paint like their young child, following motor skill level, type of painting tool (or lack of) style, mark-making, and technique as much as possible.	Connection, Observation, Mimicking, Discovery and play, Child-like exploration.
Session 3	*Tissue Paper Collages* – Texture and manipulation exploration. Parents controlled glue sticks while child had control of choosing paper color, shape, and manipulation. The dyad then traded jobs, taking turns gluing and choosing/tearing paper.	Taking turns, Boundaries and shared responsibility, Verbal Communication Skills, Teamwork, Creating ***with*** instead of just alongside one another.
Session 4	*Potato Printmaking* – Parents helped child to create "stamps" out of small potato halves. Children explored stamping their designs. Very simple directions were given to allow for open creativity and open-ended options.	Teamwork, Shared responsibility, Simple art techniques for home, Imaginative play, Creating ***with*** instead of just alongside one another.
Session 5	*Straw Painting-* Dyads were challenged to find as many ways to use straws to paint as possible (blow paint, drip, roll straw on paper etc). *Straw Sculptures* – Dyads used straws and tape to create sculptural structures	Exploration, Child-like play, Teamwork, Roles/respective jobs and ability awareness, Creating ***with*** instead of just alongside one another.
Session 6	*Group Drawing Prompts* – children and parents were encouraged to follow drawing prompts on large paper on the floor *Picture Frame Open Studio* – Dyads were prompted to choose their favorite materials and techniques that they've used over the past weeks and decorate a commemorative picture frame with those materials and techniques.	Choice-making, Teamwork, Communication, Exploration, Reinforcement, Turn-Taking, Celebration

Pre and Post-Surveys

The pre and post surveys show the most valuable quantitative data from this study (Figure 2). All parents and all elementary-aged participants completed a pre-survey at the first class and a post-survey of the same questionnaire at the last class. Elementary-aged children completed a simplified version of this survey by themselves or with the author dictating and marking the child's oral answers. Survey questions covered domains including feelings of connection between the parent and child, levels of understanding between parent and child, and comfort in communication between parent and child. Through these surveys, 56% of the study participants demonstrated growth in at least one domain between the first art session and the last art session (see Figure 1). Five out of the nine parents who participated showed an

Figure 4. Mother and daughter discussing their artwork

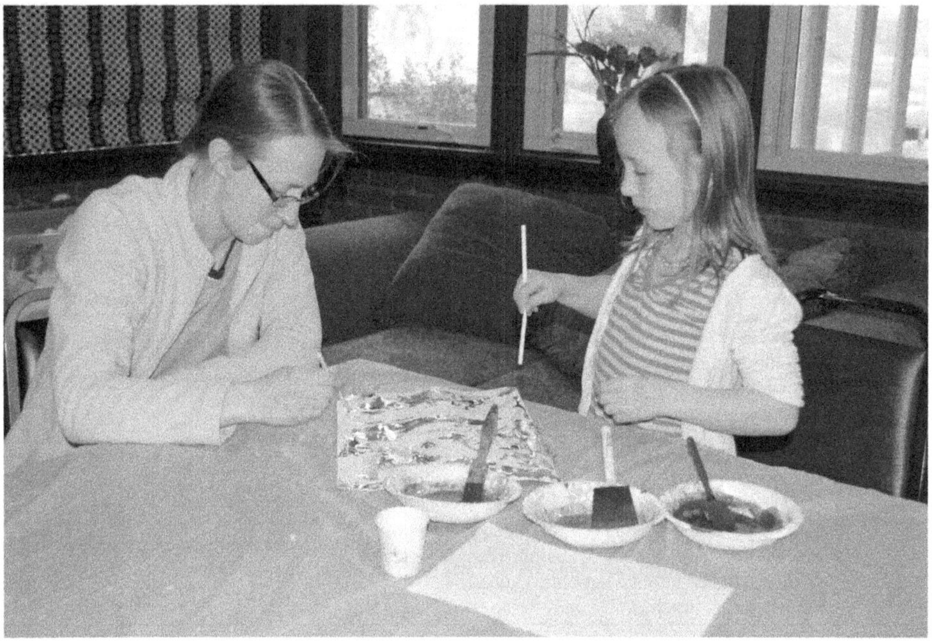

Table 2. Elementary-Aged Art Experiences

	Activity/Theme	Positive Behavior/Interaction Encouraged
Session 1	*Masking Tape Painting:* Parent and child take turns applying tape to their paper in designs and patterns of their choice. Parents were then instructed to paint like their child, following motor skill level, type of painting tool (or lack of) style, and technique. Masking tape was then removed to reveal designs and patterns.	Loosening up/Relaxation, Turn-taking, Exploration, Verbal Communication, mimicking, Child-like discovery and play, Paying attention to and connecting with child. Creating ***with*** instead of just alongside one another.
Session 2	*Tissue Paper Collages* – Dyads chose their image as a family team. Parent and child shared responsibilities by taking turns as to who controlled the glue stick/where tissue paper gets placed and glued down vs. choosing the tissue paper colors and shape.	Turn-taking, Verbal Communication Skills, Teamwork, Creating ***with*** instead of just alongside one another.
Session 3	*Straw Painting*- Dyads were challenged to find as many ways to use straws to paint as possible (blow paint, drip, roll straw on paper etc). *Straw Sculptures* – Dyads used straws and tape and were challenged to create a sculpture that resembled a vehicle or architectural structure. Parent and child were instructed to take turns and add one part at a time to their structure.	Imagination, Exploration, Childlike play, Teamwork, Roles/respective jobs and ability awareness, Creating ***with*** instead of just alongside one another.
Session 4	*Group Drawing Prompts* – children and parents were encouraged to follow drawing prompts on large paper on the floor *Picture Frame Open Studio* – Dyads were prompted to choose their favorite materials and techniques that they've used over the past weeks and decorate their frame with those materials and techniques.	Choice-making, Teamwork, Communication, Exploration, Reinforcement, Turn-taking, Celebration

increase in at least one domain on their post-assessment survey. Two out of the four elementary-aged children who completed surveys their own survey showed an increase in at least one domain. Two parents reported increases in three domains.

Open-Ended Surveys

The open-ended surveys used at the conclusion of the series of sessions provide some simple but highly valuable qualitative data through open-ended written responses. These questions focused on each of the family's experiences during and since the art sessions. Each parent was given an opportunity after the completion of the sessions to give thoughtful and reflective responses about how the sessions may or may not have affected their interactions with their child, how they may have changed any ideas about their relationship, or any changes they may have considered making in their home or in how they interact with their child . Every parent made at least one comment that implies both the need and the desire for a meaningful change in how parents in general choose to interact with their child. Many parents even voiced that they were consciously going to implement a change or already have seen changes developing in their home environment.

Some of the more valuable responses collected included comments of how the parent had a revelation about themselves in relation to their parenting approach, or came to notice something about their child for the first time. When asked about something that was learned through the experience, one parent commented "I don't sit down and actually play enough with my child." Others commented that they realized how creative their child was, or came to notice likes and dislikes they were not previously aware of.

Parents also described how things changed at home, and specified examples of growth that they had witnessed in their child. One mother wrote that she noticed her son now actively wanted her to play with him and verbalized his requests for that interaction. Another mother stated that her son was more willing to have one-on-one time with her than before. Every family commented that they had decided to make some sort of intentional change since the completion of the sessions. Many stated that they wanted to continue participating in art making experiences with their child because they recognized how enjoyable it was for them to share that quality time together. Three families also mentioned how witnessing their child be independent and try new things successfully made them feel more comfortable with allowing their child to do things for themselves and allow them to be more self-sufficient.

Figure 5. Pre and Post-Survey Results

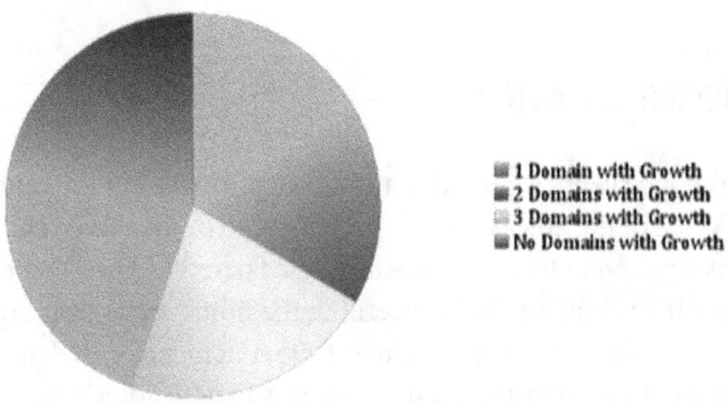

This study group was small and the sessions only met for a limited amount of time, but the growth and impact witnessed clearly indicates potential for long-term positive outcomes. Art making instances demonstrated incredibly powerful and personal emotions for each family that experienced them. These findings speak to the positive outcomes that collaborative art making experiences could foster and support in the future.

Autism, Adoption and Collaborative Art

Two families in particular reported the most powerful storytelling and most dramatic outcomes and examples of growth. The fascinating part was that in terms of stereotypical situation and environmental factors, these two families had room for the greatest amount of growth and change given that "J" was identified as an individual with autism, and "D" was adopted and both children struggle with attention skills, impulsiveness, and a high need to move and be active constantly. Despite our short time together over six weeks, growth and intentional changes were still tangibly witnessed.

Both children in question were high energy, extremely bright and creative, and had fantastic imaginations. Both mothers of these children were observed to be extremely patient, kind, and were highly in tune to their respective child's needs. However, both mothers described a desire to be able to better play with and interact with their child and did not know how to have that happen. Art making with these two families was oftentimes a bit chaotic and not always fully effective when it came to the finished project at hand, but the experience was visibly impactful. On a good day, both children would focus on the task at hand, would communicate openly and responsively with their mothers, and would both verbally explain their excitement and enjoyment of the experience. Verbal communication of impulsive desires and wants are not a strength of these children, so witnessing them take turns with tools and materials weekly, strategically plan how to build a structure out of beverage straws with their mother, and willingly engage in teamwork was unexpected and beneficial.

The verbal and written feedback from these two mothers was powerful. J's mother responded in her final survey that their interactions at home had changed since the art making sessions. She wrote about her four year old: "I noticed that J started asking me to play with him. Now he is asking constantly." It was found in talking with the mother that this is a significant change in social behavior for this child who struggles with communication and social interactions. She is joyfully accepting this change in home life dynamics and is embracing it. Similarly, D's mother wrote: "D has been more willing to sit and do an activity with me one-on-one than he was previously." In a multiple-child household, Mom was thrilled that there was now a way for her to connect with her middle child in a meaningful way and that he willingly wanted to spend this time with her.

CONCLUSION AND IMPLICATIONS

The described connection intervention provides a small step forward in the relevancy of the arts in holistic development, the value of the arts as part of the education of the whole child, and the impact of the arts supporting relationships and collaborative behaviors. There has been some valuable literature and research in the past about the visual arts being useful in the home setting for both play and educational purposes for parents and caretakers (Cohen & Gainer, 1995) but much is outdated or out of practice. New knowledge and findings would support the need for the arts in education as an integral part of fostering connection through communication skills and social awareness. Over all, the intervention further supports the validity of arts-based education and arts-based experiences as essential in the development of the whole and healthy child.

It is this authors hope that this collaborative intervention will provide experiences and tools that will foster healthy relationships within families and encourage creative play at home between children and their caregiver. In a culture so focused on technology and screen time pursuing valuable face-to-face time is so necessary. Further study is required to fully understand and appreciate the possible implications for collaborative art making on the development of deep and meaningful relationships with healthy attachments. Positive and beneficial results were certainly present with 56% of all participants reporting some form of growth in bonding and attachment behaviors and with 23% presenting meaningful qualitative data through storytelling and open reflections that inspired personal change and choices to take action for growth within their family community. Unexpected but positive results were seen that support further study of the arts and collaborating alongside individuals with autism. Longer and lasting effects would likely be seen through regular collaborative art making practice. If these small but positive results were seen from only six weeks worth of experiences, it is thrilling to think of what six months of regular collaboration in the art room could bring to relationships and families.

REFERENCES

Alexander, C. J. (2013). *Bonding assessments*. Retrieved November 10, 2015, 2015 from http://alexanderphd.com/BONDINGASSESSMENTS.html

American Music Therapy Association. (2016). *History of Music Therapy*. Retrieved from http://www.musictherapy.org/about/history/

Barone, T., & Eisner, E. W. (2012). *Arts Based Research*. Los Angeles: SAGE.

Bleakley, A., Jordan, A. B., & Hennessy, M. (2013). The relationship between parents' and children's television viewing. *Pediatrics*, *132*(2), e364–e371. doi:10.1542/peds.2012-3415 PMID:23858418

Bowlby, J. (2008). *A secure base: Parent-child attachment and healthy human development*. Basic Books.

Bretherton, I. (1992). The origins of attachment theory: John Bowlby and Mary Ainsworth. *Developmental Psychology*, *28*(5), 759–775. doi:10.1037/0012-1649.28.5.759

Cahnmann-Taylor, M., & Siegesmund, R. (2008). *Arts-based research in education: Foundations for practice*. New York: Routledge.

Cohen, E., & Gainer, R. (1995). *Art, another language for learning* (3rd ed.). Portsmouth, NH: Heinemann.

Colle, S. (2013). *Using Focusing-Oriented Art Therapy to Form Secure Attachments: A Grant Proposal Submitted in Partial Fulfillment For the Degree of Master of Arts in Marriage and Family Therapy*. Retrieved October 24, 2015, from https://scholar.google.com/citations?view_op=view_citation&continue=/scholar?hl=en&as_sdt=0,39&scilib=1&citilm=1&citation_for_view=1x9Nc4gAAAAJ:LkGwnXOMwfcC&hl=en&oi=p

Cooper, M., & Sjostrom, L. (2007). *Making art together: How collaborative art-making can transform kids, classrooms, and communities*. Beacon Press.

Corbitt, J. N. (1998). *The sound of the harvest: Music's mission in church and culture*. Grand Rapids, MI: Baker Books.

Corbitt, J. N., & Nix-Early, V. (2003). *Taking it to the streets: Using the arts to transform your community*. Grand Rapids, MI: Baker Books.

Dosamontes-Beaudry, I. (2003). *The arts in contemporary healing*. Westport, CT: Praeger.

Dunn-Snow, P., & D'Amelio, G. (2000). How Art Teachers Can Enhance Artmaking as a Therapeutic Experience Art Therapy and Art Education. *Art Education, 53*(3), 46–54. doi:10.2307/3193873

Durrani, H. (2014). Facilitating attachment in children with autism through art therapy: A case study. *Journal of Psychotherapy Integration, 24*(2), 99–108. doi:10.1037/a0036974

Giampaolo, A. (2013). *Drawing autism: parental perceptions of the impact art therapy has on communication patterns and the parent-child relationship*. Retrieved October 25th from https://dspace.smith.edu/bitstream/handle/11020/24205/GiampaoloforLibraryFinal9913.pdf?sequence=1

Grigsby, R. K. (1994). Maintaining attachment relationships among children in foster care. *Families in Society, 75*(5), 269.

Hosea, H. (2006). "The Brush's Footmarks": Parents and infants paint together in a small community art therapy group. *International Journal of Art Therapy*, 69-78. Retrieved October 28, 2015, from http://www.tandfonline.com/doi/abs/10.1080/17454830600980317#.VjA9UktFtGw

Jensen, E. (2001). *Arts with the brain in mind*. Alexandria, VA: Association for Supervision and Curriculum Development.

Kerr, C. (2008). *Family art therapy: Foundations of theory and practice*. New York: Routledge.

Levick, M. (1998). *See what I'm saying: what children tell us through their art*. Dubuque, IA: Islewest Publishing.

Levine, E. (2015). *Play and art in child psychotherapy: An expressive arts therapy approach*. London: Jessica Kingsley Publishers.

Levine, E. G. (1998). *On the play ground: Foundations of Expressive Arts Therapy: Theoretical and Clinical Perspectives*. London: Jessica Kingsley Publishers.

Lin, N. (2001). *Social capital a theory of social structure and action*. Cambridge, UK: Cambridge University Press. doi:10.1017/CBO9780511815447

Lowenstein, L. F. (2010). Attachment Theory and Parental Alienation. *Journal of Divorce & Remarriage, 51*(3), 157–168. doi:10.1080/10502551003597808

Mackenzie, J., & Hamlett, K. (2005). The Music Together program: Addressing the needs of. *Australian Journal of Music Therapy, 16*, 43.

Makin, S. R. (2000). *Therapeutic Art Directives & Resources: Activities & Initiatives for Individuals & Groups*. London: Jessica Kingsley Publishers.

Malchiodi, C. (2014). *Creative arts and play therapy for attachment problems*. New York: Guilford Publications.

Malchiodi, C. A. (2003). Art therapy and the brain. Handbook of Art Therapy, 16-24.

Malin, H. (2013). Making meaningful: Intention in children's art making. *International Journal of Art & Design Education*, *32*(1), 6–17. doi:10.1111/j.1476-8070.2013.01719.x

Maslow, A. H. (2013). *A theory of human motivation. origin 1943*. Martino Fine Books.

McNiff, S. (1998). *Art-based research*. London: Jessica Kingsley.

Mother Goose on the Loose. (2015). Retrieved from http://www.mgol.net/home/why-mgol/

Nicholson, J. M., Berthelsen, D., Abad, V., Williams, K., & Bradley, J. (2008). Impact of music therapy to promote positive parenting and child development. *Journal of Health Psychology*, *13*(2), 226–238. doi:10.1177/1359105307086705 PMID:18375628

Plante, P., & Bernèche, R. (2008). A phenomenological study addressing the reinforcement of emotional ties between parent and child through the elaboration and evaluation of dyadic art therapy groups. *Canadian Art Therapy Association Journal*, *21*(1), 18–34. doi:10.1080/08322473.2008.11432297

Ponteri, A. K. (2001). The effect of group art therapy on depressed mothers and their children. *Art Therapy: Journal of the American Art Therapy Association*, *18*(3), 148–157. doi:10.1080/07421656.2001.10129729

Potash, J., & Ho, R. T. (2011). Drawing involves caring: Fostering relationship building through art therapy for social change. *Art Therapy: Journal of the American Art Therapy Association*, *28*(2), 74–81. doi:10.1080/07421656.2011.578040

Proulx, L. (2002). Strengthening ties, parent-child-dyad: Group art therapy with toddlers and their parents. *American Journal of Art Therapy*, *40*(4), 238.

Proulx, L. (2003). *Strengthening emotional ties through parent-child-dyad art therapy: Interventions with infants and preschoolers*. London: Jessica Kingsley Publishers.

Putnam, R. D. (2000). *Bowling alone: The collapse and revival of American community*. New York: Simon & Schuster. doi:10.1145/358916.361990

Schütz, A. (1951). Making music together: A study in social relationship. *Social Research*, 76–97.

Seigel, D. (2015). *Brainstorm: the power and purpose of the teenage brain*. New York: Penguin Random House.

Stams, G. J. J., Juffer, F., & van IJzendoorn, M. H. (2002). Maternal sensitivity, infant attachment, and temperament in early childhood predict adjustment in middle childhood: The case of adopted children and their biologically unrelated parents. *Developmental Psychology*, *38*(5), 806–821. doi:10.1037/0012-1649.38.5.806 PMID:12220057

Steiner-Adair, C., & Barker, T. H. (2013). *The big disconnect: Protecting childhood and family relationships in the digital age*. Harper Business.

Thobaben, A. M. (2013). The role of art and literacy activities in Children's healing process. *Home Health Care Management & Practice*, *25*(3), 123–125. doi:10.1177/1084822313476299

U.S. Department of Health and Human Services, Administration for Children & Families. (2015). *Child Maltreatment 2013*. Retrieved from http://www.acf.hhs.gov/programs/cb/resource/child-maltreatment-2013

Van den Dries, L., Juffer, F., van IJzendoorn, M. H., & Bakermans-Kranenburg, M. J. (2009). Fostering security? A meta-analysis of attachment in adopted children. *Children and Youth Services Review*, *31*(3), 410–421. doi:10.1016/j.childyouth.2008.09.008

Weir, K. N., Lee, S., Canosa, P., Rodrigues, N., McWilliams, M., & Parker, L. (2013). Whole Family Theraplay: Integrating Family Systems Theory and Theraplay to Treat Adoptive Families. *Adoption Quarterly*, *16*(3-4), 175–200. doi:10.1080/10926755.2013.844216

Whiteland, S. (2012). *Examining visual art experiences for relationship building in shared-site locations*. Retrieved October 28, 2015, from http://digital.library.unt.edu/ark:/67531/metadc115180/m2/1/high_res_d/dissertation.pdf

Zimna, K. (2010). *Play in the theory and practice of art*. Academic Press.

KEY TERMS AND DEFINITIONS

Collaborative Art-Making: Creative play or art-making that is a collaboration or interactive teamwork between two or more individuals. For those of non-verbal age or ability, this can become a visual conversation.

Holistic: Considering the whole, defined here as referring to health. Holistic health is made up of the domains of physical, mental, emotional, and spiritual. When one domain is changed or impacted, all domains are affected.

Relationship: Relationship is defined here as the connection between individuals or the way people can become socially connected. Relationships have varying depth and intimacy that comes with intention, trust, and effort on behalf of the individuals involved.

Whole Child Development: A development and educational approach that recognizes that socio-emotional, physical, creative, and cognitive capacities are all intertwined and equally important in ensuring a child's wellbeing, learning, and growth into an adult and member of society.

APPENDIX

*Table 3. Sample Collaborative Art Making Lesson**

SESSION 1
Positive Behavior/Interaction Encouraged: Loosening up/Relaxation, Turn-taking, Exploration, Verbal Communication, Child-like discovery and play, Paying attention to and connecting with child. Creating ***with*** instead of just alongside one another.
Activity: ***Masking Tape Painting and Color Discovery (Part I)*** *Materials needed: heavy paper, masking tape, non-toxic/finger paint* • Parent and child take turns placing pieces of tape down on their *shared* piece of paper to create designs and shapes. • Encourage parent to talk with their child and to let the child have the authority to place their own tape ***(Part II)*** • Provide finger paints in primary color pairs to allow child to discover color mixing as they apply paint over their masking tape designs. • Encourage parent to finger paint alongside their child, *not* correcting or showing the child the "right way" • Remove tape at the end of the session to reveal designs and patterns left by the covered areas.

*Ideas for these interactions were inspired from the work of Lucille Proulx and her book *Strengthening Emotional Ties Through Parent-Child-Dyad Art Therapy: Interventions With Infants and Preschoolers.* To learn more or to see her original activities and art experience ideas, please read her book.

Proulx, L. (2003). *Strengthening emotional ties through parent-child-dyad art therapy: Interventions with infants and preschoolers.* London: Jessica Kingsley Publishers.

Chapter 13
Community Music Therapy Partnering With Community Musicians:
Orchestral Dialogues – Accepting Self, Accepting Others

Janelle S. Junkin
BuildaBridge International, USA

ABSTRACT

This chapter discusses the collaboration of community musicians and community music therapists working to create a community orchestral dialogues experience for youth patterned after a Middle Eastern model. The author explores the definitions of community musicians, music therapy and community music therapy, and how these definitions diverge and converge. The author explains and discusses Orchestral Dialogues: Accepting Self, Accepting Others and the learning that took place for the youth involved, as well as for the staff, both community musicians and community music therapists. The final section of the chapter provides lessons learned and implications for future collaborations for community musicians and community music therapists.

BACKGROUND: PERSONAL RELATIONSHIP TO COMMUNITY MUSIC AND MUSIC THERAPY

Music is not designed for privacy or containment – it naturally reverberates, permeates, goes through boundaries and walls. And in doing so it calls to others, attracts, gathers, connects people together. It creates community. (Pavlicevic & Ansdell, 2004, p. 16)

A 7-year old girl sits in the church pew and hears the flute played for the very first time. The sound wraps itself around her, in her and she knows, just knows, that this instrument, this sound must be made by her. Instinctively, she knows that with this instrument she can express herself in ways that words fail.

DOI: 10.4018/978-1-5225-5981-8.ch013

This child was me. There was no explanation, just an innate knowledge that I was meant to play the flute. At age 9, my flute and I began a journey that began with lessons. By age 12, I was performing in public and by age 15, I had performed in front of an audience of 300 people; I was also a member of a chamber orchestra. Throughout my childhood and youth, I always preferred to be part of a group rather than the soloist. I knew that music was my medium, and I knew I wanted to study it, but I did not want to teach or to be a performer despite being groomed for performance. I approached my band director about my relationship with music and performance when I was 16. My teacher told me about this area called "music therapy" and encouraged me to investigate this as a career. In 2001, I completed my education in music therapy and became a board-certified music therapist.

Being a both a clinical music therapist and a community musician (CM) was wonderful, but something was missing: how to connect these two passions. Then, in the fall of 2012, the answer presented itself in the form of an article describing Community Music Therapy (CoMT). Community Music Therapy was appealing as it seemed to connect the two worlds of music therapy and community musician (CM). The two main ideas of the article that resonated most with me were 1) being invited to contribute expertise to a community and 2) that the community had what it needed for its own healing. Approaching clients and community engagement through a strengths-based lens combined the clinical elements of music therapist and the training of a community musician.

Integration of self as musician, music therapist, and as someone who is knowledgeable in how those skills can interact within a community, may seem to be incongruous. There are, however, intersections of theory and practice in these two areas creating space to complement and collaborate. Finding these intersections served as an inspiration to continue to bridge the space between community musicians and music therapists. To begin to forge these connections of how exactly to complement, collaborate, and creatively work together, a shared understanding of terms is necessary.

A Shared Language

Defining Community Musician (CM)

What is a community musician? This question is not easily answered as there are several understandings of a CM, expressed through varying worldviews. The literature suggests that there are multiple ways to define a CM that include how to educate students, where to educate students, how to measure that success, and how to be present in the community. (Everett, 1997; Veblen, 2008; Walters & Shuman, 2008). Understanding the definition of CM begins with the context of the musical experience. Veblen (2008) of the Community Music Activity Commission (CMAC), under the International Society of Music Education (ISME), suggests that defining CM's includes five domains 1) Kinds of music and music making; 2) Intentions; 3) Participants; 4) Teaching, learning and interacting; and 5) Interplays between formal and informal contexts. Community musicians not only teach, but they learn and are sensitive and responsive to the contexts of the students.

Students and teachers bring their social, emotional, physical, and political contexts to their lessons. For instance, Veblen (2008) acknowledges that a student's context may be in a formal education institution, a community center, or even a lesson received on the street. Community musicians need to be aware of their own contexts, their students' contexts, and the contexts of the communities in which they work. Examples of contextualized learning include the work of Musicians Without Borders, the World Peace Orchestra, or learning that occurs in The Philadelphia School, a private school in South Philadelphia.

Each of these organizations use community musicians to teach students even as lessons and performances differ vastly in each school. Community musicians recognize that a lesson is more than just teaching a note, it is an interplay between the student, teacher, and contexts in which they exist. The pedagogical construction of a lesson by a community musician creates a foundation for how music lessons evolve educationally. It can also provide reflections from the contexts the student and teacher come and go–a metaphorical lens into the social environments in which they exist. The social environment cannot be disconnected from or discounted by the community musician in their work.

Waters and Shulman (2008) embody a liberation worldview in their description of a community artist. "The word 'community' means any group of participants who have gathered together for transformative action…" (Waters and Shulman, 2008, p. 234). This definition includes the liberation lens of transforming society through the community music expression. Liberation psychology was not the first to recognize that CM is part of transforming society. The 1960's and 70's witnessed movements by socially conscious musicians eager to be relevant in the healthiness of communities without being defined as music therapists (Ansdell, 2002). In 2001, Atkinson wrote,

Community music is a participatory music-making activity in which the community musicians work with a given community to enable them to make music which is inspired by their own interests and ideas. Some Community Music activities seek to address the issues of social difficulty experienced by the participating communities, whilst others pursue music-making for its own sake (17).

Musicians must determine their purpose in their roles as community musicians. Is it to educate, either formally or informally, prepare a group for a performance, and/or is to be a part of a societal transformation process? Answering these questions allows the musician to know her intentions, limitations and goal for being involved in the work.

Music Therapy

The American Music Therapy Association defines music therapy as:

…the clinical and evidence-based use of music interventions to accomplish individualized goals within a therapeutic relationship by a credentialed professional who has completed an approved music therapy program (2018).

A board-certified music therapist (MT) must have completed a Bachelors, Masters, Doctorate or Certificate Program at an approved school, 1200 hours of field work including a supervised internship, and passed the Board Certification Exam. Music therapists work in a variety of settings including outpatient clinics, hospitals, psychiatric hospitals, schools, community centers, prisons and others. Music therapists assess their clients, design treatment plans, and track sessions and goal progress through clinical notes. It is evident that MTs and community musicians are not the same because they do not have the same training, nor do they intervene in the community in similar manners. Music therapists approaches the individual and community with clinical goals while a community musician may approach the individual and community with educational, performance-based, or transformational goals that, inferentially, have a therapeutic effect.

Music therapists are not CM's and are quite clear in the differentiation between an MT and CM. Training ensures MT's never confuse themselves with CM's; all musical interactions are goal-driven and in the medical model, in other words provided through the lens of treating a pathology. The training of an MT clearly delineates the clinical and communal aspects of music-making. However, the emergence of community music therapy has created a bridge between these two worlds.

Community Music Therapy

CoMT falls in the field of music therapy. Ansdell (2002) traces the history of community musicians providing the basis for the CoMT definition.

However, the notion that participatory music-making can be therapeutic is as old as the existence of music, and certain participatory music organizations are starting to move into the territory traditionally occupied by music therapists – i.e. working intensively with individuals to help them overcome their pathology (Atkinson, 2001, 22).

Atkinson (2001) believes there is an inherent connection between community music and music therapy. Community music therapy combines the theoretical underpinnings of music therapy and community music. Ansdell (2002) defines CoMT as

...an approach to working musically with people in context: acknowledging the social and cultural factors of their health, illness, relationships and musics. It reflects the essentially communal reality of musicking and is a response both to overly individualized treatment models and to the isolation people often experience within society (Defining Community Music Therapy).

CoMT is understood to be an anti-model as it considers the importance of providing musical experiences that are informed by the social and cultural contexts of the participants (Ansdell, Pavlicevic, Proctor & Verney, 2002). CoMT practitioners recognize that the goal of their work is to promote health and well-being in community and that this is accomplished both with the presence of community music therapists and community musicians.

Community Music Therapy is not prescribed. Instead, it embodies, reflects and transforms the context in which it exists. It invites all who hear, who are drawn into the music, to join in and be a part of the community if even only a fleeting moment. CoMT is also musicing. Small (1999) states that "...the act of musicing [musicking] establishes in the place where it is happening a set of relationships and it is in those relationships that the meaning of the act lies." (p. 13). Musicking is not a passive hearing of the music, but an active engagement with the music, with the self, and with others. CoMT is the action of musicking together to create *musical communitas* (Pavlicevic & Ansdell, 2004).

Community Music Therapists: Community Musicians

Historically, there has been a divide between CM's and MT's as each set out to define their own areas of expertise. This has resulted in viewing one another through a lens of distrust. However, MT's and CM's need to move toward one another. The literature suggests that there is an intimate connection between CoMT's and CM's. There are shared experiences (teaching, performing, seeking well-being for communities, etc.) and opportunities for collaboration. It is necessary for the CoMT and the CM to know what drives them as well as what the community needs. Both fields bring their own skill sets, knowledge, practical experiences and creativity. Together, CoMT's and CM's can learn from one another and collaborate in community (Bonde, 2011; Shank & Schirch, 2008). It is with this foundation that the program Orchestral Dialogues: Accepting Self, Accepting Others was conceived and implemented.

ORCHESTRAL DIALOGUES: ACCEPTING SELF, ACCEPTING OTHERS

Description

Orchestral Dialogues: Accepting Self, Accepting Others is a youth orchestra project that was implemented in October 2016. It facilitates resilience, self-efficacy, a vision for youths' future, the ability to build bridges of peace and hope, and develop the skill to make music in unity. The program engages children (9–16 years old) through music and through dialogue workshops that incorporate the arts. One need the program addresses is for quality music instruction to be made available for children who might not have access due to limited resources in their home and/or in their school environments. The second need the program addresses is dialogic skills so children and adults can engage with reduced conflict in their homes, schools, and communities while bringing about opportunities for change via deep listening and responding skills.

Music and dialogue are companions in creating transformation in the areas of identity and conflict. Participation in dialogue workshops is an integral part of membership in the orchestra. Youth are engaged in dialogue to practice the skill of deep listening beyond the musical context. Listening musically– to themselves, their peers and to the conductor–during harmonic and unison music-making is a learned skill and one that can be translated into life experiences. Children have the capacity to learn about themselves and others, and to hold differing opinions and views while still living in harmony and unity. Given the pluralistic, global society (global world is redundant), unity is understood in Orchestral Dialogues as the ability to hold common goals and thoughts while acknowledging and honoring the differences of one another.

History

The host site for Orchestral Dialogues: Accepting Self, Accepting Others (Orchestral Dialogues) is BuildaBridge International (BaB), an arts intervention organization based in Philadelphia, PA. BaB's mission statement is to

*...engage creative people and the transformative power of art making to bring hope, healing and resilience to children and families living in contexts of crisis and poverty. BuildaBridge accomplishes this mission through direct arts-based afterschool and summer education and therapeutic intervention programs (Community Programs); and through training artists (The BuildaBridge Institute) in the 'BuildaBridge Classroom*SM*' a trauma-informed, hope-infused, child-centered replicable model for working with at-risk youth. BuildaBridge envisions a world where all children are resilient, experience self-efficacy, and have a vision for their future. BuildaBridge dedicates its resources to building the capacity of local communities to fulfill this vision (BuildaBridge International, 2016).*

BaB, incorporated in 2000, began its arts-based programs at a local Northeast Philadelphia church and soon expanded its' programming to several Philadelphia neighborhoods. In 2003, BaB moved its' base of operations from Northeast Philadelphia to Germantown in Northwest Philadelphia, and began providing numerous arts-based services to partner organizations, using a community based model.

BaB volunteers provide arts-based interventions where children are located (e.g., schools, after-school programs, community centers, and shelters) rather than requiring children to come to a different location. BaB believes the arts, especially arts with a purpose, help create a more just and healthy world for children. In its' 20 years of operation, BaB has partnered with community organizations that have received grants to provide arts-based interventions for survivors of torture, asylum seekers, refugees, children and families in abuse shelters, after school programs, and training for community artists.

BuildaBridge's co-founders, Dr. Vivian Nix-Early and Dr. Nathan Corbitt, envisioned a performance group (i.e., orchestra, choir, drama troupe) as the face of BaB, but did not have the necessary resources to initiate this project until September 2016. In September 2016, this author a CoMT, undertook the administrative responsibility with BaB staff, partner schools, and CM's to launch Orchestral Dialogues: Accepting Self, Accepting Others (Orchestral Dialogues). The new orchestra used music as a metaphor for healing, intentionally incorporating dialogue through intergroup contact and deep listening.

A Middle Eastern Model Adopted to the United States

The West Eastern Divan Orchestra was the inspiration for the Orchestral Dialogues initiative. Founded in 1999 by Daniel Barenboim, an Argentinian- Israeli conductor, and Edward Said, an American-Palestinian academic, the West-Eastern Divan Orchestra brought together young adults of Israeli, Palestinian, Jordanian, Lebanese, Syrian, Egyptian, Turkish, Iranian and Spanish ethnicities in an orchestral setting (Cheah, 2009). Barenboim and Said (Cheah, 2009) declared the orchestra a-political from the beginning, deciding against taking sides in the conflicts between the nations. They sought unity of sound through the music, deliberately seating people from different nationalities beside one another. Members engaged one another in dialogue and discussion about some of the conflicts occurring between nations but chose to not take a stance on the conflicts (Cheah, 2009).

However, when Israel invaded Lebanon in 2006 Barenboim and Said's widow drafted a declaration against the war and demanded all members of the orchestra sign it (Cheah, 2009). Daniel Cohen, an Israeli and former violinist in the orchestra talked about his experience of the declaration and forced signing saying that he did not agree with the declaration; since the orchestra was apolitical, it was wrong to take a political stance at that moment (Cheah, 2009). Cohen's experience in the orchestra was part of a personal journey where he encountered Palestinians, Arabs, and other Israelis struggling to make sense of their own socio-political contexts within a self-described, non-political entity. The socio-political context was never far from his mind as he created harmonic and discordant sounds with his fellow musicians (Cheah, 2009). Cohen stated that he continued to struggle to make sense of the ethnic conflicts, of what it meant to be Israeli, to be Arab, and how to discuss these things with his friends and family. Cohen explained he often felt isolated from his friends and family, unsure how to invite them into the conversation (Cheah, 2009).

It was Cohen's narrative that inspired and solidified the need for a CoMT experience involving both community musicians and community music therapists. The act of creating music with others who are different did not develop the capacity to hold the tension of differing worldview perspectives nor did it contribute to the development of language to discuss the growth that occurred for Cohen within the

West-Eastern Divan Orchestra community. CoMT's understand that dialogue or verbal processing is integral to the healing community experience. Therefore, it was necessary for Orchestral Dialogues to have both CM's and CoMT's working together to facilitate communal music making and dialogue, so that the possibilities of growth, change, music education, and the development of a community were realized. Orchestral Dialogues is possible due to the foundational work of the West Eastern Divan Orchestra and other CM's before them.

ORCHESTRA AND DIALOGUE WITH A PURPOSE

Deep Listening

Deep listening goes beyond the surface of sound. It is meaning-making from all sounds and the realization that the combinations of sounds contribute to the listening experience (Oliveros, 2005; Pavlicevic & Impey, 2013). Pauline Oliveros (2005), composer, musician, performer and teacher, coined the term *deep listening* in 1989 after realizing many performers would hear what they played, but did not listen. Oliveros (2005) stated listening was a voluntary act, one that included "...giving attention to what is perceived both acoustically and psychologically..." (p. xxii). Deep listening is bringing what was heard to the conscious to expand and heighten the interaction between self and other (sound and people). Music therapist Pavlicevic and ethnomusicologist Impey (2013) used the framework of deep listening to discuss the importance of the intersection between dialogue and listening in cultural, social and political spaces. All aspects of self, individual, and collective listening were required to successfully engage in deep listening (Oliveros, 2005; Pavlicevic & Impey, 2013).

Transformative Dialogue

Transformative dialogue included the following two steps: first, moving from blame towards responsibility, self-expression, affirmation, self-reflexivity, and, second, the co-creation of a new reality (Gergen, Mcnamee & Barrett, 2001). Moving from blame toward responsibility encouraged setting aside the self's worldview as the only truth and making space for varying worldviews. Self-expression recognized our "...inner thoughts and feelings are essential to who we are; they virtually define us..." (Gergen, Mcnamee & Barrett, 2001, p. 703). Participants in transformational dialogue needed the space to share their inner thoughts and feelings with others, but they also had to learn to *listen* to one another's inner thoughts and feelings. This could be related to the skill of deep listening as the listener witnesses the other and makes meaning for themselves and others through the dialogic exchange (Gergen, Mcnamee & Barrett, 2001; Oliveros, 2005).

Affirmation is not considered agreement, rather an acknowledgment of being heard and listened to (Gergen, Mcnamee & Barrett, 2001). The listener considered what the other said; not dismissing it demonstrated that what was said mattered. Improvisation was important as dialogue was not scripted. Dialogue developed naturally and organically with a facilitator modeling responses and interactions (Gergen, Mcnamee, & Barrett, 2001). Self-reflexivity, like deep listening, was considered the call to silence, to reflect on self, on what was heard, and to examine one's self for the grey areas within that welcomed differing opinions and worldviews (Gergen, Mcnamee, Barrett, 2001; Oliveros, 2005). Ultimately, the process of transformative dialogue resulted in co-creating a new world, a world that welcomed and explored varying ideas, opinions, and worldviews (Gergen, Mcnamee, Barrett, 2001).

Lessons Learned

During 2016-2017, the pilot year, Orchestral Dialogues was co-conducted by Dr. Najib Wong and D'Angelo Virgo, who is the current conductor. The children received weekly private lessons from Dr. Najib Wong, D'Angelo Virgo, Dr. Janelle Junkin, MT-BC, and Adam Barth, the instrumental specialist on staff. Wong, Virgo, and Barth are educators and CM's who received training in trauma-informed approaches to music and collaborated with Dr. Junkin, the CoMT on staff. Dr. Junkin facilitated monthly dialogue workshops that were music-inspired. Orchestral Dialogues began in November 2016 with monthly 4-hour rehearsals on weekends and monthly 2-hour dialogue workshops on weekends. During the first five months of the program, Dr. Junkin received Institutional Review Board (IRB) permission from Drexel University to conduct an ethnographic study was conducted to determine if and how children learn deep listening skills during orchestral rehearsals and translate them into transformative dialogue skills. The results of this study were Dr. Junkin's (2017) dissertation that has yet to be published.

The results of this study showed that the children learned, the families learned, the CM's learned, the CoMT learned, and the dialogue workshop facilitator learned; the whole community learned together. The results of this study revealed the four necessary aspects of a successful learning and translation of skills: Adult Modeling, Role Playing, Orchestra as Analogy for Components of Dialogue, and Community Building through Collaboration. In five short months, the 13 children who participated in Orchestral Dialogues demonstrated that they had learned the basic skills of deep listening and transformative dialogue, although they had demonstrated limited implementation of these skills outside of the Orchestral Dialogues space. The children could describe what deep listening and transformative dialogue were and how to use them within the orchestral setting, however, when asked to discuss how they might employ these skills in their homes, schools or neighborhoods, the children were unable to articulate this.

Informally, the results showed Orchestral Dialogues could serve as a model bringing CM's and CoMT's together with the same purpose but differing expertise in achieving the skill development. As a CoMT, I witnessed, taught, and coordinated the program with the lens of a music therapist. Though I had never considered the children, parents, or staff through a pathological lens, I did view the program through the lens of a clinician and incorporated my training as a music therapist into my work as a CM. I was aware of group dynamics, family dynamics, and the interpersonal experiences of the children, families and staff as a clinician. This resulted in my ability to assess the group experience quickly and work with the staff to respond in a manner that was clinically informed and contextual in nature.

Likewise, the CM's brought their own areas of expertise in teaching, group lessons, conducting an orchestra, and arranging music. These CM's taught the CoMT new ways to encounter the Orchestral Dialogues experience, resulting in dialogue amongst the staff about refining our program, choosing music, and how to best teach the skills of deep listening and transformative dialogue. The CM's were open to the clinical perspective, shared their own perspective and together the staff involved the children and families in the co-creation of Orchestral Dialogues.

Reflecting on how and why the model of bringing together CoMT's and CM's worked, the following underpinnings were critical to the relationship and successful implementation of Orchestral Dialogues. The relationship, between CM and CoMT, acknowledged and strengthened the connections between staff, the music, the children and families. The understanding between the CM's and CoMT was key and ensured that Orchestral Dialogues resulted in the co-creation of community through humility, curiosity, and respect.

To successfully work with one another, it was imperative that CM's and the CoMT approach each other with humility, creating space for each person's level of knowledge, expertise, and experience. My personal experience, knowledge, and expertise as a CoMT did not negate that of the CM's experience, and vice versa. This humility was extended to the children and families, as well. Yes, we were the trained musicians, but this did not discount the contributions of the children and family to the co-creation of our community. Instead, it served as an aspect of it.

As staff, there was a need to be curious about ourselves, each other, the music and the community. Orchestral Dialogues was only a theoretical concept until the community began creating together. Each of us had ideas of what the program *might* be, but none of us knew with certainty how the community would form. Approaching the program with curiosity allowed us to both hold and release our ideas and presumptions, so that the actuality of the program could come into existence. Not only did the children learn deep listening and transformative dialogue skills, but so too, did the staff. We listened to ourselves, to one another, and to the music, we engaged in dialogue, and we worked together to co-create a new reality within an orchestral experience. It was not driven by the traditional hierarchical understandings of conductor and musicians, but one that was driven by the acknowledgment and respect for the expertise and learning brought by the staff and the students alike.

We respected one another, the music, the children, the families, and the community. As CoMT's and CM's, we showed respect for each other professionally and personally as we listened, learned, and helped one another. As musicians we recognized that the act of creating and making music was therapeutic in and of itself. We respected the entity of music as a participant in the community. We demonstrated respect for the children as we actively involved them in the formation of the community, in the learning process, and in our openness to learn from them. We respected the families of the children by inviting them to attend and participate in the rehearsals with their children, by learning basic music making during lessons, and in active participation in the dialogue workshops. Our community included the families as much as the participating children.

Finally, we respected the new community that emerged. Based on our initial rehearsal in November 2016, in our wildest dreams we would never have predicted what the community would be like or how it would look. Through humility, curiosity and a relationship to the music, we participated in the co-creation of the community that is Orchestral Dialogues. This community was dynamic and experienced conflict. We worked through that conflict undergirded by the presence of CoMT's and CM's who demonstrated that creative collaboration across disciplines can result in community. Our interdisciplinary work served as a metaphor for the children and families who saw that humility, curiosity and respect are needed to successfully create a musical and dialogic community. We all learned that we must listen with intention, responding out of respect and humility, so that community is not only possible, but thrives.

Implications for CoMT's and CM's

As I wrote this chapter the question I felt a deep-seated need to answer why the need exists to work together. The answer, based on my research, clinical training, identity as a musician, and my experiences is that CoMT's and CM's need one another to contribute to strong, cohesive, and holistic communities. We need to learn from one another rather than viewing each other as potential threats or through a lens that promotes one level of training above another. Collaboration means creating space for each person's expertise while understanding one another's weaknesses and strengths. Community music therapists and community musicians need to facilitate and nurture the emerging community's participation in the musical experience. This can only be accomplished through creative collaboration.

It must be said that, as a music therapist, I will always caution the CM against making statements that they, too, are music therapists. Unless the CM has undergone the educational and training aspects of a music therapy program and is board certified, this claim cannot be made. I also recognize and appreciate that music can both be *in* therapy (as used by a music therapist) and *as* therapy (as used by a community musician). This distinction has the possibility to serve as a foundation for more CoMT's and CM's to collaboratively work together. When we do, the creative possibilities are endless. Music is our shared soundscape, and our mutual respect for it and one another can lead to the co-creation of community.

REFERENCES

American Music Therapy Association. (2018). *The American Music Therapy Association*. Retrieved from https://www.musictherapy.org/

Ansdell, G. (2002). Community music therapy & the winds of change. *Voices: A World Forum for Music Therapy*, *2*(2). doi: 10.15845/voices.v2i2.83

Ansdell, G. (2004). Rethinking music and community: theoretical perspectives in support of community music therapy. In M. Pavlicevic & G. Ansdell (Eds.), Community Music Therapy (pp. 65–90). Philadelphia, PA: Jessica Kingsley Publishers.

Ansdell, G. (2005, November). Being who you aren't; Doing what you can't: Community music therapy & the paradoxes of performance. *Voices: A World Forum for Music Therapy*, *5*(3). Retrieved from normt.uib.no/index.php/voices/article/view/229/173

Atkinson, J. (2001). *Survey of Community Music in the UK*. Unpublished report for the Speedwell Trust.

Baine, S. (2013). Music therapy as an anti-oppressive practice. *The Arts in Psychotherapy*, *40*(1), 1–5. doi:10.1016/j.aip.2012.09.003

Bergh, A., & Sloboda, J. (2010). Music & art in conflict transformation: A review. *Music & Arts in Action*, *2*(2), 1–16.

Black-Gutman, D., & Hickson, F. (1996). The relationship between racial attitudes and social-cognitive development in children: An Australian study. *Developmental Psychology*, *32*(3), 448–456. doi:10.1037/0012-1649.32.3.448

Blakemore, S. J., & Choudhury, S. (2006). Development of the adolescent brain: Implications for executive function and social cognition. *Journal of Child Psychology and Psychiatry, and Allied Disciplines*, *47*(3–4), 296–312. doi:10.1111/j.1469-7610.2006.01611.x PMID:16492261

Bonde, L. O. (2011). Health musicking – Music therapy or music and health? A model, empirical examples and personal reflections. *Music & Arts in Action*, *3*(2), 1–21.

Buhrmester, D. (1990). Intimacy of friendship, interpersonal competence, and adjustment during preadolescence and adolescence. *Child Development*, *61*(4), 1101–1111. doi:10.2307/1130878 PMID:2209180

Cheah, E. (2009). *An orchestra beyond borders: Voices of the West-Eastern Divan Orchestra*. Brooklyn, NY: Verso.

Corbitt, J. N., & Nix-Early, V. (2003). *Taking it to the streets using the arts to transform your community*. Grand Rapids, MI: Baker Books.

Curtis, S. L. (2012). Music therapy and social justice: A personal journey. *The Arts in Psychotherapy*, *39*(3), 209–213. doi:10.1016/j.aip.2011.12.004

DeNora, T. (2005). The pebble in the pond: Musicing, therapy, community. *Nordic Journal of Music Therapy*, *14*(1), 57–66. doi:10.1080/08098130509478126

Fock, E. (1997). Music – intercultural communication? Micro musics, world music and multicultural discourse. *Institute of Folklore*, 55–65. Retrieved from http://www.nordicom.gu.se/sites/default/files/kapitel-pdf/6_055_066.pdf

Gergen, K. J., Mcnamee, S., & Barrett, F. (2001). Toward transformative dialogue. *International Journal of Public Administration*, *7*(8), 697–707. Retrieved from http://works.swarthmore.edu/cgi/viewcontent.cgi?article=1411&context=fac-psychology

Hicks, T. (2001). Another look at identity-based conflict: The roots of conflict: the roots of conflict in the psychology of consciousness. *Negotiation Journal*, *17*(1), 35–45. doi:10.1111/j.1571-9979.2001.tb00225.x

Junkin, J. S. (2017). *Orchestral-dialogues: Accepting self, accepting others-translating deep listening skills to transformative dialogue skills*. Drexel University.

Kenny, C. B. (1982). *Mythic artery: The magic of music therapy*. Atascadero, CA: Ridgeview Publishing Company.

Lederach, J. P. (2014). *The little book of conflict transformation*. New York, NY: Good Books.

Ma, Y.-Y. (2016). *A new way of thinking is possible, a new consciousness – perhaps a new enlightenment – that brings the arts and science back together*. Retrieved from https://www.silkroadproject.org/about-us

Moore, D. G., Burland, K., & Davidson, J. W. (2003). The social context of musical success: A developmental account. *British Journal of Psychology*, *94*(4), 529–549. doi:10.1348/000712603322503088 PMID:14687460

O'Grady, L., & McFerran, K. (2007). Community music therapy and its relationship to community music: Where does it end? *Nordic Journal of Music Therapy*, *16*(1), 14–26. doi:10.1080/08098130709478170

Oliveros, P. (2005). *Deep listening: A composer's sound practice*. Lincoln NE: iUniverse.

Pavlicevic, M., & Impey, A. (2013). Deep listening: Towards an imaginative reframing of health and well-being practices in international development. *Arts & Health: An International Journal for Research. Policy & Practice*, *5*(3), 238–252. doi:10.1080/17533015.2013.827227 PMID:25729413

Powell, H. (2004). A dream wedding: from community music to music therapy with a community. In M. Pavlicevic & G. Ansdell (Eds.), Community Music Therapy (pp. 167–185). Philadelphia, PA: Jessica Kingsley Publishers.

Procter, S. (2011). Reparative musicing: Thinking on the usefulness of social capital theory within music therapy. *Nordic Journal of Music Therapy*, *20*(3), 242–262. doi:10.1080/08098131.2010.489998

Proctor, S. (2004). Playing politics: Community music therapy and the therapeutic redistribution of music capital for mental health. In M. Pavlicevic & G. Ansdell (Eds.), Community Music Therapy (pp. 214–230). Philadelphia, PA: Jessica Kingsley Publishers.

Shank, M., & Schirch, L. (2008). Strategic arts-based peacebuilding. *Peace and Change*, *33*(2), 217–242. doi:10.1111/j.1468-0130.2008.00490.x

Small, C. (1999). *Musicking: The meanings of performing and listening*. New York, NY: Music Library Association.

Stige, B. (2002, November). The relentless roots of community music therapy. *Voices: A World Forum for Music Therapy*, *2*(3). Retrieved from https://www.voices.no/index.php/voices/article/view/98/75

Stige, B. (2003). *Elaborations toward a notion of community music therapy*. Oslo: Unipub AS.

Stige, B. (2006). On a notion of participation in music therapy. *Nordic Journal of Music Therapy*, *15*(2), 121–138. doi:10.1080/08098130609478159

Stige, B., & Aaro, L. E. (2012). *Invitation to community music therapy*. New York, NY: Routledge Taylor and Francis Group.

Stige, B., Ansdell, G., & Elefant, C. (2010). *Where music helps: community music therapy in action and reflection*. Burlington, VT: Ashgate Publishing Company.

Vaillancourt, G. (2012). Music therapy: A community approach to social justice. *The Arts in Psychotherapy*, *39*(3), 173–178. doi:10.1016/j.aip.2011.12.011

Veblen, K. K. (2008). The many ways of community music. *International Journal of Community Music*, *1*(1), 5–21. doi:10.1386/ijcm.1.1.5_1

Watkins, M., & Shulman, H. (2008). *Toward psychologies of liberation*. New York, NY: Palgrave Macmillan. doi:10.1057/9780230227736

Willson, R. B. (2009). The parallax worlds of the West-Eastern Divan Orchestra. *Journal of the Royal Musical Association*, *134*(2), 319–347. doi:10.1080/02690400903109109

KEY TERMS AND DEFINITIONS

Harmony: The simultaneous combination of tones that blend and sound pleasing to the ear.
Unity: Musically, this term refers to a group of musicians playing the same note at the same time.

Section 5
Arts-Based Post-Traumatic Growth Assessments

As tools and strategies are gained to assist in our care for others, it is important to assess the effects of our work. Arts-based Post-traumatic Growth Assessments help us to understand how our work benefits others and can help us better guide our groups toward healing. These assessments also aid in the continued improvement of our programming, and help us build concrete data that we may later find useful. There are many methods for measuring success and growth in arts based work, several of which can be found in these next chapters.

Chapter 14
A Creative Approach to Assessment:
Applications in Youth Spiritual Development

Callie B. Dean
Eastern University, USA

ABSTRACT

This chapter explores the suitability of an arts-based approach to the spiritual assessment of adolescents. Spirituality is a notoriously difficult concept to define, much less to measure. However, many practitioners in both religious and secular settings are increasingly concerned about promoting spiritual development among the youth that they serve. Some quantitative assessment tools already exist to measure youth spirituality; however, these may be of limited practical use within real-world contexts. Complete instructions and rubrics for two assessment activities are provided, followed by sample responses and a discussion about how to use the results and extend the activities for maximum impact. Initial research suggests that these and similar activities show great promise as qualitative instruments, which can elicit deeper understandings of adolescents' experiences of transcendence and ability to make meaning out of life circumstances.

INTRODCUTION

This chapter introduces and describes an arts-based approach to spiritual assessment, which can be applied by practitioners in community-based youth development settings. The activities presented in this chapter are designed to be used both in trauma-specific contexts (e.g. counseling and support groups) and in general youth development settings (e.g. after-school programs). Therefore, the basic approach of this chapter combines the principles of positive youth development and trauma-informed care, maintaining that all youth-serving organizations can benefit from adopting a trauma-informed approach. Developing and using trauma-informed assessment tools is one essential component of trauma-informed care. Arts-based activities and assessment instruments – which rely primarily on nonverbal, symbolic language as

DOI: 10.4018/978-1-5225-5981-8.ch014

a starting point – show promise in helping trauma survivors process their experiences. Such tools seek to empower youth by elevating their own voice and perspective within the assessment process.

Indicators of spirituality include resilience, optimism, a sense of purpose, and the positive use of adversity (Lippman et al., 2009; Mariano & Damon, 2008; Zohar & Marshall, 2004). Developing and strengthening these traits can be crucial in helping a person to heal from trauma and, ultimately, to thrive. For this reason, it is important that youth workers – even those in non-religious settings – be equipped with tools to better understand, assess, and promote healthy spiritual development among the youth whom they serve.

The objectives of this chapter include the following:

- To present a model for youth programming that integrates the key features of positive youth development and trauma-informed care.
- To describe the role of spirituality within holistic youth development.
- To articulate the benefits of adopting an arts-based approach to spiritual assessment.
- To describe two different assessment activities that demonstrate the practical application of this approach.

SETTING THE STAGE: POSITIVE YOUTH DEVELOPMENT AND TRAUMA-INFORMED CARE

In recent years, positive youth development (PYD) has emerged as an approach to youth-based programming, aiming to "[create] a larger framework that promotes positive outcomes for all young people" (National Research Council, 2002, p. 3). As opposed to a risk prevention approach (which aims to minimize negative outcomes), PYD seeks to empower youth to develop both personal and social assets that promote holistic wellbeing and long-term success. The National Research Council (2002) has identified eight key features of positive youth development programs: physical and psychological safety; appropriate structure; supportive relationships; opportunities to belong; positive social norms; support for efficacy and mattering; opportunities for skill building; and integration of family, school, and community efforts.

Programs that employ a PYD approach may include schools, after-school programs, community organizations, and spiritual institutions (churches, synagogues, mosques, etc.). Participation is generally open to a wide range of youth, who may or may not disclose a history of trauma; and most programs are staffed by youth workers who lack a formal background in therapy or counseling. However, most if not all of these programs are – either knowingly or unknowingly – serving survivors of trauma. Therefore, it is essential that the programs be intentionally designed to support trauma survivors and promote healing and growth.

Adopting a trauma-informed approach requires program-wide commitment and a shift in organizational culture, policies, and procedures. According to the Substance Abuse and Mental Health Services Association (2014), a trauma-informed approach is one that:

- **Realizes** the prevalence and impact of trauma.
- **Recognizes** the signs and symptoms of trauma.
- **Responds** appropriately by incorporating trauma-informed principles throughout the system.
- **Resists re-traumatization** of clients and staff alike.

The six governing principles of trauma-informed care include the following: safety; trustworthiness and transparency; peer support; collaboration and mutuality; empowerment, voice, and choice; and cultural, historical, and gender issues (SAMHSA, 2014).

There is a good deal of overlap between the principles of a trauma-informed approach and the key features of positive youth development (see Table 1). Both approaches list safety first—recognizing that physical and emotional safety is foundational for any kind of growth (post-traumatic or otherwise). The other components only underscore the importance of creating safe spaces for participants. For example, establishing appropriate limits and rules helps provide students with a sense of predictability and control. Creating a supportive atmosphere and promoting positive social norms both contribute to an emotionally safe space for students.

Both approaches also operate from an empowerment-based approach, with the ultimate goal of having students take ownership of their own development and/or healing process. Implicit in the integration of these approaches is the assumption that youth are capable of leading their own development and making the changes necessary to heal themselves. Therefore, while staff and other caring adults may offer guidance and support, they are not superior to the youth themselves—who should increasingly take on leadership roles and have a meaningful voice in programming and organizational decisions.

Table 1. An integration of trauma-informed care and positive youth development

Principles of Trauma-Informed Care (SAMHSA, 2014)	Features of Positive Youth Development (NRC, 2002)	Indicators of an Integrated Approach
Safety	Physical and psychological safety	Utmost care is taken to ensure that facilities, policies, and programming promote both physical and emotional safety for youth and staff alike.
Trustworthiness and Transparency	Appropriate Structure	Appropriate limits, rules, and expectations are communicated clearly so that participants always know what to expect.
Peer Support	Supportive Relationships	Caring, close relationships are recognized as the foundation for building trust, establishing a safe space, and promoting growth.
Cultural, Historical, and Gender Issues	Opportunities to belong Positive Social Norms	The program supports both individual and group identity formation through the promotion of positive social norms. A culturally competent approach ensures that all youth are meaningfully included and integrated into the program and that their specific gender, racial, ethnic, and cultural needs are met.
Empowerment, Voice, and Choice	Support for Efficacy and Mattering Opportunities for Skill Building	The program values youths' strengths, experiences, and capacity for growth—and empowers youth to gain the skills necessary to make a real difference, both in their own lives and in their community
Collaboration and Mutuality	Integration of Family, School, and Community Efforts	All members of the community – youth, staff, volunteers, family members, schools, churches, etc. – value each other and work together to promote youth development.

In recent years, there have been some attempts to intentionally incorporate trauma-informed care into PYD, particularly within child welfare systems. The Brevard Family Partnership (2017) launched an initiative in 2012 to transform its local child welfare system into a trauma-informed community of practice—one including the Department of Child and Family Services, various non-profit organizations, counselors, law enforcement agencies, and school systems. The Brevard Family Partnership's framework states that positive youth development should be an outcome of trauma-informed care. Other systems – most notably, the Massachusetts Child Trauma Project – have used an integrated model to train and equip a variety of service providers throughout their systems (Fraser et al, 2014). However, even outside of trauma-specific settings, an integration of the two approaches may well provide the most optimal context for all youth to develop and thrive.

Spirituality and Positive Youth Development

Many practitioners, particularly in non-religious settings, balk at the idea of discussing spiritual development as an explicit program goal. This is because spirituality and religion frequently are conflated, both in existing literature and in popular discourse. The two often correlate; but the large number of individuals who identify as "spiritual but not religious" (e.g. Barna, 2017) serves as a reminder that this correlation is not absolute. Giesenberg (2007) sums up the dichotomy between religion and spirituality as it is commonly understood: spirituality is "being," and religion is "doing." That is to say, religion is bound up in the trappings, doctrines, and rituals of an organized community of faith. Researchers have measured religiosity and religiousness by looking at factors like organizational affiliation, doctrinal allegiances, church attendance, and participation in communal practices (Good & Willoughby, 2006; King, Clardy, & Ramon, 2013). Spirituality, on the other hand, tends to be more individualized, subjective, and not confined to any particular religion. Fields as diverse as anthropology, psychology, and nursing all conceptualize spirituality differently (Giesenberg, 2007). However, one common theme that runs throughout these definitions is transcendence—that is, a significant connection to something larger than the self (whether it be to nature, to humanity, or to a deity).

Indicators of spirituality are vast and varied. Some researchers argue that purpose is the most important indicator (Mariano & Damon, 2008), while others recommend focusing on humility as the chief virtue of a positive spirituality (Scarlett, 2008). Positive youth development practitioners operationalize spirituality as it relates to established developmental assets such as optimism, resilience, and pro-social values (Lippman et al., 2009). Brown (1998) found that non-religious spiritual development could be facilitated through stillness as well as activity; through deep reflections on identity and emotions; through developing relationships; and through creative and artistic experiences.

King et al.'s (2013) study of adolescent spiritual exemplars identified three key components of a well-developed spirituality: transcendence, fidelity, and behavior. Transcendence, as described above, refers to one's personal sense of connection to something divine or absolute. Adolescents often express a simultaneous sense of connection to God and other people. Fidelity refers to one's "commitment to beliefs, worldviews, and values" (p. 14), as indicated by one's ability to derive meaning from life experiences. Finally, behavior refers to an individual's commitment to an intentional way of living that is informed by his/her belief system (King et al, 2013).

Though spirituality and religion are distinct concepts, most people's spirituality is informed by their religious background (or lack thereof). For example, a boy who grows up in an Evangelical Christian household will most likely identify God as his main source of transcendence; will make meaning of his life experiences through a Judeo-Christian worldview based on the specific doctrines he has been taught; and may live out his beliefs through actions such as attending church, abstaining from alcohol, or reading his Bible daily. On the other hand, a girl from a non-religious household may connect with "humanity in general" as her main source of transcendence; may adhere, consciously or unconsciously, to principles of secular humanism; and live out her beliefs through behaviors such as serving in her community or advocating for social justice. (This is a broad generalization, of course; and even individuals from similar religious backgrounds may experience spirituality in vastly different ways).

In Fowler's (1981) seminal Stages of Faith model, the word "faith" is used rather than spirituality, but the concept is similar. According to Fowler, faith is "an active mode of being and committing, a way of moving into and giving shape to our experiences of life…Faith is our way of discerning and committing ourselves to centers of value and power that exert ordering force in our lives" (p. 24). Fowler places particular emphasis on the importance of meaning-making as humans progress through the life cycle, noting that the specific meanings that people construct are based upon their centers of value, images of power, and "the master stories that we tell ourselves and by which we interpret and respond to the events that impinge upon our lives" (p. 277). People from all religious and cultural traditions all must engage in this same dynamic meaning-making process (although the specific centers of values, images of power, and master stories that they draw upon may appear to be vastly different).

The Stages of Faith model draws upon the theories of Eriksen, Piaget, and Kohlberg in order to construct a structural stage theory of faith development across the life cycle. As in the major developmental theories, the initial stages of faith development (Stages 0-2) correspond roughly with the age spans and cognitive ability levels through which all people progress. However, development past these stages is not automatic; and people can become "stuck" at any stage between 2 through 6. Therefore, although Stage 3, for example, is considered to be the "adolescent" faith, some people may not reach this stage until adulthood; and others may never fully make the transition.

Adolescence is a time of rapid change and growth within all of the developmental systems. According to Eriksen (1963), identity formation is the major developmental task of adolescence, with special regard to the development of familial, vocational, and societal roles. A young person must learn to integrate all of the inner and outer changes by developing a core (albeit multidimensional) identity. Adolescence is a both a critical and opportune time for spiritual development because spirituality is so closely linked to identity formation and purpose. During adolescence, a person's cortex becomes mature enough – for the first time – to be able to truly regulate his/her emotions, attention, and behaviors. Adolescents also have heightened critical thinking skills that enable them to think abstractly about spiritual concepts (King, 2008; King et al., 2013; National Research Council, 2002).

Positive youth development is predicated on the idea that youth programs must be rooted in a holistic view of human development; recognizing that all the major developmental systems (cognitive, emotional, social, etc.) work together. Traditionally, spirituality has not been included among the major developmental dimensions; but theorists are increasingly looking at spiritual development through this systems perspective as well (Giesenberg, 2007; King, 2008). Spiritual development is an essential aspect of healthy human development throughout the life cycle; therefore, it is important to promote healthy spiritual development among our youth in the same way that we promote their physical and cognitive development.

Both spirituality and religiosity have been correlated with a wide variety of positive outcomes for youth, such as academic success, abstention from risky behaviors, and the development of positive relationships (Good & Willoughby, 2006). Churches, synagogues, and other spiritual institutions are particularly well poised to promote positive identity formation, a high capacity for meaning-making, and a variety of internal and external developmental assets. Certain doctrinal statements and creeds, for example, may help youth to form their identity in relation to a transcendent entity (i.e. "chosen people"; "sons and daughters of God"; "beloved"; "body of Christ") (Good & Willoughby, 2006; King, 2008). Such theological narratives facilitate the process of meaning-making by offering a framework to which young people are able to connect their own emerging sense of purpose and identity.

Being able to make sense of a painful experience is widely considered to be an essential component of resilience. For survivors of trauma, the arts can be a particularly useful tool for making meaning. Grossman et al. (2006) identified creative expression and spirituality, as well as cognitive reasoning and altruism, as valid strategies for meaning making. In multiple qualitative studies, both visual arts and expressive writing (poetry; journaling; etc.) have been shown to help trauma survivors reconstruct a positive identity and make meaning of their experiences (Stuckey & Nobel, 2002).

Exemplary development, or "thriving," is often measured by an individual's ability and willingness to contribute to the larger community: family, school, community, and civil society. Religious institutions often explicitly promote such contributions as a way to live out one's faith, and may offer specific opportunities for youth to participate and contribute (King, 2008; Mariano & Damon, 2008). The mores and morals of religious institutions often promote internal assets and positive values, such as honesty, integrity, and a sense of purpose. Finally, the specific focus of a religious youth program may nurture the development of assets like conflict resolution, social justice, or creative activities.

Community-based youth programs, both secular and faith-based, may not be able to offer quite as coherent a framework across the ideological, social, and transcendent dimensions as a spiritual institution (church, mosque, temple, etc.) can. However, these organizations and programs can still nurture spiritual development by connecting students with both a sense of tradition and purpose and by helping youth make meaning of their experiences based on their morals and values (King, 2008). Depending on the perceptions of both youth and community stakeholders, non-religious programs may decide to use alternative language to describe their goals—language such as "inner character development," "identity formation," or "developmental assets."

Arts-Based Assessment

Assessment is the process of gathering, analyzing, and interpreting evidence in order to better understand an individual, institution, or program. A key aspect of assessment involves using data in order to improve a particular program, curriculum, or intervention. There are two basic types of assessments:

- Formative assessments are conducted before or during a program in order to determine the need for a program, guide the planning process, or to change and improve the program while it is going on. For example, one might survey parents to find out what their felt needs are; conduct a pre-test of students to find out what they already know about a given subject; or ask students questions about a program to discover how they are benefiting from the experience.
- Summative assessments are conducted at the end of a program or intervention in order to gauge how well it has met its goals and objectives. For example, students might take a posttest or prepare a presentation to demonstrate their learning; or participants could take a survey that would measure changes in behaviors and attitudes as a result of a given program.

The discipline of assessment is widely established in fields such as therapy and education. In clinical practice, for example, therapists often conduct formative assessments to inform the development of a treatment and/or therapy plan. In education, regular assessments (usually in the form of graded assignments and tests) are scheduled to demonstrate the extent of students' learning and to highlight areas that might need remediation or further instruction.

Assessments can also be incorporated within the larger field of program evaluation, which is the systematic process of collecting and analyzing data in order to determine the efficiency, effectiveness, and/or impact of a given program. For example, the program evaluation process may include a preliminary needs assessment, which aims to determine the level of unmet needs within a given community or organization. An outcomes-based evaluation, on the other hand, may incorporate both formative and summative assessments in order to determine to what extent participants have changed as a result of a particular intervention or program.

In contexts where there is not already a strong culture of evaluation, program leaders and staff may resist efforts to incorporate regular assessments and evaluation into their practice. Some staff are worried that the process will end up feeling like a high-stakes performance review, in which any failures will be broadcast for the world to see and could even jeopardize the program's very existence. Others have practical concerns about the effects of assessment on their clients. They might argue that, within the context of a relationally focused program, it would feel unnatural and jarring to incorporate test-taking on a regular basis. Furthermore, for youth and adults who struggle with test anxiety, even filling out a simple questionnaire can trigger panic as they try to figure out what "the right answer" is. Finally, some staff members argue that it is impossible to measure their program's success, or that quantitative measures can only go so far in describing the impact their program has had on participants' lives.

None of these objections are good enough reasons to avoid evaluation altogether. Arts-based assessment, among other non-traditional methodologies, may even offer some remedies to some of these common objections. Some have argued that evaluation and assessment is most effective when it is seamlessly integrated into the regular programming of an organization or entity (Edenloff, 2011). Drawing a picture or performing a skit feels more natural, more fun, and less stressful for participants than taking a test or survey would. It is hoped that program staff could use arts-based assessment tools easily, without any specialized training in evaluation. Because arts activities can be used both as assessment tools and as teaching tools, facilitators can build upon such activities within a programmatic context, using the results of their assessments to guide their pedagogical approach and objectives.

Arts-based assessment methodologies offer additional benefits, as well. The arts serve as a window into a different way of knowing than traditional evaluation methodologies. Each artistic discipline (music; visual arts; dance; theatre) has its own symbolic language and way of representing the world. By starting with an image instead of a category, the arts allow for a wider range of perspectives and interpretations; encouraging participants to express insights that they cannot articulate in words (especially those related to abstract concepts like spirituality). Therefore, arts-based methodologies can be valuable in gathering, and even quantifying, information about a participant's experiences and perceptions. Practically, this also means that the arts can be a particularly useful, and equalizing, tool in reaching participants with limited cognitive or verbal ability; those from differing socioeconomic backgrounds; those with emotional problems; and those who have experienced trauma. Bloom (2010) writes, "The [trauma] victim experiences and remembers the trauma in nonverbal, visual, auditory, kinesthetic, visceral, and feeling ways, but is not able to 'think' about it or process the experience in any way" (p. 76). The arts speak the same "language" as the stored memories and can therefore offer trauma survivors a powerful outlet and path toward healing.

Organizational leaders may find that using arts-based assessments allow them to share their findings more creatively with their stakeholders—people including parents, volunteers, donors, a board of directors, and the students themselves. Particularly when the outcomes of a given program are nebulous or difficult to measure, it is tempting to become stuck in a rut of simply reporting outputs: that is, the activities that happened in a given program and/or the number of students in attendance. However, an arts-based approach can help program stakeholders to explore and measure more abstract outcomes. If assessments are done regularly using a standardized rubric, it may be possible to aggregate and quantify some of these changes by, for example, tracking the number of spiritual assets reported by students; or by tracking the changes in the way they make meaning of a given event from the beginning to the end of a program. Sometimes, of course, sharing students' artwork directly with stakeholders (with the students' permission) can communicate a program's impact far better than words or statistics ever could.

In designing an arts-based assessment from scratch, one should ask the following questions:

1. **What is being assessed?** Some topics are not suitable for an arts-based approach. A traditional survey, for example, is probably the best fit for understanding students' daily habits and behaviors. However, if the topic is qualitative in nature and based in students' perceptions and experiences (e.g. how they view their neighborhood; how they feel when they are at their after-school program), an arts activity might be an effective method of data collection.
2. **Will the assessment be conducted individually or with a group?** Some art activities, such as mosaics, murals, and skits, naturally foster teamwork and group reflection; these communal projects also lend themselves well to public presentations. However, a group activity may discourage some participants from expressing their own opinions, whereas an individual art project promotes personal reflection and engagement. There may be other practical limitations to consider (how much time is allotted for the assessment?) as well as concerns about students' emotional safety (will they feel comfortable sharing with their peers?)
3. **What art project is most suitable for this assessment?** Youth workers may be able to adapt existing activities from the realms of art, music, and drama therapy, though they should not attempt to use them clinically without the proper credentials. If feasible, it may be helpful to pilot an arts activity – alongside its accompanying rubric, checklist, or other analysis tool – with just a few students to see whether it will elicit useful data about the selected indicators.

Spiritual Assessment: Challenges and Opportunities

Given the important role of spiritual development in promoting adolescents' thriving, it would follow that youth workers should seek to understand and assess their students' experiences of spirituality. The goal of spiritual assessment, then, is to determine how an individual experiences transcendence, makes meaning of his/her experiences, and lives out his/her beliefs. The process can also encompass the identification of needs, hopes, and resources that may inform the individual's spiritual development. Traditional surveys and questionnaires have already proven to be effective at measuring adolescents' behaviors and habits (church attendance; prayer and spiritual disciplines; service projects) quantitatively. Such instruments may also seek to understand adolescents' experiences of transcendence and fidelity, but they tend to be limited to very specific items that the youth is both aware of and able to articulate.

Arts-based assessment activities, on the other hand, are perhaps best suited for helping participants express these other two aspects of spirituality. An arts-based approach goes further than simply assessing for the *presence* of transcendence within a youth's life; it instead offers a thick, qualitative description of *how* the youth perceives and experiences that transcendence. The arts can be particularly useful in better understanding adolescents' intrinsic meaning-making capacity, even when they themselves are not fully aware of this capacity.

There is currently is no consensus about the best way to assess and measure spiritual development. Practitioners and researchers from different disciplines may have different motivations for assessing spirituality: A nurse, for example, might be interested in the way religious beliefs should inform a patient's healthcare; whereas a psychologist might seek to understand the way in which a research participant conceptualizes his/her spirituality. In fact, the most pragmatically useful assessment tools have originated in the field of chaplaincy, where spirituality is directly related to a treatment plan that includes personalized interventions and outcomes (LaRocca-Pitts, 2009).

Most spiritual assessment tools can be divided into two categories: those based on a "belief" framework and those based on a "resource" framework. The belief framework is an older model, more closely associated with religion, and measures spirituality in terms of belief in God or a higher power. The second main category of spiritual assessment approaches, the "resource framework," is less driven by a specific religious tradition and is more concerned with how participants utilize aspects of their spirituality to make meaning from their experiences. Grossoehme (2008) defines spiritual resources as "those values, beliefs and practices which the patient already possesses and brings with them to understand their experience, and which can be enlisted to aid them in healing from their brokenness" (p. 72). Resources can be contrasted with spiritual needs, which are "those elements of their brokenness, or beliefs or practices which prevent them from feeling whole" (p. 72). Specific spiritual resources might include a positive God-image, strong familial relationships, and hope; spiritual needs may be manifested through feelings of loneliness, shame, or blame for life problems. The majority of tools developed for the clinical setting operate from a resource framework, using the identification of spiritual assets as a way to enhance health care treatment plans. The Child/Adolescent Screening Tool (CAST) (Grossoehme, 2008), and the Religiosity and Spirituality Scale for Youth (RaSSY) (Hernandez, 2011) are two examples of adolescent-specific instruments that focus on spiritual resources. The resource framework supports a developmental approach with its implication that people can gain resources as they progress through their life cycle.

Because spiritual development is constructed as being a process, in many ways a process-oriented evaluation methodology is most suitable for spiritual assessment. Because the arts are often correlated with strong existing emotions, an arts-based approach is primed to promote transcendence through the assessment process itself. Therefore, the very act of participating in an arts-based assessment activity can promote spiritual development for students. In one collage activity that combined music and visual art, many students expressed a definite progression of thought from beginning of the project to the end—with the last part of their collages seeming to be particularly important to the students themselves. The activity appeared to give youth the chance to gain a better understanding their own thoughts and beliefs as they found ways to express these creatively.

While an arts-based assessment activity can be facilitated by non-academic laypeople, the interpretation of data relies on in-depth, complex involvement with participants in the art-making process. The flexibility of this approach allows for nuanced understandings of spirituality but may require facilitators to be able to interpret multiple layers of data. Developing rubrics or checklists ahead of time can standardize the assessment process and help the facilitator both to interpret the data and to focus on the most important indicators.

Many arts-based assessment activities are derived from the fields of therapy and education, and all could be expanded upon within a real-world youth development setting. Youth workers would do well to incorporate assessment fully into their pedagogical approach. For example, a lesson on purpose might begin by asking students to draw a picture of what they think it means to live out their purpose (see Figure 1). Their pictures would then serve as a springboard for group discussion. As the students draw and discuss, the facilitator would pay attention to particular factors, including the following:

- **Students' Ability to Respond Easily to the Prompt:** Those who struggle to come up with a personal answer to the prompt may not possess as strong a sense of purpose as those who quickly come up with several examples.
- **Descriptions/Depictions of Transcendent Experiences:** Students may reference their main source of transcendence as determining their purpose: a deity; relationships with family or friends; a sense of connection with all of humanity, nature, or art.
- **Students' Sense of Intentionality:** Students with a less-developed understanding of purpose might speak primarily in the present tense of things that they already like or do. Students with a more mature sense of purpose would be more likely to speak in the future tense of their intentions to "accomplish something meaningful to the self" (Mariano & Damon, 2008, p. 212).

Ultimately, all of these observations would work together to assess each youth's initial understanding of purpose. The facilitator could adjust his/her educational activities to meet the needs of participating students and reach them at their most appropriate level of spiritual development. This use of assessment could be seen as eliciting "critical awareness," upon which specific intervention and educational strategies

Figure 1. Sample artistic response to the prompt, "I am living out my purpose when..."

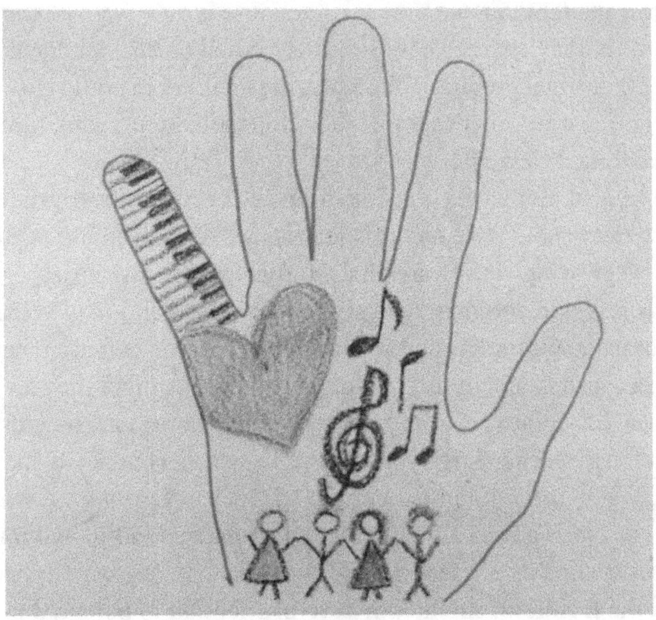

can be based (Corbitt & Nix-Early, 2003, p. 67). At the end of the experience or lesson, students could even complete the assessment exercise again, so that the facilitator (and/or the students themselves) could see how their answers changed and how well they were able to incorporate the new ideas presented.

This shift requires facilitators to see their role, and the process of assessment, through a different lens. Neither assessment tools nor lesson plans themselves can be viewed as static, stand-alone activities. Especially in the context of real-world programming, both assessment and pedagogy must be dynamic enough to effectively interact with one another, as well as with the youths' lived experiences, in order to effect change in their attitudes and practices. Such changes, therefore, will ultimately increase the program's overall effectiveness.

ARTS-BASED ASSESSMENT ACTIVITIES

The following two activities were designed to assess particular aspects of spiritual development and were tested in church-based youth group settings that already had long-standing, positive group dynamics in place. If students are meeting for the first time, or if they have had ongoing conflicts or tension, the facilitator will likely need to do additional work in order to establish a healthy rapport. Icebreaker activities can be helpful in setting the tone for the rest of the session.

When using an arts-based assessment activity, it is important to clearly state one's expectations at the outset of the activity. This gives students a sense of predictability and control – which, in turn, creates an emotionally safe space for all participants. If the group has a covenant of behavioral and/or relational expectations, the facilitator can use this as a guiding document and continue to refer to it as needed. Otherwise, it might be wise to let the group to write down their own expectations and "rules" at the beginning of the session.

Another consideration relates to the interpretation of the artistic product. In general, it is recommended that students be able to choose whether, and to what extent, they might wish to share their work with their peers. If students know that they will have to talk about their drawings to others, they might choose a different subject matter than one they might choose if they were to know that they would have control over whether or not they share. That said, it is crucial to take students' own explanations into account when assessing their final product. Therefore, the facilitator should ensure that all students have the chance to explain their artwork in a way that feels comfortable to them, through a written response or some sort of individual interview afterwards.

The facilitator should also emphasize the importance of process over product, in order to prevent students from feeling anxiety about the final artistic product. As Lowenfeld & Brittain (1987) famously pointed out, adolescents' growing self-awareness can manifest as insecurity, criticism, and frustration about their own art. They tend to compare their work with others and may become anxious about their ability to fit in with their peers. Silliness and humor can be common defense mechanisms, as teens try to laugh off their self-consciousness about their art and/or the subject that they are portraying. The facilitator must judge whether the silliness is at an appropriate level or if the students need to be redirected.

Another common defense mechanism is for students to simply shut down and refuse to participate or respond to the prompt. While this could be a normal adolescent response, it is also a classic symptom of trauma. Due to changes in the brain's functioning, a traumatized individual may literally be unable to process an experience of trauma or revisit the painful memory in any way. When working in a trauma-informed environment, the facilitator should pay careful attention to potential triggers—and in order to avoid re-traumatizing the youth, should never force any student to participate. Some topics are obviously sensitive and have a higher likelihood of upsetting participants (e.g. death, violence, sexual experiences, sexual orientation), but even seemingly routine questions could trigger a traumatic response. For example, a student who has experienced abuse or neglect might have difficulty with questions about his/her family background. If a student becomes upset during the assessment process, the facilitator should stop, attend to his/her immediate needs, and help to re-establish a sense of safety before continuing (SAMSHA, 2015).

Activity 1: Illuminative Art

Developed and described by Spouse (2000), illuminative art is a technique that uses a visual art exercise as a prompt to promote reflection about a specific topic. Students' oral and written responses are critical to understanding how they have been able to make meaning of their experiences, but the art-making process serves as a necessary guiding device. For this particular activity, students were given the choice of two prompts: "Draw a spiritual experience" or "draw an experience that had a significant impact on your life." In their drawings, students were asked to depict their chosen experience from two perspectives: external (what actually happened) and internal (what it felt like). After completing the activity, all students had the opportunity to share their images with the group. Then they filled out a confidential worksheet to describe their drawings, answering the questions below:

- What happened during the experience you depicted?
- What did this experience feel like to you?
- How do you think that this experience has affected your life, and the person you have become?

Because the focus group participants did not necessarily share any particular life experience, this prompt was designed to be intentionally vague. In another context, it may be helpful to provide a more specific prompt. For example, in a grief support group, possible prompts might be to draw "a picture of the funeral" or "a time when you missed the person who died," from both the internal and external perspectives. The prompt could also be altered in order to specifically highlight a particular aspect of the rubric by focusing on particular experiences related to families and friends (relational resources) or coping mechanism (religious coping).

Assessment

This prompt is particularly well suited to assess students' meaning-making capacity, coping, and relational resources. Use the checklist in Table 2 to identify any of the indicators referenced by the youth in their drawing. The left-hand column represents indicators of spiritual deficits, while the right-hand column represents spiritual assets. In general, the more boxes that are checked on the right-hand side, the better equipped a student might be with spiritual assets that can help them develop a lasting sense of resilience, purpose, and/or hope. Please note that this checklist is not exhaustive, and other issues may arise during this prompt that may need to be addressed separately.

Table 2. Assessment checklist for the illuminative art activity

Relational Resources	
□ Student talks about unsupportive or dysfunctional family dynamics. □ Students' peers are not supportive and/or exert a negative influence on him/her.	□ Student refers to strong, loving family relationships. □ Student mentions strong, supportive friendships.
Meaning Making	
□ Student expresses a lack of hope or purpose, or a general feeling that life will not get better.	□ Student is able to explain a lesson that he/she learned from the experience. □ Student can explain how an experience of adversity affected him/her positively. □ Student expresses a sense of purpose, calling, or service as a result of the experience.
Religious Coping	
□ Student mentions negative coping mechanisms in times of adversity, like turning to drugs, becoming depressed, or withdrawing from people. □ Student expresses unresolved anger or frustration towards God or a religious community.	□ Student reports turning to God or another higher power during the experience. □ Student mentions finding comfort in religious rituals or disciplines (i.e. prayer; scripture study) during the experience. □ Student refers to the support of a religious community during the experience.

DISCUSSION

Layla was an 11th grade student who was extremely involved in her church youth group. She attended regularly, volunteered in the church nursery, and was seen as a leader by her peers. After hearing the prompt, she immediately began working on a two-sided drawing that depicted her grandmother's suicide (see Figure 2). As she explained her drawing to the group, she said, "[The aftermath of my grandmother's suicide] was spiritual because no one knew what we were feeling as a whole. The only person we could turn to was God. People judged our family and pointed fingers, saying, you know, this isn't right. My mother went into a deep depression, and started doing drugs. I lived most of my life without my mother. I got picked on a lot, and was different from other kids." In Layla's written response to the question, "How has this experience affected your life?" she wrote, "I think I matured faster and developed a tuffer [sic] skin."

An individual's meaning-making capacity is demonstrated by his/her ability to craft narratives that spin an experience of adversity in a positive light: Zohar and Marshall (2004) list "positive use of adversity" as a spiritual asset that is indicated by the ability to see "a bright side" in difficult situations (Loc. 2262). The RaSSY (Hernandez, 2011) operationalizes this positive use of adversity through questionnaire items such as "When bad things happen, I try to figure out what lesson God is trying to teach me" and "When something bad happens, I know God is trying to make me stronger" (p. 37). Although these items operate from a theistic perspective, the basic premise remains true even in a non-theistic context: Spiritual development involves the ability to find the good, learn a lesson, or craft meaning from situations of crisis. Even though Layla described her friends and family as being unsupportive during this time – potentially a significant spiritual deficit – she nonetheless was able to draw upon deep spiritual assets to cope – and even thrive – after grandmother's death.

Figure 2. Layla, an 11th grade female, chose to depict her grandmother's suicide.

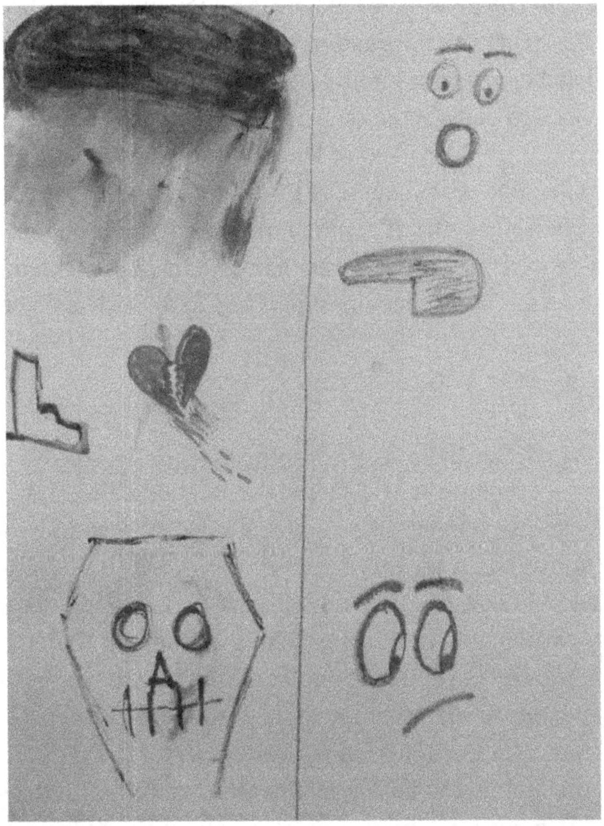

Many youth, like Layla, made the choice to depict experiences of adversity, even though the prompt did not specifically ask them to do so. Because of the nature of the experiences depicted, many chose not to share verbally, meaning that their written responses provided the only explanation of the visual art. If time had permitted, it would have been preferable to meet with students individually to allow them to process out loud in a safe setting.

The artwork created during this activity attests to the fact that adolescents are in the process of developing the ability to think symbolically. Younger adolescents tended to respond to the prompt with extremely concrete images; three different seventh graders, for example, created diagram-like drawings, with verbal labels, to explain the sequence of events and dialogue that comprised their experiences. These youth were much more concerned with depicting what actually happened than what their experiences had felt like.

Older adolescents, on the other hand, are more capable of creating highly abstract, symbolic images. Some older youth focused almost exclusively on their personal feelings about the experience without making any reference to what actually happened. Most, however, used a combination of concrete and symbolic imagery. They drew recognizable objects (sports equipment; chairs; tables) to depict the external perspective on their experiences, and mixed personal symbols with easily recognizable ones, such as hearts and teardrops, in order to convey their feelings.

Visual art activities like this one tend to be best suited for individual engagement and reflection – though, of course, it would also be possible to incorporate community art projects (such as murals and mosaics) into program assessment and evaluation efforts. One strength of visual art is that it allows youth to use both personal and communal symbols that have meaning for them; however, it is important to give participants the chance to explain the meaning of their work, either in verbally or in writing, to avoid misinterpretation. Spouse (2000) talked at length about creating space for supplementary verbal explanations; and a small anecdote will show why this recommendation is so important. At one point, a student drew a picture of herself on the edge of a cliff, which the researcher initially associated with feelings of desperation or depression. However, as the participant explained her drawing to the group, she said that she felt like she was on the edge of giving her life to God, and she looked forward to taking "a leap of faith."

Activity 2: Mad Libs

This activity was based on a common music therapy technique called lyric analysis, through which students listen to and analyze the meaning of a song and may subsequently be guided through a song-writing intervention. The song chosen for this exercise was "Restless" by Switchfoot because it is rich with concrete imagery, and although it addresses spiritual themes, it is not explicitly theistic. In fact, when discussing the song, participants were asked who they thought the "you" to whom the song was addressed might represent. Several participants guessed God, but others guessed a lover.

For the activity itself, students received a copy of the lyrics to the song "Restless"; as they listened to the song, they were instructed to circle or underline the lyrics that stood out to them. Then they worked together to create a group illustration of the images that they had heard in the song. This group drawing was used as the jumping-off point for a brief discussion about the meaning of the song. Participants were then asked to create and draw a symbol that would represent their own relationship with God, and to rewrite the chorus of "Restless" using words to describe this relationship. Students received the opportunity afterward to share their rewritten songs with the rest of the group.

Different songs could, of course, be used to assess other aspects of spirituality; and variations of the prompt could be adapted for other settings. In music therapy, songs are often chosen based on themes and/or life issues that are presented in the lyrics (e.g. loneliness; loss; self-questioning; friendship; acceptance). Youth may also respond well to the works of a particular artist if they view that artist as a role model or if they connect with some aspect of his/her life story. Grocke & Wigram (2007) offer a list of songs that have been found suitable for lyric analysis in music therapy, noting that "clients will interpret songs in different ways, based on their own views of the song, and it is this dynamic that makes the method therapeutically valuable" (p. 160).

Assessment

This prompt allows students to use metaphors to depict both their sense of self and their relationships in the world. More than simply an assessment of *whether* participants experience transcendence, this activity can begin to form a deeper picture of *how* participants understand their experiences of transcendence.

Use the checklist in Table 3 to identify any of the indicators referenced by the youth in order to identify the major themes that define their relationship to a higher power. Please note that this checklist is not exhaustive, and that other issues may arise during this prompt that need to be addressed separately.

DISCUSSION

The worksheet prompt, as with all arts-based prompts, serves as the "container" for the assessment: that is, a concrete focal point, with defined parameters, which creates a safe space for participants to engage with the topic. All of the youth seemed to enjoy listening to the song and were able to both identify lyrics that stood out to them and draw images from the song immediately afterward. Some students, however, initially seemed unsure about their ability to create a song about their relationship with God. Ultimately, though, the task-based nature of the worksheet, with its specific instructions and fill-in-the-blank format, made the process seem much less overwhelming. A few students even remarked, "Oh, I can do that!"

Once again, the youth's use of symbolism tended to vary with age. Younger students were more likely to use conventional religious symbols (e.g. cross; churches), while older students invented new ways of conceptualizing their relationship with God (e.g. a compass; a brick wall; a cliff). It is worth noting that this progression in the use of symbolism seems to support the general structure of Fowler's faith development theory, in which the progression of faith development is increasingly individuative. Adolescents may move from a mythic or conventional understanding of faith (i.e. the cross as the chief symbol of one's relationship with God) to a more self-reflective faith (i.e. the creation of a personal symbol).

Similarly, the categories included in the above checklist explore some of these developmental shifts. The theme "Love and Praise" generally implies a relational view of God, while "Purpose and Self-Worth" is directly related to the adolescent developmental task of understanding one's identity and role within society. Students whose responses fell into the latter category referred to their own attributes of strength and power, often in conjunction with being created or having a higher calling.

Rob, a ninth grader, drew a spray paint can to represent his relationship with God, which was characterized by both of the above themes (see Figure 3). He explained, "God's spraying us in the direction he wants us to go. Like, he might send [another student] to play the drums and [another student] to go to college and become an engineer." He wrote, "I am a spray can. I am wonderfully created, I am difrent [sic], I am loved, I am prasing [sic] you."

Table 3. Assessment checklist for the Mad Libs activity

Love and Praise	☐ Student says that they love God. ☐ Student feels loved by God. ☐ Student focuses on positive, praiseworthy characteristics or actions of God.
Purpose and Self-Worth	☐ Student focuses on his/her own attributes as having purpose. ☐ Student believes that s/he was created by God for a higher calling or purpose.
Faith and Trust	☐ Student expresses a willingness to believe in, trust, or rely on God.
Uncertainty, Change, and Crisis	☐ Student's faith is actively developing or growing as a result of a major life change or crisis. ☐ Student appears to be struggling in his/her relationship with God ☐ Student asks questions of God. ☐ Student directs anger, grief, or doubt toward God.
Other	☐ *List any other notable features of the student's artwork:*

Figure 3. Rob, a ninth grade male, used a can of spray paint to symbolize his relationship with God.

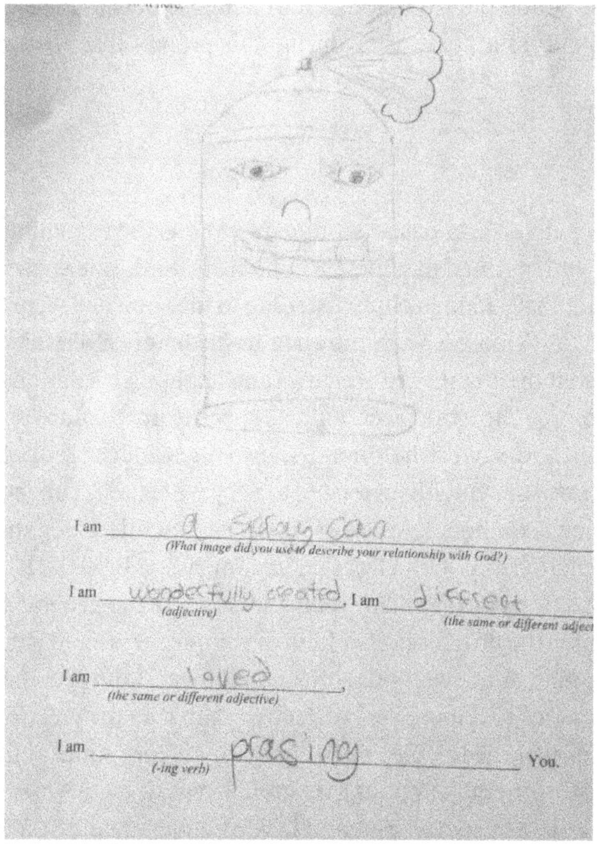

It is important to note that "Uncertainty, Change, and Crisis" is not necessarily a negative category, although the facilitator must interpret youth responses carefully in order to accurately assess the participant's level of spiritual development. This theme can, in fact, be indicative of an actively developing faith. Fowler (1981) writes, "Growth and development in faith…result from life crises, challenges, and the kinds of disruptions that theologians call revelation" (p. 101). John, a 12th grader, chose a finger trap to represent his relationship with God; using the words "stretching" and "pulling" to depict a dynamic, changing faith (see Figure 4). He defined his relationship as one of trusting and seeking to understand God (Faith and Trust) in the midst of uncertainty.

On the other hand, Marissa, a 10th grader, wrote, "I am a lost traveler. I am broken, I am broken, I am broken, I am needing You." To accompany her lyrics, she drew a girl standing beside a map with roads crossing each other and spiraling around each other (see Figure 5). A building with a cross (presumably a church) was located in the middle of the map, but was not easily accessible from the main road. The task, presumably, for the youth worker would be to provide both John and Marissa with a safe space to explore their changing spirituality. For Marissa particularly, it would be important to offer guidance and stability as she moved toward wholeness (regardless of whether her spiritual development process ultimately led her toward the church/organized religion, or away from it).

Figure 4. John, a 12th grade male, depicted his relationship with God with the image of a finger trap.

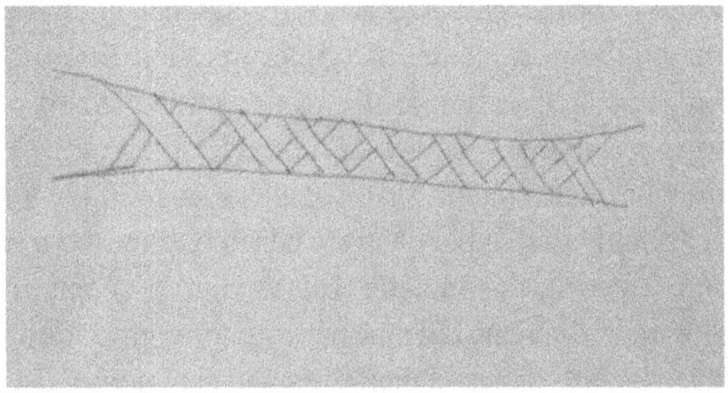

Figure 5. Marissa, a 10th grade female, drew a map.

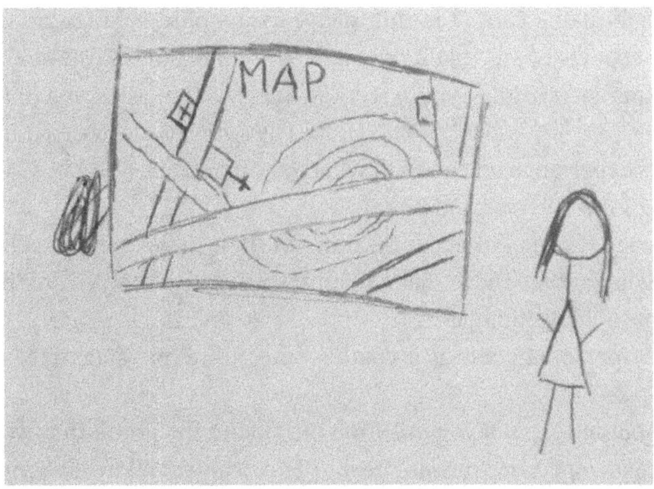

CONCLUSION

Youth workers should consider using an arts-based approach to assessment and program evaluation when they wish to:

- Explore qualitative topics, such as spiritual development, which cannot be adequately captured through traditional surveys.
- Integrate the assessment process into their regular curriculum or programming.
- Reach students with differing cognitive and/or language abilities.
- Engage youth and stakeholders in new ways.

Arts-based assessments are well suited for organizational contexts whose approach combines positive youth development and trauma-informed care. Because arts-based evaluation instruments are inherently subjective, the facilitator must rely on students' own interpretations in order to accurately understand their perspectives. Therefore, this approach amplifies the youth's own voices to the adults who serve them, providing an empowering and equalizing experience for the youth. Youth workers may choose to go one step further and involve youth intentionally at every stage of the evaluation process, allowing them to assess themselves explicitly and make changes based on their own results.

The specific activities presented in this chapter aim to elicit a deeper, more complex understanding of youth spiritual development than has been accessible through traditional surveys. Though some PYD organizations work directly with licensed therapists and social workers who can apply assessment results to create specific treatment plans, most youth workers will use their results primarily to guide programming decisions. It is important to check in with students to understand, among other things, how they perceive transcendence; make meaning of their life experiences; and live out their beliefs. For organizations that serve the same youth for multiple years, completing regular assessments will provide a glimpse of how these aspects of spirituality change over time and in response to specific programs or interventions. In analyzing their results, youth workers may want to ask some of the following questions:

1. Does this student's experience line up with what our organization teaches? If not, how can we better impart our organization's values and beliefs?
2. How can we help our students to make meaning of their life experiences?
3. What does our organization believe that a mature spirituality should look like? What are we doing to help our students achieve that goal?
4. Am I achieving my personal goals as a youth worker? Are my students learning what I am trying to teach them?
5. What spiritual resources can our organization provide to the youth that we serve?
6. What are my students' specific spiritual needs? How can we address them?

The arts themselves show great potential for facilitating spiritual development. First, their symbolic language gives them *ideological* power to support the beliefs, stories, and values of an individual or community. Second, they derive *social* power from their ability to bring people together within the therapeutic, research, or community context. Finally, the very experience of art-making has *transcendent* power to connect the artist with a renewed vision for his/her own life, purpose, and creative potential. Therefore, arts-based assessments can serve as a catalyst for spiritual development—particularly if strengthened with proper follow-up from the facilitator.

Ultimately, developing innovative and collaborative ways to assess adolescent spirituality will also unlock new ways of understanding and improving the broader context of positive youth development. Both the process and the products of art-making reveal new possibilities and new ways of knowing, for youth workers as well as for the youth themselves. As assessment and pedagogical tools, the arts remain flexible and dynamic enough to transcend many different boundaries; to speak to participants' deepest experiences; and to promote spiritual transformation among those who are willing to create.

REFERENCES

Barna, G. (2017, April 6). *Meet the "Spiritual but Not Religious."* Barna Group. Retrieved from https://www.barna.com/research/meet-spiritual-not-religious

Bloom. (2011). Bridging the black hole of trauma: The evolutionary significance of the arts, part 2: The arts and evolution—What is art for? *Psychotherapy and Politics International, 9*(1), 67-82. doi:10.1002/ppi.229

Brevard Family Partnership. (2017). *Brevard youth thrive: Protective and promotive factors for healthy development and well-being*. Retrieved from http://brevardfp.org/brevard-youth-thrive/

Brown, E. (1998). Things of the Spirit: Spiritual, moral, social, and cultural development. *Support for Learning, 13*(4), 157–162. doi:10.1111/1467-9604.00081

Corbitt, J. N., & Nix-Early, V. (2003). *Taking it to the streets: Using the arts to transform your community*. Grand Rapids, MI: Baker Books.

Edenloff, J. (2011). *Arts-based evaluation tools for community arts programs: A case study of Art City's 'Green Art' in Winnipeg, Manitoba (Unpublished thesis)*. Winnipeg, Manitoba: University of Manitoba. Retrieved from http://mspace.lib.umanitoba.ca/handle/1993/4893

Eriksen, E. (1993). *Childhood and society*. New York: W. W. Norton & Company Ltd. (Original publication 1963)

Fowler, J. W. (1981). *Stages of faith: The psychology of human development and the quest for meaning*. New York, NY: HarperCollins Publishers.

Fraser, J. G., Griffin, J. L., Barto, B. L., Lo, C., Wenz-Gross, M., Spinazzola, J., ... Bartlett, J. D. (2014). Implementation of a workforce initiative to build trauma-informed child welfare practice and services: Findings from the Massachusetts Child Trauma Project. *Children and Youth Services Review, 44*, 233–242. doi:10.1016/j.childyouth.2014.06.016

Giesenberg, A. (2007). *The phenomenology of preschool children's spirituality (Unpublished thesis)*. Brisbane, Australia: Queensland University of Technology. Retrieved from http://eprints.qut.edu.au/16519/1/Anna_Giesenberg_Thesis.pdf

Good, M., & Willoughby, T. (2006). The role of spirituality versus religiosity in adolescent psychosocial adjustment. *Journal of Youth and Adolescence, 35*(1), 41–55. doi:10.100710964-005-9018-1

Grocke, D., & Wigram, T. (2007). *Receptive methods in music therapy*. Philadelphia, PA: Jessica Kingsley Publishers.

Grossman, F. K., Sorsoli, L., & Kia-Keating, M. (2006). A gale force wind: Meaning making by male survivors of childhood sexual abuse. *The American Journal of Orthopsychiatry, 76*(4), 434–443. doi:10.1037/0002-9432.76.4.434 PMID:17209711

Grossoehme, D. H. (2008). Development of a spiritual screening tool for children and adolescents. *The Journal of Pastoral Care & Counseling, 62*(1), 71–85. doi:10.1177/154230500806200108 PMID:18572542

Herndandez, B. C. (2011). *The Religiosity and Spirituality Scale for Youth: Development and initial validation (Unpublished dissertation)*. Baton Rouge, LA: Louisiana State University. Retrieved from http://etd.lsu.edu/docs/available/etd-10142011-115001/unrestricted/hernandez_diss.pdf

King, P. E. (2008). Spirituality as Fertile Ground for Positive Youth Development. In R. M. Lerner, R. W. Roeser, & E. Phelps (Eds.), *Positive youth development & spirituality: From theory to research* (pp. 55–73). West Consohocken, PA: Templeton Foundation Press.

King, P. E., Clardy, C. E., & Ramon, J. S. (2013). Adolescent spiritual exemplars: Exploring spirituality in the lives of diverse youth. *Journal of Adolescent Research*, *28*(5), 1–27. doi:10.1177/0743558413502534

LaRocca-Pitts, M. (2009). In FACT, chaplains have a spiritual assessment tool. *Australian Journal of Pastoral Care and Health*, *3*(2), 8–15. Retrieved from http://www.pastoraljournal.findaus.com/pdfs/ar2.pdf

Lippman, L. H., Moore, K. A., & McIntosh, H. (2009). *Positive indicators of child well-being: A conceptual framework, measures, and methodological issues*. Innocenti Working Paper No. 2009-21. Florence, Italy: Innocenti Research Centre (UNICEF). Retrieved from http://www.unicef-irc.org/publications/pdf/iwp_2009_21.pdf

Lowenfeld, V., & Brittain, W. L. (1987). *Creative and mental growth*. Upper Saddle River, NJ: Prentice Hall. (Original work published 1949)

Mariano, J. M., & Damon, W. (2008). The role of spirituality and religious faith in supporting purpose in adolescence. In R. M. Lerner, R. W. Roeser, & E. Phelps (Eds.), *Positive youth development & spirituality: From theory to research* (pp. 210–230). West Consohocken, PA: Templeton Foundation Press.

National Research Council and Institute of Medicine. (2002). *Community programs to promote youth development*. Washington, DC: National Academy Press.

Scarlett, W. G. (2008). Spirituality and positive youth development: The problem of transcendence. In R. M. Lerner, R. W. Roeser, & E. Phelps (Eds.), *Positive youth development & spirituality: From theory to research* (pp. 42–54). West Consohocken, PA: Templeton Foundation Press.

Spouse, J. (2000). Talking pictures: Investigating personal knowledge through illuminative art-work. *Nursing Times Research*, *5*(4), 253–261. doi:10.1177/136140960000500404

Stuckey, H. L., & Nobel, J. (2010). The connection between art, healing and public health: A review of current literature. *American Journal of Public Health*, *100*(2), 254–263. doi:10.2105/AJPH.2008.156497 PMID:20019311

Substance Abuse and Mental Health Services Administration. (2014). *SAMHSA's concept of trauma and guidance for a trauma-informed approach. HHS Publication No. (SMA) 14-4884*. Rockville, MD: Substance Abuse and Mental Health Services Administration.

Substance Abuse and Mental Health Services Administration. (2015, November). *A guide to GPRA data collection using trauma-informed interviewing skills*. Retrieved from https://www.integration.samhsa.gov/about-us/Trauma-InformedInterviewingManual-508.pdf

Zohar, D., & Marshall, I. (2004). *Spiritual capital: Wealth we can live by. Kindle Edition*. San Francisco, CA: Berrett-Koehler Publishers.

ADDITIONAL READING

Brevard Family Partnership. (2014). *Principles of trauma[-]informed care and positive youth development.* Center for the Study of Social Policy. Retrieved from http://brevardfp.org/wordpress/wp-content/uploads/2014/07/TIC-Booklet-Reduced.pdf

Hodge, D. R. (2005). Developing a spiritual assessment toolbox: A discussion of the strengths and limitations of five different assessment methods. *Health & Social Work, 30*(4), 314–323. doi:10.1093/hsw/30.4.314 PMID:16323723

Lerner, R. M., Roeser, R. W., & Phelps, E. (Eds.). (2008). *Positive youth development & spirituality: From theory to research.* West Consohocken, PA: Templeton Foundation Press.

Rogers, F. (2011). *Finding God in the graffiti: Empowering teenagers through stories.* Cleveland: The Pilgrim Press.

Search Institute. (2007). *40 developmental assets for adolescents.* Retrieved from http://www.search-institute.org/content/40-developmental-assets-adolescents-ages-12-18

Smith, C., & Denton, M. L. (2009). *Soul searching: The religious and spiritual lives of American teenagers.* Oxford: Oxford University Press.

KEY TERMS AND DEFINITIONS

Assessment: The process of gathering, analyzing, and interpreting evidence in order to better understand and improve a particular program, curriculum, or intervention.

Formative Assessment: The collection of data before or during a program, which helps to determine the need for a program, guide the planning process, or change the program while it is ongoing.

Meaning-Making: The way in which an individual understands and interprets life experiences and world events based on his/her worldview.

Positive Youth Development: An asset-based approach toward youth programming which incorporates and applies knowledge of developmental systems in order to maximize positive outcomes for youth.

Summative Assessment: The collection of data at the end of a program or intervention in order to better understand its outcomes and impact.

Transcendence: A sense of connection to something larger than the self – such as to nature, humanity, art, or a deity.

Chapter 15
Beyond Words:
Arts-Based Assessment of Post-Traumatic Growth

Suet Ferng Tan
Eastern University, Singapore

ABSTRACT

Post-traumatic growth is an intangible yet a very real and possible phenomenon. Conventional measurement of post-traumatic growth relies on formal self-assessed questionnaires and interviews which may be challenging to administer and sustain in the long course of the healing process. This chapter builds upon the post-traumatic growth inventory designed by authors Tedeschi and Calhoun and proposes an arts-based assessment for post-traumatic growth. This may offer a more organic approach to the measurement of growth and it may be utilized by caregivers and counselors in a safe, non-clinical environment. The results from this research demonstrate the effectiveness and depth of arts-based assessment both as a standalone as well as a complementary tool that can be used alongside other forms of assessment to measure growth.

INTRODUCTION

During a traumatic experience, the left hemisphere (that controls linear processing and language function) tends to be inhibited while the right hemisphere (that controls sensory-perceptual experience) is stimulated (Van der Kolk, 1994). People who suffer from post-traumatic stress replay their traumatic memories through the sensory and imaging storage area of the brain's right hemisphere (Lanius et al., 2004). This may explain why healers or shamans, through generations, used experiences that engaged the brain's right hemisphere such as drumming, dance and imagery for healing (Jacobson-Levy, 2013).

DOI: 10.4018/978-1-5225-5981-8.ch015

BACKGROUND

Trauma and Brain

During a traumatic experience, the dominant hemisphere (likely to be the left brain) which controls linear processing and language function tends to be inhibited while the non-dominant hemisphere (which controls the sensory-perceptual experience) is stimulated (Van der Kolk, 1994). Lanius et al. (2004) confirmed that people who experienced a traumatic event and are suffering from post-traumatic stress replay their traumatic memories through the sensory and imaging storage area of the brain's right hemisphere. Thus, through generations, healers or shamans used experiences that engaged more fully the brain's right hemisphere such as drumming, dance, and the use of symbols that appeared in the person's dreams, art, and imagery (Jacobson-Levy, 2013) for healing.

In the absence of cultural rituals in our postmodern world, the arts may serve as an effective platform where traumatic narratives may be expressed, and where community bonds may be forged in a safe space. On the other hand, conventional counseling or talk therapy may not attain its desired effectiveness in facilitating healing since the traumatized person has likely lost most connection with the brain's left hemisphere, and therefore may find it hard to process the situation through words. The traumatic experience is likely to be articulated in an entirely different language – the language of the nonverbal and of the enacted (Bloom, 2010). Whether it is through verbal or nonverbal expressions, many researchers and authors in the field of trauma recovery spell out the need for one to tell his or her story of the trauma. Through this, the person is able to reconcile the right hemisphere with the left. In doing so, the person can categorize, order or place the traumatic experience in a meaning that is associated with the past, and relegate it to the past as a memory (Bloom, 2010). If not, the traumatic experience will remain unmetabolized, unintegrated and continues to have an existence in the non-dominant hemisphere reality. The experience may continue haunting the person in the form of nightmares, flashbacks and behavioral re-enactments (Bloom, 2010). Until some other experiences occur to permit to permit a reordering of reality and incorporation of the trauma into a new sense of meaning, the haunting will continue and the person may develop all kinds of secondary behaviors in an attempt to cope with this continuing problem. In fact, addictions, compulsive behaviors, behavioral reenactments, anxieties, phobias, depression, and a variety of physical symptoms may manifest due to a failure to cope with their trauma in healthy ways (Bloom, 2010).

To facilitate healing and give trauma a new meaning, the arts may be a good and safe platform for one to "re-tell" his or her traumatic experience. As such, arts-based assessment may also be a relevant approach in evaluating post-traumatic growth.

Arts and Healing

Art acts as a bridge between the two hemispheres of the brain. For example, the melody within a piece of music works on the right hemisphere while the lyrics work on the left (Huey-Heck & Kalnin, 2006). The bridging process requires both hemispheres to function in an integrated, active manner and this helps one to make sense of and deal with the traumatic memories.

Research has shown that creative processes such as journaling can help to improve the physical health of trauma survivors (Bloom, 2010). Music has also been found to help cancer patients in increasing their sense of control, increasing immunity, reducing pain, anxiety and other psychological and physical symptoms (Stuckey & Nobel, 2010). Some studies also found that dance and movement programs help to improve body image, shoulder function and increase quality of life among breast cancer survivors (Sandel, Judge, Landry, Faria, Ouellette & Majczak, 2005).

Among all its other functions, art is able to help people express experiences that may be too difficult to put into words. Often, words may be woefully inadequate when it comes to describing the spiritual experience that art offers. It is the process of art making that is transformational. It teaches, guides and encourages one to seek deeper spirituality (Huey-Heck & Kalnin, 2006). The process of art making helps one to explore the meanings of past, present and future, thereby integrating the traumatic experience into one's life story and giving it meaning (Stuckey & Nobel, 2010).

The process of art-making also helps to encourage verbal communication among a group of participants, form communities, facilitate cathartic release, and reveal unconscious materials and symbols that cannot be expressed through words (Stuckey & Nobel, 2010). This is a vital step towards post-traumatic growth. Overall, the arts can engage trauma survivors on multiple levels: the cognitive, emotional, social and biological, and this may bring about holistic healing since trauma also affects the bereaved persons in just as many aspects.

Post-Traumatic Growth

Post-traumatic growth refers to a change in people that goes beyond an ability to resist and not be damaged by highly stressful circumstances. It involves a movement beyond pre-trauma levels of adaptation (Tedeschi & Calhoun, 2004a). This means that the development of individuals in some areas would surpass what was present before the struggle. Post-traumatic growth is not simply a return to the baseline, but an experience of improvement that may be found to be deeply profound (Tedeschi & Calhoun, 2004a). A common expression would be the survivor becomes "a stronger person" after the trauma.There is a body of literature suggesting that people exposed to even the most traumatic events may perceive some good emerging from their struggle with tragedies such as rape, incest, bereavement, cancer, HIV infection, heart attacks, natural disasters, combat and the Holocaust (Tedeschi & Calhoun, 1996). Existing research also reveals that people who are less capable physically or psychologically tend to register greater growth than those who are more capable (Tedeschi & Calhoun, 2004a). This is because people with stronger coping capacities will be less challenged by trauma, and researchers posit that the struggle with trauma is crucial for post-traumatic growth (Tedeschi & Calhoun, 2004a). In fact, the often lengthy process during which distress persists may actually be important for the maximum degree of post-traumatic growth to occur. This period keeps the cognitive processing active and eventually helps individuals to make sense of and accommodate the traumatic events (Tedeschi & Calhoun, 2004a).

Though post-traumatic growth is possible even in the toughest of situations, Tedeschi & Calhoun (2004b) cautioned that there is still a need to promote a respect for the difficulty of trauma recovery. Clinicians are encouraged to use interventions that facilitate post-traumatic growth with care, and yet not to create expectations for post-traumatic growth in all trauma survivors.

Areas of Post-Traumatic Growth

Tedeschi & Calhoun (2004b) asserted that growth emerging from the struggle with trauma can be described by five major domains: seeing new possibilities, changed relationships, holding the paradoxical view of being both stronger yet more vulnerable, a greater appreciation for life, and changes in the individual's spiritual and existential domain. Based on these five domains, Tedeschi & Calhoun (1996) developed a post-traumatic growth inventory that comprises 21 items, measuring the individual's perception of positive changes after a traumatic life experience. These five domains include relating to others, new possibilities for life, personal strength, spiritual change, and appreciation of life.

While citing the main categories of growth, Tedeschi & Calhoun (2004b) admitted that it is possible that individuals may experience significant changes in their lives that do not readily fit within these broad categories. The Robitschek (1998) Personal Growth Initiative Scale, for example, focuses on taking personal ownership of one's decisions and future development. This chapter utilizes both the Tedeschi & Calhoun's (1996) Post-traumatic Growth Inventory as well as the Robitschek's (1998) Personal Growth Initiative Scale to assess growth.

Factors Leading to Growth

As mentioned, not everyone who experiences trauma will experience personal growth. Some of the factors that lead to growth are cognitive processing, emotional coping, and disclosure within supportive relationships (Tedeschi & Calhoun, 2004b). Calhoun, Tedeschi, Cann and Hanks termed such vital relationships as "expert companionship" (2010, p. 136). Though Calhoun (2010) positioned the expert companion as a clinician working with the bereaved, this concept may be applied to non-clinical settings too.

The expert companion should possess a few attributes such as having humility and respect for the bereaved persons. He or she should show respect for the beliefs and experiences of the bereaved persons, and must be willing to explore these beliefs and the doubts about them (Calhoun et al., 2010). The expert companion also exhibits constancy and does not rush the bereaved persons into attaining expectations set by friends and family. He or she can tolerate the fact that bereavement can be a longer-termed process than what is desired by those who surround the bereaved. The expert companion is a constant in spite of oscillations in the grief experience of the individual (Stroebe & Schut, 1999). In addition, the expert companion should be a non-judgmental listener and show tolerance of strange, non-rational or ambiguous talk by the bereaved persons. He or she must possess the courage to listen to unpleasant stories of death, despair or other traumatic details that the bereaved persons may carry with them (Calhoun et al., 2010).

More importantly, the expert companion has to appreciate the paradox that is presented by the traumatic experience, or by the bereaved person. The companion needs to realize that post-traumatic growth often unfolds in the process of grief itself (Calhoun et al., 2010). While loved ones and companions hope to see the bereaved person come out of his or her grief in the shortest time possible, the companions should realize that amidst the vulnerability displayed by the bereaved person, strength will emerge. Amidst doubtful questioning, new insights may arise. Amidst the desperate need for support, independence can be achieved (Calhoun et al., 2010). Thus, expert companions should be patient in the process, and continue to believe in the good that arises from the struggle with grief or trauma.

No one, especially the bereaved person, would want to hear anything about how the loss can produce something good. This may be especially so at the onset of the traumatic experience. During that period, it may be cruel to the bereaved person to receive comments such as "there must be a reason why this happened". Expert companions should grant the bereaved person time to grieve instead of pointing them to an immediate solution. They need to realize that it is the struggle with grief, and not the actual loss itself, that produces growth (Calhoun et al., 2010). It is what happens afterward, not the event itself, that is valued (Tedeschi & Calhoun, 2004b).

Based on research, other factors that could contribute to growth include optimism (Updegraff & Marshall, 2005; Hart, Vella & Mohr, 2008). Updegraff and Marshall (2005) identify two forms of optimism: generalized (or dispositional) optimism and situation-specific optimism. Generalized optimism is defined as an individual's inherent belief that the future holds positive outcomes, while situation-specific optimism refers to one's beliefs that positive outcomes will result from a particular event (Updegraff & Marshall, 2005; Urcuyo, Boyers, Carver, Antoni, 2005). Hart et al. (2005) discovered through research that improved benefit finding helps in reduced depression, leading to positive affect.

Existing literature also finds that religiosity or spirituality are among the top predictors of post-traumatic growth (Znoj, 2006). Religiosity and spirituality are relied upon as a coping mechanism, a means for self-regulation, as well as to serve as a framework for meaning (Tedeschi & Calhoun, 1996; Urcuyo et al. 2005; Calhoun et al., 2010). It seems that spirituality that leads to the construction of new meaning is linked more directly to post-traumatic growth. Some literature refers to this cognitive processing as "rumination" or the change of schemas (Tedeschi & Calhoun, 2004a). Many writers refer to rumination as recurrent positive or negative event-related thinking. Tedeschi & Calhoun (2004a) asserted that while trauma survivors are likely to report intrusive thoughts and images that are distressing in the initial aftermath of the trauma, such cognitive processing may change in quality over time. The acknowledgement of loss, regret, realization of unattained goals, and deliberate disclosure of the traumatic experience through verbal or non-verbal means can lead to post-traumatic growth (Tedeschi & Calhoun, 2004a).

Often, with the help of a supportive community, the bereaved person can disengage, or give up certain goals and basic assumptions while at the same time persisting in building new schemas, goals, and meanings. However, when friends and family do not wish to hear from the bereaved person, cognitive processing may be inhibited, and past research reports that there is less post-traumatic growth (Tedeschi & Calhoun, 2004a). Having discussed the factors that would facilitate growth, it is important to highlight that post-traumatic growth is both a process and an outcome (Tedeschi & Calhoun, 2004a).

Arts-Based Assessment

Most of the research on the role of arts in healing was conducted within hospitals rather than community settings (Stuckey & Nobel, 2010). There is a need for more research on the arts, healing and post-traumatic growth at the non-clinical, community level so that care and assessment may be administered not just by art therapists, but by counselors and caregivers.

Arts-based approaches use the arts to explore, understand and represent human action and experience (Savin-Baden & Major, 2013). In fact, arts-based methods make use of a larger spectrum of creative intelligence and communications, and generate important information that often feels more accurate, original, and intelligent than more conventional methods (McNiff, 2007).

This chapter describes the use of the artistic process in two folds: to facilitate healing as well as to assess post-traumatic growth. The process of art-making offers an excellent platform for data collection and analysis in a more organic and less clinical approach compared to conventional questionnaires or interviews. The use of arts-based inquiry allows one to observe and assess growth in the context of informal, authentic everyday living. The way the artist or participant creates or interacts with the art

Figure 1. Model of post-traumatic growth.

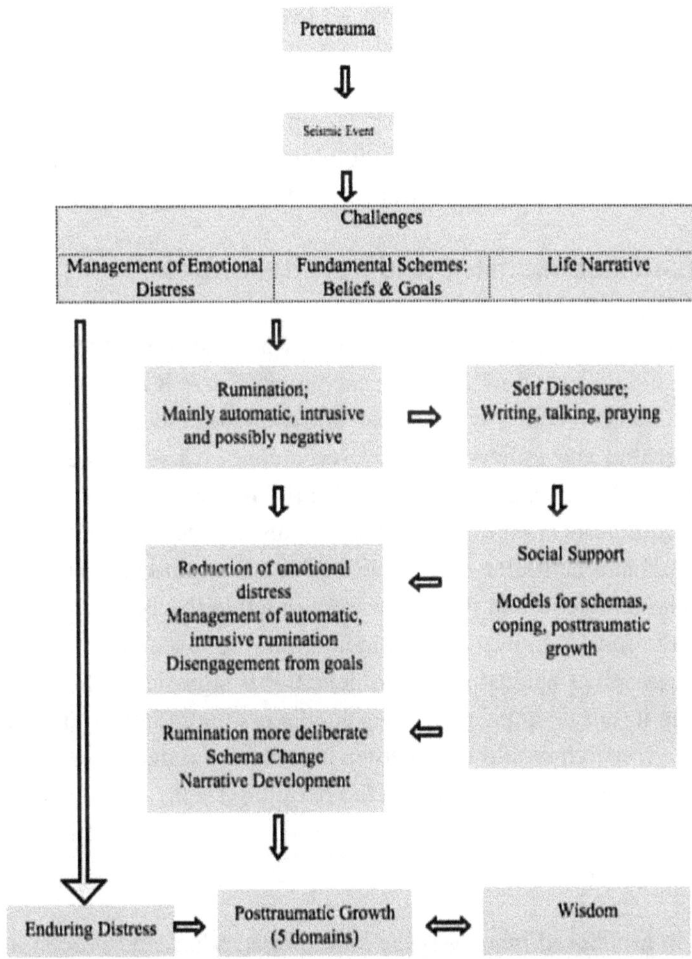

piece speaks of the way he or she approaches life. McNiff (2007) highlighted that the way we treat the most mundane or apparently inconsequent experiences may have the most to offer in suggesting social transformation. One of the most valuable features of arts-based research might be its potential in offering different ways to approach the most serious problems that we face in the world today.

Though Tedeschi and Calhoun (1996; 2004a) relied mainly on a simple self-report questionnaire that asked people to rate their post-traumatic growth in five domains, they highlighted that the questionnaire approach may be complemented by one that focuses on the presence of growth themes within narrative accounts of traumatic events themselves. There are two growth themes that signify transformation: the acknowledgement of the disequilibrating impact of the traumatic event on the self, as well as the construction of a positive ending for the story that provides coherence and resolution. (Pals & McAdams, 2004) There are also factors that may influence the narrative construction of the traumatic event that in turn affects post-traumatic growth. Factors such as personality traits (e.g. the openness to feelings, talking to others, praying, journaling) may help to move the bereaved person towards positive self transformation (Tedeschi & Calhoun, 2004a; Pals & McAdams, 2004). The arts provide a good platform for narrative construction in a safe space. The process of art making allows one to discover about oneself and learn about life from a safe distance through the use of metaphors, stories or analogies. The participants at the art sessions may safely retreat, hide or use their art pieces as the centre of discussion instead of putting themselves at the foreground to be subjected to scrutiny and judgment. While discussing their art pieces, the participants allow others to speak into their life in a non-threatening way. They, in turn, may share more freely and construct new meanings or schemas of their traumatic experience in a gradual, non-intimidating manner. Overall, the arts have the ability to convey personal and communal values, and they possess the catalytic power to affect transformation (Corbitt & Nix-Early, 2003).

Using an Arts-Based Assessment and Its Challenges

Though arts-based inquiry may not have as long a history as other quantitative and scientific research, there are a few existing guidelines to how it may be carried out. First, it is good to start small, stay focused and have a clear method that can be easily described and then implemented in a systematic way. Ideally, the method can be replicated and utilized by other researchers who may want to explore the problem separately (McNiff, 2007). The researcher should keep the research simple instead of trying to do too many things. Second, facilitators should freely observe, suspend judgment, and avoid pre-empting the outcome when investigating human behavior (McNiff, 2007). Sigmund Freud highlighted the importance of pure observation and attentiveness in psychoanalytic practice (McNiff, 2007).

Third, and perhaps the most important guideline, is that the research must be useful to others. Researchers must guard themselves against self-indulgence. It is significant if a study proves to be useful to the person conducting it, but its impact on other people is a more important goal (McNiff, 2011). A guiding question for the research would be whether it generates outcomes that inform the practice of others, and whether it has a positive influence on the people served.

Challenges

One of the challenges in arts-based inquiry is the lack of a standardized procedure to follow (McNiff, 2007). What makes arts-based inquiry challenging and interesting is that it is not prescriptive, and often the "rules" of qualitative inquiry cannot be applied easily (Savin-Baden & Major, 2013). The search for a method for arts-based inquiry is often characterized by a crucible of tensions, struggles, chaos and even the destruction of cherished assumptions (McNiff, 2007). It is still a relatively new field in research, and researchers must be able to live with nuances and "create outside the lines" (McNiff, 2007, p. 39).

Another challenge in arts-based inquiry is the difficulty in working with participants who are not inclined towards artistic expression (McNiff, 2007). Participants may feel intimidated by the process and become self-conscious. In this case, the facilitation skills of the researcher are vital in helping the participants find comfort in artistic expression, and to create a safe environment for the participants to freely create and share their thoughts. Ultimately, the essence of arts-based inquiry lies within the tripartite relationship between the researcher, the participant, and art.

DEVELOPING AN ARTS-BASED ASSESSMENT

Overview

There are three components of the following arts-based assessment: written questionnaire, observations during the arts sessions (both arts-based response and non-arts-based response), and a face-to-face interview. The validity of the arts-based assessment as a tool to measure post-traumatic growth is trusted. However, the descriptive language that is conveyed via the questionnaire and interview adds another dimension of understanding to post-traumatic growth, and may potentially validate what is revealed through the participants' arts-based and non arts-based responses during art making. Similarly, the arts sessions may also serve to validate what is conveyed via the written self-report questionnaire and the verbal response via the interview. In general, it is best to administer the questionnaire before the first art session so that it can serve as a pre-test. A post-test can also be administered after the last art session to see if any growth is registered. The questions in the questionnaire found in the appendix are extracted from Tedeschi and Calhoun's (1996; 2004a) Post-traumatic Growth Inventory (5 domains of growth), as well as Robitschek's (1998) Personal Growth Initiative. These indicators were developed by the author and are used as a reference when taking notes of the observations during the art sessions. These same indicators should be applied throughout the entire assessment period to measure growth.

Illustrating the Assessment

To best illustrate the use of this arts-based assessment, a description of its use with a small group of pregnant teens is included in this chapter. The assessment took place over three weekly art making sessions of two hours each at a residential centre in Singapore called Dayspring New Life Centre. This centre houses young pregnant mothers. The girls engaged in art making based on three different themes over the weekly sessions. Each of the themes seeks to impart life's lessons and facilitate growth through the use of metaphors. The sessions and activities were sequenced in such a way that learning could be progressive. Detailed lesson plans for the three sessions are provided in the appendix.

The participants are three girls aged 18 to 20 years old. These girls were staying at the centre because they had no or little family support for their pregnancy. The art sessions were part of their recovery program at the centre. They attended other classes such as pilates, prenatal preparation sessions and counseling during their stay at the centre. Two of these participants were into their fifth month of pregnancy when they started the first art session, while the third participant had just given birth to a baby boy weeks before.

Context

Teenage pregnancy is a social taboo in an Asian context like Singapore, and is kept away from the public realm. Teenage girls who get pregnant are often taken out of school. They may stay in temporary shelters until they deliver their babies. Many parents do not want their pregnant teens to stay at home for fear of contempt and gossip.

The number of teenage pregnancies in Singapore is on the decline (The Straits Times, 2016). The rate of teenage abortion in Singapore is also declining, but the social and psychological impact that teenage mothers suffer remains difficult to understand. There is little social support for teenage mothers and this often aggravates the trauma that these girls experience. Gender discrimination may also result in females being given a more negative treatment compared to the males. Overall, the lack of family and social support may inhibit post-traumatic growth in Asian teenage mothers. Thus, the established western models of post-traumatic growth may have a different effect in the Singaporean context.

The role of cultural narratives in post-traumatic growth need to be highlighted in this study. Though the arts are able to bring about positive growth and benefits to people across cultures and age groups, culture plays a large part in shaping narrative construction and post-traumatic growth (Pals & McAdams, 2004). For example, some societies may consider some traumas so bad or so debilitating that efforts to construct stories of subsequent growth may be seen as futile from the start, illogical, and never-to-be-believed or affirmed (Pals & McAdams, 2004).

ASSESSMENT APPLICATION

Questionnaire

Prior to the first art session, participants are asked to complete the Growth Areas Questionnaire (found in the chapter appendix). The questionnaire provides a 6-point likert scale, but remains one dimensional until paired with the arts-based assessment. It is recommended that the facilitator refrain from viewing completed questionnaires until the assessment period is complete to avoid bias.

Art Session 1: Donna and Jean

(names changed to protect identity)

I was aware that the two participants might be a little lethargic after their medical check-up earlier in the day. I welcomed them to the art space with lively, cheerful music in the background. Once they arrived, they were asked to design their own name tags. Both of them only wrote their names on the card. After seeing me add graphics and designs to my card, Donna followed suit and drew a cartoon on her name tag.

We began the session by asking if there was anything they were thankful for that day. Both paused for a while and said they could not think of anything. I then rephrased the question and asked if there was anything that they liked or disliked for that day. Jean replied that there was not much that she liked or disliked for that day. She elaborated that since they were at the residential home, they just followed instructions. There was little opportunity for them to think about whether they like or dislike doing certain tasks. I next asked if there was anything that made them happy on that day. Jean immediately said it was her new born baby. Donna still struggled to think of something. Jean helped her along and said jokingly that the noodles that Donna just ate made her happy. Donna did not seem to agree, but she could not think of other things that made her happy.

After the opening talk, I started the session by asking the two participants to crack a ceramic pot using the hammer that was provided. Both of them hesitated. Jean asked if she could avoid cracking the pot because the sound of the hammer hitting the pot may cause her sleeping baby to wake up. The other participant, Donna, supported her and asked if they could avoid using the hammer. I asked how they could crack the pot without using the hammer. Jean said perhaps they could just drop the paper bag with the pot in it onto the floor. I agreed to let them try this approach. It worked. They managed to crack the pot without using the hammer.

Next, they were told the story of how a little boy (found in the chapter appendix), despite his teacher cautioning him, ran down the corridor, bumped into his classmate and dropped his pot onto the floor. At this point, I asked both Donna and Jean how they might feel if they were the boy. Jean replied, "Sad." Donna hesitated for a while and said, "Fearful". When asked what made Donna fearful for the boy, she explained that the boy might be afraid that he would be reprimanded by the teacher. After the two girls responded, I continued with the story.

In the story, the boy asked his teacher if he could get another pot for his art class but the teacher replied that there was no extra pot for him, but he could make do with what he had. I then told the two participants that the broken pot is now in their hands, and that they could do whatever they wished with the pot. Jean responded without hesitation, "What else can we do with the pot?" I replied that they could do anything they wanted using the material that was provided. Jean then said, "Ah. We can just glue the broken pieces together and mend the pot." I smiled while the girls began to start their work.

Figure 2. Sample participant pot

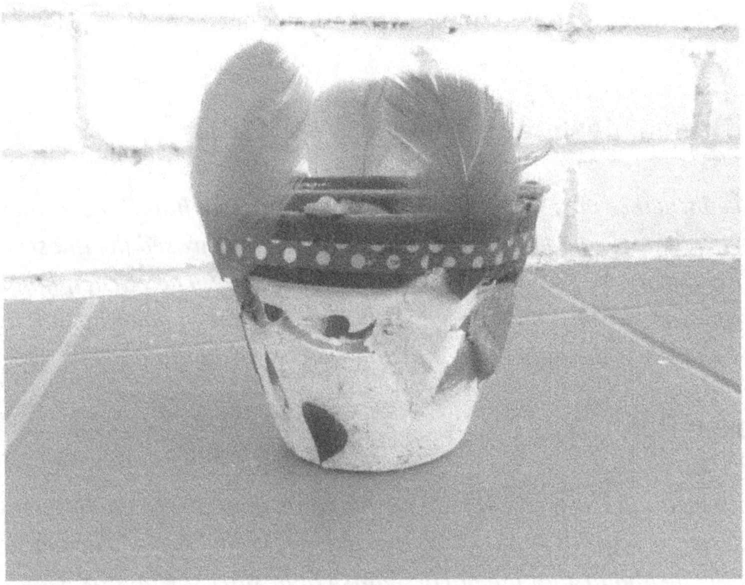

Art Session 1: Observations

The actions and speech of the participants during the art session provided much insight to their inner world. It was surprising how receptive the girls were. They were friendly and cooperative. When asked what the girls enjoyed or did not enjoy doing, Jean replied that she did not think much about that. She felt she had little choice. She would just follow instructions and do what she was told to do at the centre. It might be for this reason that the girls were mild and cooperated in all that they were asked to do for the art session. There was little resistance. Trauma survivors require a lot of support in the initial stage of recovery. When they find a pillar of support, they are receptive and treasure the support that is rendered to them. Dayspring New Life Centre was that pillar of support for the girls during this tough period of their life, and the girls reciprocated by being cooperative and agreeable to what was arranged for them at the centre. This speaks of the importance of genuine and nurturing support for trauma survivors. They can be receptive yet vulnerable during the period of recovery. Positive role models are also vital in guiding the girls on the path of recovery. Just as they are receptive to good advice, they may also be vulnerable to advice that may do more harm than good. Realising that they are "victims" of trauma, the girls showed care and concern for others in the same journey. Jean and Donna only knew each other for less than two months and yet they had learned to look after the needs of each other. It seems trauma survivors possess the ability to show concern for others and contribute to the world around them, despite facing struggles in their life.

The process of art-making and the conversations that arose during the session revealed strengths in the girls that they might not be aware of themselves. The inner strengths and potential, when affirmed, would greatly equip the girls in their journey ahead. The art experiences provided an effective and safe platform to explore, discuss and learn about life.

The first art session also showed positive signs that the girls reflected on and attempted to improve their art pieces (and likewise in life). When asked how they could have created their art pieces differently and improved on them, the girls replied immediately and pointed out at least one they could improve their art pieces.

Art Session 2: Donna, Jean, and Miki

This time, when asked whether they were thankful for anything that happened to them during the day or week, none of the participants could cite any examples. I then rephrased the question and asked if there was anything they did during the past week that made them happy. The participants still could not think of any examples. Jean was the only one who gave an example. She mentioned that the baby shower that took place the day before was the only thing that she was happy about for that week.

Story of the Broken Pot

Following our opening ritual, I shared with the participants the story of the broken pot (included in the chapter appendix). After which, I introduced the art activity for the day – "The Garden of Possibilities". The story provided the metaphor that the participants could start sowing for what they wished to reap in future.

Figure 3. Sample Participant "Garden of Possibilities"

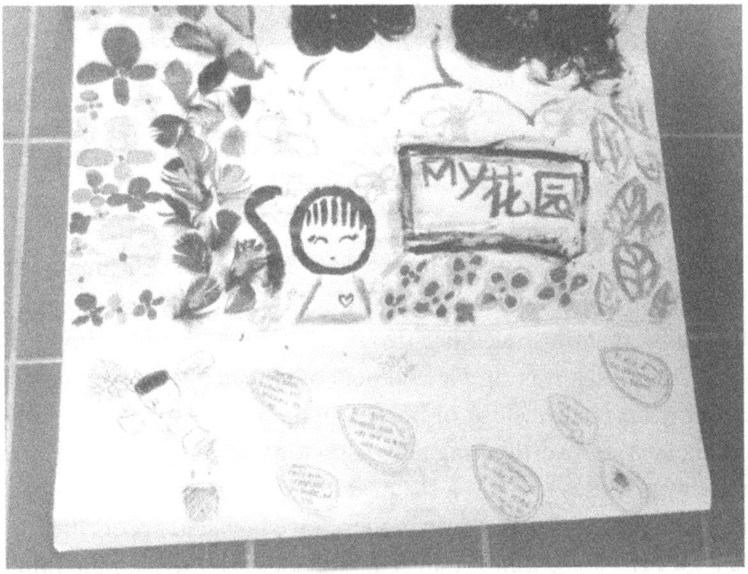

Art Session 2: Observations

This session broke the ice and a deeper connection was felt among the participants. Each one was present to share the pain of another. Each of the participants chose to be vulnerable as they shared their thoughts on what they regretted in life and what they desired for the future.

Art Session 3: Donna and Miki

The focus of the third art session was on the "weak and strong self". The metaphor is that we all have our weak and strong fronts. Just as we design our "strong" mask, we can work towards building our strengths and be strong. At the same time, being aware of our weaknesses and our "weak self" helps us to improve and avoid sinking into areas that may make us weak or bring us down.

When asked to explain what she had in mind when she designed her "weak self", Donna could not think of anything to say. When I elaborated and asked how she would think, act or say when she was "in her weak self", Donna paused and finally said that her weakness was hiding her true emotions from people and not letting others know how she felt. She would fake a smile and pretend that things were alright even if they were not, and this made her feel lousy. When asked to use a word or some phrases to describe her weak self, she replied, "Complicated". She said this word just came to her mind and she could not explain why she chose this word.

When I asked Donna about her mask, Donna gave a long pause and said she could not describe her strong self. Next, she repeated, "I do not know what to say." After a while, Donna managed to find the word "confident" to describe her strong self. When asked about her design, Donna explained that she had planned to make a simple mask, one that was not complicated so she would not "spoil the mask". Donna also said that she worked with what was available on the table. Though Donna seemed to have a plan for the design of her mask, she also appeared to have followed what Miki did. After seeing Miki paint her mask beige, Donna did likewise.

Art Session 3: Observations

Though Donna often could not find the words to describe her thoughts, she demonstrated understanding and growth through her art piece. For example, Donna mentioned that her weak self was "complicated". While working on the mask that illustrated her strong self, Donna made a choice, perhaps almost subconsciously, to design a mask that was simple and not complicated. She was seeking out a manageable and feasible way to do her art piece instead of being caught in a complicated process. In a way, Donna was aware of her weaknesses (ie. overthinking and being too complicated at times). She seemed to have started working on her weaknesses to build a stronger self.

At the same time, Donna often took reference and followed what her peers did. In the first art session, Donna tended to do or say the same things that Jean did. Likewise during the third art session, Donna followed Miki closely when working on her mask. The only time that Donna seemed to work and decide independently was during the second art session when Miki and she were working on their art pieces at separate corners of the centre. Donna could be independent and solve problems on her own. She possessed strengths that she herself might not be aware of.

Miki gave a rich description of her "weak" self. She said that when she was weak, she was "messy", "had purple hair and was not nice", "not radiant", "could only see brokenness and sadness", and "could not say nice things to people". When asked if she had other descriptions for how her weak self might think, act or speak, Miki mentioned the word "confused".

Figure 4. Sample participant mask

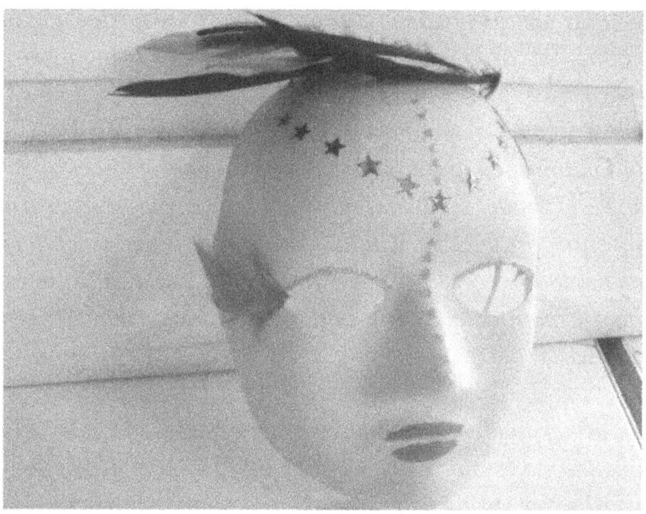

Miki worked on her mask with enthusiasm and she seemed more decisive than during the previous art session. She described her strong self as "glamorous" and "someone whom people would look up to".

Miki seemed to have low self esteem and a poor image of herself. From her description of her art piece, Miki appeared to have a strong sense of awareness of her physical and mental being. She thought lowly of her physical traits.

Post Sessions Interview

Following the third art session, an interview was conducted with the participants. Both facilitator and participants remained in the room together as safety and trust had been built over their time together. Interview questions are provided in the appendix. During the short interview, the participants seemed to be at a loss for words. The conversation did not seem as fluid compared to the discussions arising from the art sessions. Perhaps, the participants were still not comfortable in expressing their thoughts to each other, as had been assumed. The participants might also find the interview questions too open-ended so they may be at a loss as to what to focus on or express. The questions may have also seemed too distant from their current context. The participants could still be concerned about their day-to-day needs, and might be too anxious about their immediate situation to reflect on their growth or future.

While, in this particular case, the interview was not extremely useful in assessing post-traumatic growth, it did help the participants to be aware of the positive changes that had taken place. For example, all of the participants were able to articulate the strengths they had developed through their pregnancy crisis.

OBSERVATIONS AND RECOMMENDATIONS

Throughout the session, observations were made on the participants' actions and speech in correlation to growth areas on the Post-Traumatic Growth Inventory by Tedeschi & Calhoun (1996) as well as the Personal Growth Initiative scale by Christine Robitschek (1998). In general, notes were taken of positive traits indicating growth. Any blanks left on the table indicate that that particular area of growth was not observed during this session. Following the three sessions, the facilitator took note of the areas of growth that seem consistently lacking throughout the three art sessions. Using the findings, recommendations were made to the centre. The recommendations would help the centre to plan for future programs so as to enhance personal development and growth for these participants.

Recommendations

Miki might need help in gaining a healthy routine such as sleeping and eating well. Breathing exercises, taking walks or a simple workout might be useful. She needed to have more confidence in herself. Affirmations will help her to realize her strengths. Group activities may also help her to learn to trust in others and see the good in people. She loves reading and writing so journaling may help her to tell stories of her trauma and facilitate post-traumatic growth. Activities that require her to take initiative, persevere, make decisions, or those that will build her confidence will be beneficial for her.

Table 1. Sample Areas of Growth Findings

Areas of Post-Traumatic Growth	Findings
Relating to Others	Miki could relate generally well with others and she was eloquent in expressing her thoughts. However, she seemed unwilling at times to receive help from others. Perhaps she did not trust them. During the interview, she mentioned that she knew who her true friends were after her crisis. It seemed that she felt some friends did not stand by her. In addition, she often thought that people were critical or judgmental of her art piece. At the same time, she responded well to affirmations.
Personal Strengths	Miki gave herself lower scores in the area of personal strengths compared to other areas. Miki seemed to have low self esteem. In particular, she might be concerned with her physical appearance. During art sessions, it seemed that she was also afraid to try new approaches, and always chose the safe, easy route. She lacked confidence and perseverance. Miki was also aware of her past mistakes. Such an awareness might be a good first step towards building personal strengths.

SUMMARY

Arts-Based Assessment

One distinctive feature of an arts-based assessment is that it provides a much "thicker" and richer description of the subject in question compared to written questionnaires and even face-to-face interviews. In the illustration, the participants have just experienced the trauma of premarital pregnancy and are suffering from its consequences. Based on the conversations during the art session, it seemed that the participants were still in a state of confusion over their next step in life. While they had little to say about how they had grown through the crisis, they exhibited evidence of growth through their arts-based responses, more than what words could describe.

Based on analysis of the arts-based responses, it is found that they generally correspond to the findings from the questionnaire. While questionnaires may provide a quick and concise feedback in reflecting a current situation, arts-based assessment adds dimension to the understanding. They give a richer description compared to the quantitative scores that are reflected on the survey. For example, while the participants rated themselves well in the area of relating to others (ie. I put effort into my relationships), the art sessions provide a fuller picture of how that looks in real life. The participants were seen offering help to one another. They were patient in listening and used a gentle tone when speaking. Noting these details is important because affirmations may be given to the trauma survivors so as to perpetuate these good practices and attributes. Often, trauma survivors may not see these traits as strengths.

It was heartening and encouraging to see the participants grow through the art sessions. For example, Miki mentioned that she has learned to work on things from scratch, from a blank canvas. Transformation may not have to start from bold actions in life, but from the little things the participants do such as having the courage to work independently, using new material, and persevering to complete the art piece. The courage to create can be synonymous to the participants' ability to create possibilities in real life. They can translate their habits in creating art to other aspects of their life.

While it does not make sense to administer questionnaires every week, art experiences provide an organic and authentic platform to assess post-traumatic growth frequently and over a long period of time. Overall, the facilitator serves as an expert companion (Calhoun et al., 2010) who journeys with the trauma survivors. The art experiences act as a safe container where authentic and organic conversations can take place. These interpersonal interactions help the facilitator (or any other caregiver who is interested in facilitating art experiences) to assess and encourage post-traumatic growth.

CONCLUSION

Trauma can have long-lasting effects on individuals and their families. A traumatic experience, though in altered form, may pass through generations (Sutton, 2002). However conscious the adult is of the experience, and however they attempt to protect their children from it, they still have the memory of their own traumatic experience at the unconscious level (Sutton, 2002). While an "inherited" experience may be inevitable, one needs not be resigned to it. Resilience may be nurtured through sourcing help from a support group, learning coping strategies and exercising self-care. Post-traumatic growth starts from a desire for transformation.

There are different ways to assess growth. Arts-based inquiry is not aimed toward a quest for certainty, but an enhancement of perspectives (Barone & Eisner, 2011). The arts-based approach has proven to be effective and compliments the quantitative questionnaires that are commonly used to assess post-traumatic growth. Arts-based inquiry gives an added dimension to understanding personal development and growth, beyond what is expressed verbally and in written form. There are many ways to approach the subject of arts and post-traumatic growth. Through this chapter, it is hoped that more are inspired to engage in an arts-based or non-verbal approach when journeying with someone towards recovery. What is spoken or written may be only a tip of the iceberg of who someone really is, and what the inner spirit hopes to convey. Welcome to a world beyond words.

REFERENCES

Barone, T., & Eisner, E. (2011). *Arts-based Research.* Los Angeles, CA: Sage Publications, Inc.

Bloom, S. (2010). *Bridging the black hole of trauma: The evolutionary significance of the arts.* Academic Press.

Buildabridge Institute. (2013). Philadelphia: Eastern University.

Calhoun, L., Tedeschi, R. G., Cann, A. & Hanks, E. A. (2010). Positive outcomes following bereavement: Paths to traumatic growth. *Psychologica Belgica, 50*(1-2), 125-143.

Corbitt, J. N., & Nix-Early, V. (2003). *Taking it to the streets: using the arts to transform your community.* Grand Rapids, MI: BakerBooks.

Gast, D., & Ledford, J. (2014). *Single case research methodology: Applications in special education and behavioral sciences.* New York: Routledge.

Hart, S. L., Vella, L., & Mohr, D. C. (2008). Relationships among depressive symptoms, benefit-finding, optimism, and positive affect in multiple sclerosis patients after psychotherapy for depression. *Health Psychology*, *27*(2), 230–238. doi:10.1037/0278-6133.27.2.230 PMID:18377142

Huey-Heck, L., & Kalnin, J. (2006). *The Spirituality of Art*. Northstone Publishing.

Jacobson-Levy, M. (2013). *The Arts & Healing: Visual Arts* [Class handout].

Kilmer, R. P., Gil-Rivas, V., Tedeschi, R. G., Cann, A., Calhoun, L. G., Buchanan, T., & Taku, K. (2009). Use of the revised post-traumatic growth inventory for children. *Journal of Traumatic Stress*, *22*(3), 248–253. doi:10.1002/jts.20410 PMID:19462437

Lanius, R. A., Williamson, P. C., Densmore, M., Boksman, K., Neufeld, R. W., Gati, J. S., & Menon, R. S. (2004). The nature of traumatic memories: A T-T FMRI functional connectivity analysis. *The American Journal of Psychiatry*, *161*(1), 36–44. doi:10.1176/appi.ajp.161.1.36 PMID:14702248

McNiff, S. (2007). *Art-based research*. London: Jessica Kingsley Publishers.

McNiff, S. (2011). Artistic expressions as primary modes of inquiry. *British Journal of Guidance & Counselling*, *39*(5), 385–396. doi:10.1080/03069885.2011.621526

Pals, J. L., & McAdams, D. P. (2004). The transformed self: A narrative understanding of post-traumatic growth. *Psychological Inquiry*, *15*(1), 65–69.

Robitschek, C. (1998). Personal growth initiative: The construct and its measure. *Measurement & Evaluation in Counseling & Development*, *30*, 183–198.

Sandel, S. L., Judge, J. O., Landry, N., Faria, L., Ouellette, R., & Majczak, M. (2005). Dance and movement program improves quality-of-life measures in breast cancer survivors. *Cancer Nursing*, *28*(4), 301–309. doi:10.1097/00002820-200507000-00011 PMID:16046894

Stroebe, M. S., & Schut, H. (1999). The dual process model of coping with bereavement: Rationale and description. *Death Studies*, *23*(3), 197–224. doi:10.1080/074811899201046 PMID:10848151

Stuckey, H. L., & Nobel, J. (2010). The connection between art, healing, and public health: A review of current literature. *American Journal of Public Health*, *100*(2), 254–263. doi:10.2105/AJPH.2008.156497 PMID:20019311

Sutton, J. P. (2002). *Music, music therapy and trauma: International perspectives*. London: Jessica Kingsley Publishers.

Tedeschi, R., & Calhoun, L. (1996). The post-traumatic growth inventory: Measuring the positive the positive legacy of trauma. *Journal of Traumatic Stress*, *9*(3), 455–471. doi:10.1002/jts.2490090305 PMID:8827649

Tedeschi, R., & Calhoun, L. (2004a). Post-traumatic growth: Conceptual Foundations and Empirical Evidence. *Psychological Inquiry*, *15*(1), 1–18. doi:10.120715327965pli1501_01

Tedeschi, R., & Calhoun, L. (2004b). The foundations of post-traumatic growth: New considerations. *Psychological Inquiry*, *15*(1), 93–102. doi:10.120715327965pli1501_03

The Straits Times. (2016, Feb 22). *Figure at 25-year low; social workers say teens now more savvy about using contraceptives*. Retrieved from http://www.straitstimes.com/singapore/big-drop-in-number-of-teen-pregnancies

Updegraff, J. A., & Marshall, G. N. (2005). Predictors of perceived growth following direct exposure to community violence. *Journal of Social and Clinical Psychology*, *24*(4), 538–560. doi:10.1521/jscp.2005.24.4.538

Urcuyo, K. R., Boyers, A. E., Carver, C. S., & Antoni, M. H. (2005). Finding benefit in breast cancer: Relations with personality, coping, and concurrent well-being. *Psychology & Health*, *20*(2), 175–192. doi:10.1080/08870440512331317634

Van der Kolk, B. A. (1994). The body keeps the score: Memory and the evolving psychobiology of post-traumatic stress. *Harvard Review of Psychiatry*, *1*(5), 253–265. doi:10.3109/10673229409017088 PMID:9384857

Znoj, H. (2006). Bereavement and post-traumatic growth. In L. G. Calhoun & R. G. Tedeschi (Eds.), *Handbook of Post-traumatic Growth: Research and Practice* (pp. 176–196). Mahwah, NJ: Lawrence Erlbaum Associates.

KEY TERMS AND DEFINITIONS

Arts-Based Inquiry: The use of art-making processes as a way of observing and understanding the characteristics and internal processing of individuals.

Healing: The restoration of one's psychological, emotional, and physical wellbeing.

Post-Traumatic Growth: A qualitative yet observable change (to a level that surpasses pre-trauma conditions) in people who had undergone situations that overwhelm their resilience.

Trauma: A situation that stretches and overwhelms an individual's coping mechanisms.

APPENDIX

Full Lesson Plans

Numbers in brackets [ ] indicate the possible areas of growth that may be assessed through the activities. The numbers relate to the Growth Area Rubric.

Opening Exercise

Each participant is to name something they are thankful for during the past week. [5c, 5d] Tip: If they cannot think of anything, the facilitator may rephrase the question to "something happy you have done or something happy that happened to you over the past week".

Art Session 1: Broken Pot

- **Metaphor:** Beautiful mess. Brokenness does not mark the end but the start of a beautiful journey.
- **Time Required:** 1 hr 30 min
- **Material Required:**
  - Ceramic pots
  - Hammers
  - White glue (not super glue because the objective is not to mend the pot perfectly)
  - Decorative material e.g. paint, glitters, crepe paper, ribbons, feathers

Process

- **Breaking of Pot:**
  - Each participant is to break the pot in their hands using a hammer
  - Ask how the participants feel [1c]
  - Acknowledge emotions of individuals. Some may find it more difficult than others to break the pots
- **Story:**
  - Tell them of a story of a little boy. The little boy was excited and running down the corridor with a pot in hand. He was going for his art class. Before that, the teacher asked him to be careful and not to run. On his way to the art studio, he knocked into another student who was carrying a thick stack of books. The pot fell from the boy's hands.
  - Pause and ask the participants: If you were the boy, how would you feel and what would you do? [1c, 2c]
  - There was no extra pot for him. Imagine how he felt. Other students will get to do the craft, and each will bring home a beautiful pot except him. The teacher asked whether he wanted to work on the broken pieces of the pot and see how they might turn out.
- **Instructions:**
  - Today, the broken pot is in your hands. How would you like to work on the broken pieces? Use the available materials.

- Participants should take 45 minutes to work on the pot
- Facilitator will observe and take notes on the art-making process e.g. what the participants did and said.

- **Reflection:**
  - After the participants had worked on their pots, the facilitator will get the participants to present their pots to the other group members (they can give their pot a name or a title for their art piece if they wish). If they feel comfortable, they may share on the following as prompted by the Facilitator:
  - Are there any difficulties they encountered during the art-making process and how they overcame them? [2b, 2c]
  - Initially, did they think they can overcome the difficulties? What helped them to overcome their lack of confidence? [2a, 2b, 2d]
  - Name a strength that they see in themselves while working on the pot [2a]
  - What did they learn in the process? What can we learn from the "broken pieces" in our life?
- **Closure:** In our lives, we may meet with unexpected situations that may "break our lives", bring about drastic changes or cause us much disappointment. Just as how the little boy is given the choice to work on the broken pot, we too can work on the broken pieces in our lives.
- **Ask:** Just as there is available art material to mend or beautify your pot, what are the available "materials" in your lives that may help you when you meet a difficult situation? [e.g. 1a]

Art Session 2: Garden of Possibilities

- **Metaphor:** We can start sowing for what we desire to reap.
- **Time Required:** 1 hr 30 min
- **Material Required:**
  - Large pieces of white paper
  - Markers
  - Paint
  - Crayons
  - Glue
  - Magazines
  - Decorative material e.g. feathers, glitters
  - Seeds (printed on paper)

Process

Opening Story: *The Broken Pot*

A water bearer in India had two large pots, each hung on an end of a pole which he carried across his neck. One of the pots had a crack in it, and while the other pot was perfect and always delivered a full portion of water at the end of the long walk from the stream to the master's house, the cracked pot arrived only half full.

For two years, this went on daily. The bearer would deliver only one and a half pot full of water to his masters house. Of course, the perfect pot was proud of its accomplishments. But the poor cracked pot was ashamed of its imperfection. It felt miserable that it was able to accomplish only half of what it was given to him.

After two years of what it perceived to be a bitter failure, the cracked pot spoke to the water bearer, "I am ashamed of myself and I want to apologize to you."

"Why?" asked the bearer. "What are you ashamed of?"

"For these past two years, I could deliver only half my load because this crack on my side causes water to leak out. Because of my flaws, you have to do all of this work, and you don't get the full value from your efforts." the pot said.

The water bearer felt sorry for the old cracked pot, and in his compassion he said, "As we return to the master's house, I want you to notice the beautiful flowers along the path."

Indeed, as they went up the hill, the old cracked pot took notice of the sun warming the beautiful wild flowers on the side of the path, and this cheered it up somewhat. However, at the end of the trail, it still felt bad because it had leaked out half its load, and so again the cracked pot apologized to the water bearer for its failure.

The bearer said to the pot, "Did you notice that there were flowers only on your side of your path, but not on the other side? That's because I have always known about your flaw, and I took advantage of it. I planted flower seeds on your side of the path, and every day while we walk back from the stream, you've watered them. For two years, I have been able to pick these beautiful flowers to decorate my master's table. Without you being just the way you are, he would not have this beauty to grace his house."

Each of us has our own unique flaws. We're all cracked pots. Don't be afraid of your flaws. Nothing goes to waste. Something beautiful can grow from there.

- **Instructions:**
    - Seeds grow and flowers bloom. It's now time to build our garden of possibilities. What would you like to have grow in this garden? Imagine it is a future that you desire for yourself and for the people around you. How will it look?
    - Using the materials provided (e.g. scrap paper, markers, crayons, magazines, glue, glitter), design your garden of possibilities. If you have a choice and can dream of anything you want, what would you put in this garden? You can use drawings or words to illustrate the things you desire.
    - Before you start, draw a line across the paper at the bottom-third of your paper. Do not touch this portion when you design your garden.

- **Reflection:** Ask the participants to share about what they had drawn or included in their own garden. [3b, 3c, 3d, 3e]
- **Further Instructions:**
    - Why do you think you need to leave a blank space on the paper? (Allow participants to suggest answers.)
    - Now that you have drawn or designed you garden, what may be needed to allow this garden to grow well? What are the seeds that you need to plant to achieve the garden or future that you desire? [5a, 5b, 5d]
    - Participants can write or draw on the printed paper seeds and paste them on the bottom-third (ie. ground) of the drawing.
- **Reflection:**
    - Do you think what you have envisioned for the future can be attained? Why or why not? [3c, 3d, 3e, 6a, 6c, 6d, 6e]
    - What have you learned from this exercise? What is your next step? How will the people or community around you benefit? [6b, 6c, 6e, 6f]
- **Closing:** We can start sowing for what we desire to reap.

Now that you know what you desire for your future, you can take steps to reach your goals.

Art Session 3: Mask (Strong and Weak Self)

- **Metaphor:** We all have our weak and strong fronts. We can choose to be strong if we want to.
- **Time Required:** 1 hr 30 min
- **Material Required:**
    - Masks
    - Paint
    - Markers
    - Paper
    - Decorative Material e.g. glitters, feathers
- **Instructions:**
    - How do we look or behave when we are weak? [2e]
    - Draw your weak self on this piece of paper. You may use colours, drawings, or words to illustrate your weak self.
    - Participants will share what they have drawn.
    - What makes us weak? How does knowing your own weaknesses help you? [3b, 3d, 3e]

Story (adapted from Dr. Nathan Corbitt.)

Once, a family had 2 dogs – King and Fluffy. King was a strong and brave dog. It often barked at suspicious strangers and helped to guard the house. On the other hand, Fluffy was a timid dog and was always hiding behind King.

One day, their master's house was burnt down. Now that their master could no longer take care of the dogs, he decided to give them away. While King was popular and was adopted quickly, no one wanted Fluffy.

One night, some robbers intruded the half burnt down house and wanted to steal from the house while everyone was asleep.

(Stop and ask the participants to guess what may happen next.)

Some time later, the master was awakened in the middle of the night by a dog's barking. He did not think that it was Fluffy because Fluffy hardly barked that loudly. Nonetheless, he sensed that something was amiss so he got up and went outside the house to take a look. There he saw Fluffy on the ground, with blood oozing out of its body, grasping for his last breath. He also spotted the robbers from a distance and they were cursing at the dog while moving away from the house.

The master realized that Fluffy was attacked by the robbers as he tried to protect the house and the family. The master, with tears in his eyes, patted Fluffy and said, "Well done, Fluffy." Fluffy died soon after.

Tell the participants that we all may have a weak self but there is strength deep within us and this strength may arise when we are put to the test. We may feel that we are like Fluffy – timid and always trying to hide behind others to escape from our problems. However, we can also be strong like him.

- **Further Instructions:**
  - How does your strong self look?
  - Using the materials provided, design a mask based on your strong self. You may use colours, drawings, or words to illustrate your strong self.
  - How would you look, think or act when you are strong? What makes you strong?
- **Reflection:** Have the participants share about their masks (e.g. what thoughts went through their minds as they were designing their masks).
- **Closure:** When we become aware of our strengths and weaknesses, it opens the window for change and transformation. We can do things or cultivate habits to build our strengths and diminish our weaknesses.

Post Session Interview Questions

Growth Factor 1: What has changed with regards to your relationship with others after this difficult experience?
Growth Factor 2: What are some of the strengths you developed through this tough period in your life?
Growth Factor 3: Are there new directions or opportunities in life that can arise out of this situation?
Growth Factor 4: What has changed in your spiritual journey? Does this experience help you in your belief or in the way you see God?

Table 2. Pre-Session Self Reporting Questionnaire

General Well-Being						
I am able to handle my emotions	1	2	3	4	5	6
I am able to rest and eat well	1	2	3	4	5	6
Relating to Others						
A. I have people whom I can count on in times of trouble	1	2	3	4	5	6
B. I feel close to my friends and loved ones	1	2	3	4	5	6
C. I am willing to express my emotions	1	2	3	4	5	6
D. I have compassion for others	1	2	3	4	5	6
E. I put effort into my relationships	1	2	3	4	5	6
F. I learned that people are wonderful	1	2	3	4	5	6
G. I need others to help me in my life	1	2	3	4	5	6
Personal Strength						
A. I feel that I can rely on myself most of the time	1	2	3	4	5	6
B. I know I can handle difficulties	1	2	3	4	5	6
C. I can accept that things may not work out well sometimes	1	2	3	4	5	6
D. I discover that I am stronger than I thought I was	1	2	3	4	5	6
E. I can accept my flaws and failures.	1	2	3	4	5	6
New Possibilities						
A. I developed or found new interests and hobbies	1	2	3	4	5	6
B. I can see a new direction in my life	1	2	3	4	5	6
C. I am able to better things in the future	1	2	3	4	5	6
D. There are new opportunities for me	1	2	3	4	5	6
E. I am more willing to make changes in my life	1	2	3	4	5	6
Spiritual Change						
A. I have a better understanding of spiritual matters	1	2	3	4	5	6
B. I am stronger in my faith now	1	2	3	4	5	6
Appreciation of Life						
A. I know what is important in my life	1	2	3	4	5	6
B. I value my life	1	2	3	4	5	6
C. I appreciated each new day	1	2	3	4	5	6
D. I appreciate things in my environment	1	2	3	4	5	6
Taking Ownership						
A. I know how to change specific things that I want to change in my life	1	2	3	4	5	6
B. I have a good sense of where I am headed in my life.	1	2	3	4	5	6
C. If I want to change something in my life, I initiate the transition process	1	2	3	4	5	6
D. I know what I need to do to get started toward reaching my goals	1	2	3	4	5	6
E. I have a specific action plan to help me reach my goals	1	2	3	4	5	6
F. I know what my unique contribution to the world might be	1	2	3	4	5	6
G. I know how to lead a balanced life	1	2	3	4	5	6

Tedeschi & Calhoun, 1994 & 2004a; Robitschek, 1998.

Table 3. Growth Areas Observation Table

Area of Growth	Possible Art or Non Art Response
1. Relating to Others	
A. I have people whom I can count on in times of trouble	Allow people to help them, sense of community, not isolated, mention people who are available to help them
B. I feel close to my friends and loved ones	Mention details about friends/family members, express closeness verbally or through body language
C. I am willing to express my emotions	Expression of emotions during conversations/activities
D. I have compassion for others	Volunteer or render help to others
E. I put effort into my relationships	Makes effort to encourage, affirm, or help others, listen when others talk, expression of care
F. I learned that people are wonderful	Express awareness of the strengths in others. Believe that there is goodness in people
G. I need others to help me in my life	Express the need for help or having others in their life during conversations or in their actions
2. Personal Strength	
A. I feel that I can rely on myself most of the time	Taking initiative to do things and solve problems on their own. In the instance of the broken pot, solve problems or make their own decision regarding their art piece without assistance.
B. I know I can handle difficulties	Showing confidence, courage, determination, or perseverance.
C. I can accept that things may not work out well sometimes	Show acceptance instead of frustration or having a sense of regret. Comfortable with uncertainties, willing to work around obstacles.
D. I discover that I am stronger than I thought I was	Show awareness of the strengths they possess, mention incidents where they are surprised at how well they cope or how they manage to overcome difficulties.
E. I can accept my flaws and failures.	Happy and feel glad about themselves regardless of how well they do. If mistake is made during creation, work continues either around the mistake or incorporates the mistake.
3. New Possibilities	
A. I developed or found new interests and hobbies	Express new found interest or hobbies, ask questions about their new interests, show interest and look forward to the next art session.
B. I can see a new direction in my life	Able to express the new goals or outlook, indication of change from 'old' life. Try new ways to approach the art piece, use of new materials.
C. I am able to better things in the future	Expression of hope or the ability to do better things in future. Attempts to improve the art piece.
D. There are new opportunities for me	Expression of the new opportunities/people/experience they encounter.
E. I am more willing to make changes in my life	Expression of the desire and willingness to make changes in artwork.
4. Spiritual Change	
A. I have a better understanding of spiritual matters	Expression of awe, wonder, curiosity, purpose, and appreciation of things. Demonstrates faith and awareness of higher power in artwork or in conversation. Mention things or feelings deriving from the non-physical realm.

continued on following page

Table 3. Continued

Area of Growth	Possible Art or Non Art Response
B. I am stronger in my faith now	Expression of trust and hope in higher power, as well as optimism.
5. Appreciation of Life	
A. I know what is important in my life	Show awareness of what is important to them. Recognition and expression of life's priorities. Sets an aim for the art piece at the start. Prioritizes certain steps, choice of materials.
B. I value my life	Expression of joy, satisfaction, and anticipation in life through art making, values one's art piece and takes good care of it.
C. I appreciate each new day	Expression of gratitude. Appreciate the given art material and the final art piece.
D. I appreciate things in my environment	Expression of gratitude for the environment in artwork. Express appreciation/delight in the little things. Takes care of the environment, e.g. helps to clean up.
6. Taking Ownership	
A. I know how to change specific things that I want to change in my life	Expression of awareness or resolution to make changes in artwork or life. Have a plan in mind and set out to make changes in the art piece.
B. I have a good sense of where I am headed in my life.	Expression of clear direction in life or in art work. Sets an aim for the final art piece and work towards it.
C. If I want to change something in my life, I initiate the transition process	Express willingness to ignite change in artwork. Takes initiative to modify or obtain certain art material.
D. I know what I need to do to get started toward reaching my goals	Identification of the next concrete step and work towards the goal. Evidence of planning and awareness that processes are involved.
E. I have a specific action plan to help me reach my goals	Can list the steps to achieve goals. Following the plan in mind and executing it.
F. I know what my unique contribution to the world might be	Expression of connection between self and the community/world. Create a new usage for found objects, e.g. broken pot.
G. I know how to lead a balanced life	Expression of awareness of the importance of balance. Open to using different art materials, content of art piece is balanced and not extreme. Focus on rebuilding, reconstructing, as well as beautifying artwork.

Growth Factor 5: In what way has this experience helped you to appreciate life or approach life differently?

Growth Factor 6: Do you feel that you are in control of your future? In what way(s) can you shape your future?

Which art activity did you like best and why?

How do you think the art sessions have helped you?

Compilation of References

ABColombia. (2010). *Caught in the crossfire: Colombia's indigenous peoples*. Retrieved from www.abcolombia.org.uk

Alcorn, N. (2008). *Violated: Mercy for sexual abuse*. Enumclaw, WA: Winepress Publishing.

Alexander, C. J. (2013). *Bonding assessments*. Retrieved November 10, 2015, 2015 from http://alexanderphd.com/BONDINGASSESSMENTS.html

American Dance Therapy Association. (2014). *About Dance/Movement Therapy*. Retrieved from: http://adta.org/About_DMT

American Music Therapy Association. (2016). *History of Music Therapy*. Retrieved from http://www.musictherapy.org/about/history/

American Music Therapy Association. (2018). *The American Music Therapy Association*. Retrieved from https://www.musictherapy.org/

American Psychiatric Association. (2013). *Diagnostic and statistical manual of mental disorders* (5th ed.). Arlington, VA: American Psychiatric Publishing.

American Psychological Association. (2014). *Trauma*. Retrieved from: http://www.apa.org/topics/trauma/index.aspx

American Psychological Association. (n.d.). *Recovering Emotionally from Disaster*. Retrieved from http://www.apa.org/topics/trauma/index.aspx

Amsden, J. & VanWynsberghe, R. (2005). Community mapping as a research tool with youth. *SAGE Publications*, *3*(4), 357-381. DOI: 10.1177/1476750305058487

Anderson, T., & Milbrandt, M. (2004). *Art for Life: Authentic instruction in art*. Columbus, OH: McGraw-Hill.

Andrzejewski, C. E. (2008). *A Holistic Investigation of Teacher Identity, Knowledge, and Practice* (Doctoral Dissertation). Ohio State University. Retrieved October 5, 2011, from http://etd.ohiolink.edu/send-pdf.cgi/Andrzejewski%20Carey%20Ellen.pdf?osu1217014454

Annual. (n.d.). *BuildaBridge*. Retrieved May 1, 2012, from http://www.buildabridge.org/programs/institute-programs/annual

Ansdell, G. (2002). Community music therapy & the winds of change. *Voices: A World Forum for Music Therapy*, *2*(2). doi: 10.15845/voices.v2i2.83

Ansdell, G. (2004). Rethinking music and community: theoretical perspectives in support of community music therapy. In M. Pavlicevic & G. Ansdell (Eds.), Community Music Therapy (pp. 65–90). Philadelphia, PA: Jessica Kingsley Publishers.

Ansdell, G. (2005, November). Being who you aren't; Doing what you can't: Community music therapy & the paradoxes of performance. *Voices: A World Forum for Music Therapy*, *5*(3). Retrieved from normt.uib.no/index.php/voices/article/view/229/173

Anttila, E. (2003). *A Dream Journey to the Unknown: Searching for Dialogue in Dance Education* (Doctoral dissertation). Theatre Academy, Department of Dance and Theatre Pedagogy.

Arkin, L. C. (1994). Dancing the Body: Women and Dance Performance. *Journal of Physical Education, Recreation & Dance*, 65.

Atkinson, J. (2001). *Survey of Community Music in the UK.* Unpublished report for the Speedwell Trust.

Baer, R. A., Smith, G. T., & Allen, K. B. (2004). Assessment of mindfulness by self-report: The Kentucky inventory of mindfulness skills. *Assessment*, *11*(3), 191–206. doi:10.1177/1073191104268029 PMID:15358875

Baine, S. (2013). Music therapy as an anti-oppressive practice. *The Arts in Psychotherapy*, *40*(1), 1–5. doi:10.1016/j.aip.2012.09.003

Bandura, A. (1994). Self-efficacy. In V. S. Ramachaudran (Ed.), *Encyclopedia of human behavior, 4* (pp. 71–81). New York: Academic Press.

Banitt, S. P. (2012). *The trauma tool kit: Healing PTSD from the inside out.* Wheaton, IL: Quest Books.

Barna, G. (2017, April 6). *Meet the "Spiritual but Not Religious."* Barna Group. Retrieved from https://www.barna.com/research/meet-spiritual-not-religious

Barone, T., & Eisner, E. (2011). *Arts-based Research.* Los Angeles, CA: Sage Publications, Inc.

Barone, T., & Eisner, E. W. (2012). *Arts Based Research.* Los Angeles: SAGE.

Barrett, T. (1997). *Talking About Student Art.* Worcester, MA: Davis Publications.

Barrett, T. (2011). Experiencing art with the ill, the elderly, and their caregivers. *Teaching Artist Journal*, *9*(2), 90–100. doi:10.1080/15411796.2011.556565

Bartenieff, I. (2002). Body movement: Coping with the environment. New York, NY: Routledge.

Basile, K. C., Smith, S. G., Breiding, M. J., Black, M. C., & Mahendra, R. (2014). *Sexual Violence Surveillance Uniform Definitions and Recommended Data Elements, Version 2.0.* Center for Disease Control.

Basting, A. (2006). Arts in dementia care: This is not the end...it's the end of this chapter. *Generations (San Francisco, Calif.)*, *30*(1), 16–20.

Bath, H. (2008). The three pillars of trauma-informed care. *Reclaiming Children and Youth*, *17*(3), 17–21. Retrieved from https://reclaimingjournal.com/sites/default/files/journal-article-pdfs/17_3_Bath.pdf

Bath, H. (2015). The three pillars of traumawise care: Healing in the other 23 hours. *Reclaiming Children and Youth*, *23*(4), 5–11.

Beaton, R. D., & Murphy, S. A. (1995). Working with People in Crisis; Research Implications. In *Compassion fatigue: Coping with secondary traumatic stress disorder in those who treat the traumatized.* New York, NY: Brunner/Mazel.

Beck, M. (2001). *Finding your own North Star.* New York, NY: Three Rivers Press.

Beck, M. (2008). *Steering by starlight.* New York, NY: Rodale.

Behrens, G. A. (2014). *Arts in healing panel: Neurobiology of trauma and the arts* (PowerPoint slides). Retrieved from https://plus.google.com/u/1/communities

Behrens, G. A. (2014, May 26). *Art in healing panel: Neurobiology of trauma and the arts* [PowerPoint Slides].

Bell, C. E., & Robbins, S. J. (2007). Effect of Art Production on Negative Mood: A Randomized, Controlled Trial. *Art Therapy: Journal of the American Art Therapy Association, 24*(2), 71-75.

Bell, H., Kulkarni, S., & Dalton, L. (2003). Organizational prevention of vicarious trauma. *Families in Society, 84*(4), 463–470. doi:10.1606/1044-3894.131

Bell, J. S. (2002). Narrative Inquiry: More Than Just Telling Stories. *TESOL Quarterly, 36*(2), 207. doi:10.2307/3588331

Beltrán, R., & Begun, S. (2014). 'It is medicine': Narratives of healing from the Aotearoa Digital Storytelling as Indigenous Media Project (ADSIMP). *Psychology and Developing Societies, 26*(2), 155–179. doi:10.1177/0971333614549137

Bergh, A., & Sloboda, J. (2010). Music & art in conflict transformation: A review. *Music & Arts in Action, 2*(2), 1–16.

Bernstein, G. (2010). *Add more –ing to your life*. New York, NY: Harmony Books.

Bernstein, G. (2016). *The universe has your back*. Carlsbad, CA: Hay House.

Bernstein, G. (2018). *Judgment detox*. New York, NY: North Star Way.

Bird, J. L., & Wanner, E. T. (2015). Research as curriculum inquiry: helping college students with anxiety. In V. C. X. Wang (Ed.), *Handbook of research on scholarly publishing and research methods* (pp. 273–295). Hershey, PA: Information Science Reference. doi:10.4018/978-1-4666-7409-7.ch014

Bird, J. L., Wanner, E. T., Urenda, R., & Perry, R. (2015). Multigenre medicine. In J. L. Bird (Ed.), *Innovative collaborative practice and reflection in patient education* (pp. 1–19). Hershey, PA: Information Science Reference. doi:10.4018/978-1-4666-7524-7.ch001

Black-Gutman, D., & Hickson, F. (1996). The relationship between racial attitudes and social-cognitive development in children: An Australian study. *Developmental Psychology, 32*(3), 448–456. doi:10.1037/0012-1649.32.3.448

Blakemore, S. J., & Choudhury, S. (2006). Development of the adolescent brain: Implications for executive function and social cognition. *Journal of Child Psychology and Psychiatry, and Allied Disciplines, 47*(3–4), 296–312. doi:10.1111/j.1469-7610.2006.01611.x PMID:16492261

Bleakley, A., Jordan, A. B., & Hennessy, M. (2013). The relationship between parents' and children's television viewing. *Pediatrics, 132*(2), e364–e371. doi:10.1542/peds.2012-3415 PMID:23858418

Bloom, S. (2010). *Bridging the black hole of trauma: The evolutionary significance of the arts*. Academic Press.

Bloom. (2011). Bridging the black hole of trauma: The evolutionary significance of the arts, part 2: The arts and evolution—What is art for? *Psychotherapy and Politics International, 9*(1), 67-82. doi:10.1002/ppi.229

Bloom, S., & Farragher, B. (2013). *Restoring Sanctuary: A New Operating System for Trauma-Informed Systems of Care*. Oxford University Press. doi:10.1093/acprof:oso/9780199796366.001.0001

Blume, L. B. (2003). Embodied (by) Dance: Adolescent De/constructions of body, sex and gender in Physical Education. *Sex Education, 3*(2), 95–103. doi:10.1080/14681810309035

Bober, T., & Regehr, C. (2006). Strategies for reducing secondary or vicarious trauma: Do they work? *Brief Treatment and Crisis Intervention, 6*(1), 1–9. doi:10.1093/brief-treatment/mhj001

Boje, D. M. (1991). Learning story telling: Storytelling to learn management skills. *Journal of Management Education, 49*(2), 279–294. doi:10.1177/105256299101500302

Bonde, L. O. (2011). Health musicking – Music therapy or music and health? A model, empirical examples and personal reflections. *Music & Arts in Action, 3*(2), 1–21.

Bourassa, D. (2012). Examining self-protection measures guarding adult protective services social workers against compassion fatigue. *Journal of Interpersonal Violence, 27*(9), 1699–1715. doi:10.1177/0886260511430388 PMID:22203624

Bowlby, J. (2008). *A secure base: Parent-child attachment and healthy human development.* Basic Books.

Boyd Webb, N. (2004). *Mass trauma and violence: helping families and children cope.* New York: Guilford Press.

Bretherton, I. (1992). The origins of attachment theory: John Bowlby and Mary Ainsworth. *Developmental Psychology, 28*(5), 759–775. doi:10.1037/0012-1649.28.5.759

Brevard Family Partnership. (2017). *Brevard youth thrive: Protective and promotive factors for healthy development and well-being.* Retrieved from http://brevardfp.org/brevard-youth-thrive/

Brittian, A. S., O'Donnell, M., Knight, G. P., Carlo, G., Umana-Taylor, A. J., & Roosa, M. W. (2013). Associations between adolescent's perceived discrimination and prosocial tendencies: The mediating role of Mexican American values. *Journal of Youth and Adolescence, 42*(3), 328–341. doi:10.1007/s10964-012-9856-6 PMID:23152074

Bromet, E., Karam, E., Koenen, K. C., & Steine, D. J. (2018). *Trauma and posttraumatic stress disorder: Global perspectives from the WHO world mental health surveys.* Academic Press.

Brown, B. (2011, January). *Brené Brown: The power of vulnerability* (Video File). Retrieved from https://www.youtube.com/watch?v=iCvmsMzlF7o

Brown, B. (2015). *Rising strong.* New York, NY: Spiegel & Grau.

Brown, B. (2017). *Braving the wilderness.* New York, NY: Random House.

Brown, E. (1998). Things of the Spirit: Spiritual, moral, social, and cultural development. *Support for Learning, 13*(4), 157–162. doi:10.1111/1467-9604.00081

Brubaker, N. D. (2009). Negotiating Authority in an Undergraduate Teacher Education Course: A Qualitative Investigation. *Teacher Education Quarterly*, 99–118.

Brummel, S. (1989). Developing an intergenerational program. *Journal of Children in Contemporary Society., 20*(3–4), 119–133. doi:10.1300/J274v20n03_13

Brydon-Miller, M., Kral, M., Maguire, P., Noffke, S., & Sabhlok, A. (2011). *Jazz and the Banyan tree: roots and riffs on participatory action research. ResearchGate.* Retrieved from ResearchGate.

Buffington, M. (2007). The big idea: Service-learning and art education. *Art Education, 60*(6), 40–44.

Buhrmester, D. (1990). Intimacy of friendship, interpersonal competence, and adjustment during preadolescence and adolescence. *Child Development, 61*(4), 1101–1111. doi:10.2307/1130878 PMID:2209180

Buildabridge Institute. (2013). Philadelphia: Eastern University.

BuildaBridge. (2015). *Our Core Philosophy.* Retrieved from http://buildabridge.org/about-us/our-core-philosophy/

Burton, B., & Dunn, C. (n.d.). Ethics of Care. *Encyclopedia Britannica.* Retrieved from https://www.britannica.com/topic/ethics-of-care

Bussing-Birks, M. (n.d.). *Mental Illness and Substance Abuse.* Retrieved from https://www.nber.org/digest/apr02/w8699.html

Cahnmann-Taylor, M., & Siegesmund, R. (2008). *Arts-based research in education: Foundations for practice.* New York: Routledge.

Caldwell, K., Gray, J., & Wolever, R. Q. (2013). The process of patient empowerment in integrative health coaching: How does it happen? *Global Advances in Health and Medicine: Improving Healthcare Outcomes Worldwide*, *2*(3), 48–57. doi:10.7453/gahmj.2013.026 PMID:24416672

Calhoun, L., Tedeschi, R. G., Cann, A. & Hanks, E. A. (2010). Positive outcomes following bereavement: Paths to traumatic growth. *Psychologica Belgica, 50*(1-2), 125-143.

Cameron, C. A., Pinto, G., & Tapanya, S. (2014). Scaffolding one Thai youth's drawing toward resilience. *Culture and Psychology*, *20*(4), 453–476. doi:10.1177/1354067X14551293

Cameron, J. (1998). *The right to write.* New York, NY: Tarcher/Putnam.

Cameron, L. (2018). *The mindful day.* Washington, DC: National Geographic.

Camilleri, V. A. (2007). *Healing the inner city child: Creative arts therapies with at-risk youth.* London: Jessica Kingsley Publishers.

Carter, C. (2015). *The sweet spot.* New York, NY: Ballantine.

Caxaj, S.C. (2015). Indigenous storytelling and participatory action research: allies toward decolonization? Reflections from the People's International Health Tribunal. *Global Qualitative Nursing Research*, 1-12. DOI: 10.1177/2333393615580764

Centers for Disease Control and Prevention. (2011). *"Health Related Quality of Life." Health Related Quality of Life Surveillance Program.* Retrieved from http://www.cdc.gov/hrqol/hrqol14_measure.htm

Chavkin, N. F., & Gonzalez, J. (2000). Mexican immigrant youth and resiliency: Research and promising programs. *ERIC Digests.* Retrieved from www.eric.ed.gov

Cheah, E. (2009). *An orchestra beyond borders: Voices of the West-Eastern Divan Orchestra.* Brooklyn, NY: Verso.

Chung, S. K. (2007). Art education technology: Digital storytelling. *Art Education, 60*(2), 17–22.

Clandinin, D. J., & Connelly, F. M. (2000). *Narrative inquiry.* San Francisco, CA: Jossey-Bass.

Clark, E. (2004). *Around the Corporate Campfire.* Sammamish, WA: C&C Publishing.

Clason, J., Johansson, F., & Mortberg, E. (2015). Individual cognitive therapy for professional actors with performance anxiety. *Ann Depress Anxiety*, *2*(6), 1066.

Clement, J. (2007). *Reforming Dance Pedagogy: A Feminist Perspective on the Art of Performance and Dance Education.* University of South Florida Scholar Commons, Paper 673.

Cobley, P. (2001). *Narrative.* London: Routledge.

Coe, D., & Strachan, J. (2002). Writing Dance: Tensions in Researching Movement or Aesthetic Experiences. *International Journal of Qualitative Studies in Education: QSE*, *15*(5), 497–511. doi:10.1080/09518390220000l9795

Cohen, E., & Gainer, R. (1995). *Art, another language for learning* (3rd ed.). Portsmouth, NH: Heinemann.

Colle, S. (2013). *Using Focusing-Oriented Art Therapy to Form Secure Attachments: A Grant Proposal Submitted in Partial Fulfillment For the Degree of Master of Arts in Marriage and Family Therapy*. Retrieved October 24, 2015, from https://scholar.google.com/citations?view_op=view_citation&continue=/scholar?hl=en&as_sdt=0,39&scilib=1&citilm=1&citation_for_view=1x9Nc4gAAAAJ:LkGwnXOMwfcC&hl=en&oi=p

Conner, J. (2008). *Writing down your soul*. San Francisco, CA: Conari.

Cooper, M., & Sjostrom, L. (2007). *Making art together: How collaborative art-making can transform kids, classrooms, and communities*. Beacon Press.

Corbitt, J. N. (1998). *The sound of the harvest: Music's mission in church and culture*. Grand Rapids, MI: Baker Books.

Corbitt, J. N., & Nix-Early, V. (2003). *Taking it to the streets using the arts to transform your community*. Grand Rapids, MI: Baker Books.

Corbitt, J. N., & Nix-Early, V. (2003). *Taking it to the streets: Using the arts to transform your community*. Grand Rapids, MI: Baker Books.

Corbitt, J. N., & Nix-Early, V. (2003). *Taking it to the Streets: Using the Arts to Transform your Community*. Grand Rapids, MI: Baker Books.

Corbitt, J. N., & Nix-Early, V. (2003). *Taking it to the streets: using the arts to transform your community*. Grand Rapids, MI: BakerBooks.

Cori, J. L. (2007). *Healing from trauma: A survivor's guide to understanding your symptoms and reclaiming your life*. New York, NY: Marlowe & Co.

Culberston, R. (1995). Embodied Trauma, Re-establishing the Self. *New Literary History*, *26*(1).

Curry, N. A., & Kasser, T. (2005). Can coloring mandalas reduce anxiety? *Art Therapy: Journal of the American Art Therapy Association*, *22*(2), 81–85. doi:10.1080/07421656.2005.10129441

Curtis, S. L. (2012). Music therapy and social justice: A personal journey. *The Arts in Psychotherapy*, *39*(3), 209–213. doi:10.1016/j.aip.2011.12.004

Cutler, C. V., & Huntsberry, R. (2007). Creative Listening: Overcoming Fear in Life & Work. Lincoln, NE: iUniverse.

Dalebout, K. (2016). *Let it out*. Carlsbad, CA: Hay House.

Dalebroux, A., Goldstein, T. R., & Winner, E. (2008). Short-term mood repair through art-making: Positive emotion is more effective than venting. *Motivation and Emotion*, *32*(4), 288–295. doi:10.100711031-008-9105-1

Danielewicz, J. (2001). *Teaching selves identity, pedagogy, and teacher education*. Albany, NY: State University Of New York Press.

Dayton, T. (2007). *Emotional sobriety: From relationship trauma to resilience and balance*. Deerfield Beach, FL: Health Communications, Inc.

De Petrillo, L. D., & Winner, E. (2005). Does art improve mood? A test of a key assumption underlying art therapy. *Art Therapy: Journal of the American Art Therapy Association*, *22*(4), 205–212. doi:10.1080/07421656.2005.10129521

Delaney, B. & Scheiber, D. (n.d.). *Surviving the shadows: A journey of hope into post-traumatic stress*. Naperville, IL: Sourcebooks, Inc.

Dell, C. (1970). *A primer for movement description: Using effort-shape and supplementary concepts*. New York, NY: Dance Notation Bureau Press.

Dell, C. (1977). *A primer for movement description using effort-shape and supplementary concepts* (Rev. ed.). New York: Dance Notation Bureau Press.

Delue, C. (1999). Physiological effects of creating mandalas. *Medical Art Therapy with Children*, 33-49.

Denning, S. (2011). *The leader's guide to storytelling: Mastering the art and discipline of business narrative*. San Francisco, CA: Jossey-Bass.

DeNora, T. (2005). The pebble in the pond: Musicing, therapy, community. *Nordic Journal of Music Therapy*, *14*(1), 57–66. doi:10.1080/08098130509478126

Devilly, G. J., Gist, R., & Cotton, P. (2006). Ready! Fire! Aim! The status of psychological debriefing and therapeutic interventions: In the work place and after disasters. *Review of General Psychology*, *10*(4), 318–345. doi:10.1037/1089-2680.10.4.318

Dolan, G., & Naidu, Y. (2013). *Hooked: How leaders connect, engage and inspire with storytelling*. John Wiley & Sons. [Kindle Edition]. Retrieved from http://www.amazon.com/dp/

Dosamontes-Beaudry, I. (2003). *The arts in contemporary healing*. Westport, CT: Praeger.

Drake, J. E., & Winner, E. (2012). Confronting sadness through art-making: Distraction is more beneficial than venting. *Psychology of Aesthetics, Creativity, and the Arts*, *6*(3), 255–261. doi:10.1037/a0026909

Drake, J., Coleman, K., & Winner, E. (2011). Short term mood repairs through art: Effects of medium and strategy. *Art Therapy: Journal of the American Art Therapy Association*, *28*(1), 26–30. doi:10.1080/07421656.2011.557032

Duarte, N. (2010). *Resonate*. Hoboken, NJ: John Wiley & Sons.

Duckworth, A. (2016). *Grit*. New York, NY: Scribner.

Dufrene, P. (1991). Utilizing the arts for healing from a Native American perspective: Implications for creative Arts therapies. *Canadian Journal of Native Studies*.

Duncum, P. (2001). Visual culture: Developments, definitions, and directions for art education. *Studies in Art Education*, *42*(2), 101–112. doi:10.2307/1321027

Dunn-Snow, P., & D'Amelio, G. (2000). How Art Teachers Can Enhance Artmaking as a Therapeutic Experience Art Therapy and Art Education. *Art Education*, *53*(3), 46–54. doi:10.2307/3193873

Durrani, H. (2014). Facilitating attachment in children with autism through art therapy: A case study. *Journal of Psychotherapy Integration*, *24*(2), 99–108. doi:10.1037/a0036974

Dutton, J., & Heaphy, E. (2003). The power of high quality connections. In K. Cameron, J. Dutton, & R. Quinn (Eds.), *Positive organizational scholarship* (pp. 263–278). San Francisco, CA: Berrett-Koehler.

Dyer, B. (2010). Ruminations of a Road Traveled Towards Empowerment: Musing Narratives of Teaching, Learning, and Self-realization. *Research in Dance Education*, *11*(1), 5–18. doi:10.1080/14647891003653393

Eddy, M. (2002). Somatic Practices and Dance: Global Influences. *Dance Research Journal*, *34*(2), 46–62. doi:10.2307/1478459

Edenloff, J. (2011). *Arts-based evaluation tools for community arts programs: A case study of Art City's 'Green Art' in Winnipeg, Manitoba (Unpublished thesis)*. Winnipeg, Manitoba: University of Manitoba. Retrieved from http://mspace.lib.umanitoba.ca/handle/1993/4893

Elliot, D. E., Bejelajac, P., Fallot, R. D., Markoff, L. S., & Glover Reed, B. (2005). Trauma- Informed or Trauma- Denied: Pricincples and Implementation of Trauma- Informed Services for Women. *Journal of Community Psychology*, *33*(4), 461–477. doi:10.1002/jcop.20063

Ellsworth, E. (1989). Why Doesn't This Feel Empowering? Working Through the Repressive Myths of Critical Pedagogy. *Harvard Educational Review*, *59*(3), 297–325. doi:10.17763/haer.59.3.058342114k266250

Emerson, D., & Hopper, E. (2011). *Overcoming trauma through yoga: Reclaiming your body*. Berkeley, CA: North Atlantic Books.

Emunah, R. (2017). From behind the scenes to facing an audience in self-revelatory performance. In S. Penkzik, R. Emunah, & R. J. David (Eds.), *The Self In Performance: Autobiographical, Self-Revelatory, and Autoethnographic Forms of Therapeutic Theatre* (pp. 37–53). Palgrave Macmillian.

Enayati, A. (2015). *Seeking serenity*. New York, NY: New American Library.

Eriksen, E. (1993). *Childhood and society*. New York: W. W. Norton & Company Ltd. (Original publication 1963)

Erikson, E. H. (1995). *Childhood and Society*. London: Vintage.

Evans, J. F. (2010). Introducing wellness & writing connections conference papers. In J. F. Evans (Ed.), *Wellness & Writing Connections* (pp. 3–10). Enumclaw, WA: Idyll Arbor, Inc.

Faigin, D. A., & Stein, C. H. (2015). Community-based theater and adults with psychiatric disabilities: Social activism, performance and community engagement. *American Journal of Community Psychology*, *55*(1-2), 148–163. doi:10.100710464-014-9695-6 PMID:25520209

Farrelly-Hansen, M. (2001). Nature. In *Spirituality and art therapy: Living the connection* (pp. 137–158). London: J. Kingsley Publishers.

Fearnside, L., Bereza, M., & McConn, G. (2015). Using photography to foster intergenerational understanding. *Journal of Visual Literacy*, *34*(2), 70–80. doi:10.1080/23796529.2015.11674730

Feder, B., & Feder, E. (1998). *The art and science of evaluation in the arts therapies: How do you know what's working?* Springfield, IL: Charles C. Thomas Publishers, LTD.

Feldman, C., & Kornfield, J. (2015, April). Symposium conducted at the National Storytelling Network, Kansas City, MO.

Felton, P., & Clayton, P. (2011). Service-Learning. *New Directions for Teaching and Learning*, *128*(128), 75–84. doi:10.1002/tl.470

Figley, C. R. (1995). *Compassion fatigue: Coping with secondary traumatic stress disorder in those who treat the traumatized*. New York, NY: Brunner/Mazel.

Figley, C. R. (2002). Compassion fatigue: Psychotherapists' chronic lack of self care. *Journal of Clinical Psychology*, *58*(11), 1433–1441. doi:10.1002/jclp.10090 PMID:12412153

Fincher, S. (2014). *Psychology of the mandala*. Retrieved from http://creatingmandalas.com/psychology-of-the-mandala

Fincher, S. F. (1991). *Creating mandalas: For insight, healing, and self-expression*. Boston, MA: Shambhala.

Fischman, D. (2009). Therapeutic relationship and kinesthetic empathy. In S. Chaiklin & H. Wengrower (Eds.), *The art and science of dance/movement therapy: Life is dance* (pp. 33–53). New York, NY: Routledge.

Fisher, W. R. (1989). Clarifying the narrative paradigm. *Communication Monographs*, *56*(1), 55–58. doi:10.1080/03637758909390249

Fitzgerald, F. S. (1925). *The great Gatsby*. New York, NY: Scribner.

Fletcher, J. (1998). Relational practice: A feminist reconstruction of work. *Journal of Management Inquiry*, *7*(2), 163–186. doi:10.1177/105649269872012

Fletcher, J. (1999). *Disappearing acts: Gender, power, and relational practice at work*. Cambridge, MA: The MIT Press.

Fock, E. (1997). Music – intercultural communication? Micro musics, world music and multicultural discourse. *Institute of Folklore*, 55–65. Retrieved from http://www.nordicom.gu.se/sites/default/files/kapitel-pdf/6_055_066.pdf

Fortin, S. (1998). *Somatics: A Tool for Empowering Modern Dance Teachers. In Dance, power, and difference: critical and feminist perspectives on dance education* (pp. 49–74). Champaign, IL: Human Kinetics.

Foundations Recovery Network. (n.d.). *The Connection Between Mental Illness and Substance Abuse*. Retrieved from https://www.dualdiagnosis.org/mental-health-and-addiction/the-connection/

Fowler, J. W. (1981). *Stages of faith: The psychology of human development and the quest for meaning*. New York, NY: HarperCollins Publishers.

Fraser, J. G., Griffin, J. L., Barto, B. L., Lo, C., Wenz-Gross, M., Spinazzola, J., ... Bartlett, J. D. (2014). Implementation of a workforce initiative to build trauma-informed child welfare practice and services: Findings from the Massachusetts Child Trauma Project. *Children and Youth Services Review*, *44*, 233–242. doi:10.1016/j.childyouth.2014.06.016

Freidman, M. J. (2016). *PTSD history and overview*. Retrieved from https://www.ptsd.va.gov/professional/ptsd-overview/ptsd-overview.asp

Freire, P. (2000). Pedagogy of the oppressed (30th ann. ed.). New York: Continuum.

Freire, P. (1970). *Pedagogy of the Oppressed*. New York, NY: Bloomsbury Academic.

Freire, P. (1974). Conscientisation. *Cross Currents*, *24*(1), 23–31.

Gapp, K., Bohacek, J., Grossmann, J., Brunner, A. M., Manuella, F., Nanni, P., & Mansuy, I. M. (2016). Potential of environmental enrichment to prevent transgenerational effects of paternal trauma. *Neuropsychopharmacology*, *41*(11), 2749–2758. doi:10.1038/npp.2016.87 PMID:27277118

Gast, D., & Ledford, J. (2014). *Single case research methodology: Applications in special education and behavioral sciences*. New York: Routledge.

Gauthier-Pin, S. (Writer/Performer). (2017, November 4). *Finding my voice: A musical montage* (Video File). Live performance in St. Thomas of Canterbury Church, Long Beach, CA. Retrieved from https://www.youtube.com/watch?v=Dq_r7ODbj2U

Geist, J. H. (2014). *Overview of Trauma and Stress Related Disorders*. Retrieved from https://www.merckmanuals.com/professional/psychiatric-disorders/anxiety-and-st ressor-related-disorders/overview-of-trauma-and-stressor-related-disorders

Gergen, K. J., Mcnamee, S., & Barrett, F. (2001). Toward transformative dialogue. *International Journal of Public Administration*, *7*(8), 697–707. Retrieved from http://works.swarthmore.edu/cgi/viewcontent.cgi?article=1411&context=fac-psychology

Germer, C. K. (2009). *The Mindful path to self-compassion*. New York, NY: The Guilford Press.

Giampaolo, A. (2013). *Drawing autism: parental perceptions of the impact art therapy has on communication patterns and the parent-child relationship*. Retrieved October 25th from https://dspace.smith.edu/bitstream/handle/11020/24205/GiampaoloforLibraryFinal9913.pdf?sequence=1

Giesenberg, A. (2007). *The phenomenology of preschool children's spirituality (Unpublished thesis)*. Brisbane, Australia: Queensland University of Technology. Retrieved from http://eprints.qut.edu.au/16519/1/Anna_Giesenberg_Thesis.pdf

Glazer, H. R., & Stein, D. S. (2010). Qualitative research and its role in play therapy research. *International Journal of Play Therapy*, *19*(1), 54–61. doi:10.1037/a0017933

Godman, H. (2018). *Regular exercise changes the brain to improve memory, thinking skills.* Retrieved from http://www.dhs.pa.gov/cs/groups/webcontent/documents/document/s_002537.pdf

Goetz, T. (n.d.). *Movement matters - Brain dance workshop*. Retrieved from http://www.artstime.org/infors/documents/braindance_handoutgoetz.pdf

Goldberg, B. (1996). *Room to write*. New York, NY: Tarcher/Putnam.

Goldberg, N. (1986). *Writing down the bones*. Boston, MA: Shambhala.

Goldberg, N. (1990). *Wild mind.* New York, NY: Bantam.

Goldberg, N. (2007). *Old friend from far away*. New York, NY: Free Press.

Goldberg, N. (2013). *The true secret of writing*. New York, NY: Atria.

Goleman, D., Boyatzis, R., & McKee, A. (2002). *Primal Leadership: Unleashing the Power of Emotional Intelligence* [Kindle DX Version]. Retrieved from Amazon.

Good, J. (2003). Storytelling builds compassionate communities. *Edmonton Journal*. Retrieved from https://search.proquest.com/docview/252999613

Goodill, S. W. (2005). *An introduction to medical dance/movement therapy*. London: Jessica Kingsley Publishers.

Good, M., & Willoughby, T. (2006). The role of spirituality versus religiosity in adolescent psychosocial adjustment. *Journal of Youth and Adolescence*, *35*(1), 41–55. doi:10.100710964-005-9018-1

Gore, J. M. (1993). *The Struggle for Pedagogies: Critical and Feminist Discourses as Regimes of Truth*. New York: Routledge.

Grant, H. (2008). American Indians: Working with American Indians and historical trauma. *Illness, Crisis & Loss*, *16*(2), 125–136. doi:10.2190/IL.16.2.c

Green, J. (1998). *Engendering Bodies: Somatic Stories in Dance Education*. Annual Meeting of the American Educational Research Association. Retrieved November 3, 2011, from http://www.eric.ed.gov/PDFS/ED432552.pdf

Green, J. (2008). *American Body Pedagogies: Somatics and the Cultural Construction of Bodies in the Institution of Higher Education*. Retrieved October 5, 2011, from http://content3.bestthinking.com/s/1/thinkers/864/media/75cd883e-c887-4589-b101-5a0d3b901bdc.pdf

Grigsby, R. K. (1994). Maintaining attachment relationships among children in foster care. *Families in Society*, *75*(5), 269.

Grobstich, A. (2011). *Building social capital through intergenerational art participation: An analysis on trends in generational social capital* (Master of Arts dissertation). The American University. Retrieved from Dissertations & Theses. (AAT 1497652)

Grocke, D., & Wigram, T. (2007). *Receptive methods in music therapy*. Philadelphia, PA: Jessica Kingsley Publishers.

Grossman, F. K., Sorsoli, L., & Kia-Keating, M. (2006). A gale force wind: Meaning making by male survivors of childhood sexual abuse. *The American Journal of Orthopsychiatry*, *76*(4), 434–443. doi:10.1037/0002-9432.76.4.434 PMID:17209711

Grossoehme, D. H. (2008). Development of a spiritual screening tool for children and adolescents. *The Journal of Pastoral Care & Counseling*, *62*(1), 71–85. doi:10.1177/154230500806200108 PMID:18572542

Grotberg, E. H. (1995). *A guide to promoting resilience in children: Strengthening the human spirit.* Retrieved from http://resilnet.uiuc.edu/library/grotb95b.html

Grotberg, E. H. (1996). *The international resilience project: Research and application.* Retrieved from http://resilnet.uiuc.edu/library/grotb96a.html

Grotberg, E. H. (2006). *Implications of the shift from diagnosis and treatment to recovery and resilience for research and practice.* Retrieved from http://resilnet.uiuc.edu/library/grotberg2006_implications-diagnosis-recovery-georgeton.pdf

Gruwell, E. (2007). Teach with your heart. New York, NY: Broadway.

Gruwell, E., & the The Freedom Writers. (1999). The Freedom Writers diary. New York, NY: Broadway.

Guggenheim Museum, R. (n.d.). *Visitor Studies, Evaluation & Audience Research.* Retrieved from http://www.artsedsearch.org/summaries/educational-research-the-art-of-problem-solving

Gulliver, Griffiths, K. M., & Christensen, H. (2010). Perceived barriers and facilitators to mental health help-seeking in young people: A systematic review. *BMC Psychiatry*, *10*(1), 113. doi:10.1186/1471-244X-10-113 PMID:21192795

Gyllensten, A. L., Skar, L., Miller, L., & Gard, G. (2010). Embodied Identity: A Deeper Understanding of Body Awareness. *Physiotherapy Theory and Practice*, *26*(7), 439–446. doi:10.3109/09593980903422956 PMID:20649495

Halprin, D. (n.d.). *Tamalpa Institute - Our Philosophy - Statement by Co-Founder Daria Halprin.* Tamalpa Institute. Retrieved October 20, 2011, from http://www.tamalpa.org/about/philosophy.html

Handler, J. (2013). *Braving the fire.* New York, NY: St. Martin's Griffin.

Hanna, J. L. (1988). *Dance and stress: Resistance, reduction and euphoria.* New York, NY: AMS Press, Inc.

Hanna, T. (1972). *Bodies in revolt: a primer in somatic thinking.* New York: Dell.

Hanna, T. (1988). *Somatics: Reawakening the mind's control of movement, flexibility, and health.* Cambridge, MA: Da Capo Press.

Hari, J. (2015, January 20). *The likely cause of addiction has been discovered, and it is not what you think.* Retrieved from: http://www.huffingtonpost.com/johann-hari/the-real-cause-of-addicti_b_6506936.html

Harris, D. A. (2007). Pathways to embodied empathy and reconciliation after atrocity: Former boy soldiers in a dance/movement therapy group in Sierra Leone. *Intervention (Amstelveen, Netherlands)*, *5*(3), 203–231. doi:10.1097/WTF.0b013e3282f211c8

Harris, J., & Kim Barnes, B. (2006). Leadership storytelling. *Industrial and Commercial Training*, *38*(7), 350–353. doi:10.1108/00197850610704534

Hart, S. L., Vella, L., & Mohr, D. C. (2008). Relationships among depressive symptoms, benefit-finding, optimism, and positive affect in multiple sclerosis patients after psychotherapy for depression. *Health Psychology*, *27*(2), 230–238. doi:10.1037/0278-6133.27.2.230 PMID:18377142

Haugk, K. C. (2000). *When and how to use mental health resources.* St. Louis, MO: Stephen Ministries.

Haven, K. (2007). *Story proof: The Science behind the startling power of story*. Westport, CT: Greenwood Publishing Group.

Haviland, V. S., Gere, A. R., Buehler, J., & Dallavis, C. (2009). Making the Journey Toward Cultural Competence With Poetry. *Multicultural Perspectives*, *11*(1), 19–26. doi:10.1080/15210960902743870

Hawthorne, N. (1955). The scarlet letter. New York, NY: Washington Square Press. (Original text published 1850).

Healing through storytelling. (2015). *The New Indian Express*. Retrieved from http://proxy.stu.edu:2048

Heard, G. (1995). *Writing toward home*. Portsmouth, NH: Heinemann.

Heifetz, R. A. (1994). *Leadership without easy answers*. Cambridge, MA: The Belnap Press of Harvard University Press.

Heise, D. (2014, May). Steeling and resilience. *Art Education*, 26–30.

Helm, H. M. (2011). *Managing vicarious trauma and compassion fatigue*. Retrieved from http://www.lianalowenstein.com/artcile_helm.pdf

Henderson, P. G. (2012). *Empirical study of the healing nature of artistic expression: Using mandalas with the positive emotions of love and joy* (Unpublished doctoral dissertation). Texas A & M University.

Henderson, E. C. (2000). *Understanding addiction*. Jackson, MS: University Press of Mississippi.

Henderson, P., Rosen, D., & Mascaro, N. (2007). Empirical study on the healing nature of mandalas. *Psychology of Aesthetics, Creativity, and the Arts*, *1*(3), 148–154. doi:10.1037/1931-3896.1.3.148

Herndandez, B. C. (2011). *The Religiosity and Spirituality Scale for Youth: Development and initial validation (Unpublished dissertation)*. Baton Rouge, LA: Louisiana State University. Retrieved from http://etd.lsu.edu/docs/available/etd-10142011-115001/unrestricted/hernandez_diss.pdf

Heydon, R. (2007). Making meaning together; Multi-modal literacy learning opportunities in an inter-generational art programme. *Journal of Curriculum Studies*, *39*(1), 35–62. doi:10.1080/00220270500422665

Hicks, T. (2001). Another look at identity-based conflict: The roots of conflict: the roots of conflict in the psychology of consciousness. *Negotiation Journal*, *17*(1), 35–45. doi:10.1111/j.1571-9979.2001.tb00225.x

Hoffman-Kipp, P. (2008, Summer). Actualizing Democracy: The Praxis of Teacher Identity Construction. *Teacher Education Quarterly*.

Hosea, H. (2006). "The Brush's Footmarks": Parents and infants paint together in a small community art therapy group. *International Journal of Art Therapy,* 69-78. Retrieved October 28, 2015, from http://www.tandfonline.com/doi/abs/10.1080/17454830600980317#.VjA9UktFtGw

Howard, J. (1991). Entertainment spiritual warmth of storytelling art attracts listeners. *Las Vegas Review Journal*. Retrieved from https://search.proquest.com/docview/259857659

Huey-Heck, L., & Kalnin, J. (2006). *The Spirituality of Art*. Northstone Publishing.

Hughes, D. A. (2013). *8 keys to building your best relationships*. New York, NY: W.W. Norton.

Hutzel, K., Russell, R., & Gross, J. (2010). Eighth-graders as role models: A service-learning art collaboration for social and emotional learning. *Art Education*, *63*(4), 12–18.

Innella, V. (2010). Curriculum and the gallery space: A service-learning partnership. *Art Education*, *63*(3), 46–51.

Irving, M. C. (1995). *Natalistic art in therapy theory: Working with birth and prenatal issues through art*. The Union Institute.

Jacobson-Levy, M. (2013). *The Arts & Healing: Visual Arts* [Class handout].

Jaffer, Z. (2015). *Healing our wounds through storytelling*. Retrieved from http://proxy.stu.edu:2048

Jain, S., & Cohen, A. K. (2013). Fostering resilience among urban youth exposed to violence: A promising area for interdisciplinary research and practice. *Health Education & Behavior*, *40*(6), 651–662. doi:10.1177/1090198113492761 PMID:23818463

Jensen, E. (2001). *Arts with the brain in mind*. Alexandria, VA: Association for Supervision and Curriculum Development.

Johns Hopkins Medicine. (n.d.). *Mental Health Disorder Statistics*. Retrieved from https://www.hopkinsmedicine.org/healthlibrary/conditions/mental_health_disorders/ment

Johnson, D. H. (1983). *Body: Recovering Our Sensual Wisdom*. Berkeley, CA: North Atlantic Books.

Johnson, L. (1998). *Two parts textbook, one part love*. New York, NY: Hyperion.

Junkin, J. S. (2017). *Orchestral-dialogues: Accepting self, accepting others-translating deep listening skills to transformative dialogue skills*. Drexel University.

Kaur, R. (2015). *Milk and honey*. Kansas City, MO: Andrews McMeel Publishing.

Kelso, P. T. (2003). Behind the Curtain: The Body, Control, and Ballet. *Edwardsville Journal of Sociology*, *3*(2). Retrieved April 2, 2012, from http://www.siue.edu/sociology/EJS/v32kelso.htm

Kenny, C. B. (1982). *Mythic artery: The magic of music therapy*. Atascadero, CA: Ridgeview Publishing Company.

Kerr, C. (2008). *Family art therapy: Foundations of theory and practice*. New York: Routledge.

Killian, K. D. (2008). Helping till it hurts? A multimethod study of compassion fatigue, burnout, and self-care in clinicians working with trauma survivors. *Traumatology*, *14*(2), 32–44. doi:10.1177/1534765608319083

Kilmer, R. P., Gil-Rivas, V., Tedeschi, R. G., Cann, A., Calhoun, L. G., Buchanan, T., & Taku, K. (2009). Use of the revised post-traumatic growth inventory for children. *Journal of Traumatic Stress*, *22*(3), 248–253. doi:10.1002/jts.20410 PMID:19462437

King, P. E. (2008). Spirituality as Fertile Ground for Positive Youth Development. In R. M. Lerner, R. W. Roeser, & E. Phelps (Eds.), *Positive youth development & spirituality: From theory to research* (pp. 55–73). West Consohocken, PA: Templeton Foundation Press.

King, P. E., Clardy, C. E., & Ramon, J. S. (2013). Adolescent spiritual exemplars: Exploring spirituality in the lives of diverse youth. *Journal of Adolescent Research*, *28*(5), 1–27. doi:10.1177/0743558413502534

Kirmayar, L. J., Gone, J. P., & Moses, J. (2014). Rethinking historical trauma. *Transcultural Psychiatry*, *51*(3), 299–319. doi:10.1177/1363461514536358 PMID:24855142

Kirylo, J., & Boyd, D. (2017). *Paulo Freire: His Faith*. Boston, MA: Spirituality and Theology. doi:10.1007/978-94-6351-056-1_7

Kivnick, H. Q., & Erikson, J. M. (2010). The arts as healing. *The American Journal of Orthopsychiatry*, *53*(4). doi:10.1111/j.1939-0025.1983.tb03405.x PMID:6638153

Kleim, B., & Westphal, M. (2011). Mental health in first responders: A review and recommendation for prevention and intervention strategies. *Traumatology, 17*(4), 17–24. doi:10.1177/1534765611429079

Knox, D., Kimuna, S., & Zusman, M. (2005). College student views of the elderly: Some gender differences. *College Student Journal, 39*(1), 14–16.

Kodish, B. I. (2001). *Back pain solutions: How to help yourself with posture-movement therapy and education.* Pasadena, CA: Extensional Publishing.

Korn, R. (2010). *Educational research: The art of problem solving.* New York: Solomon.

Kouri, H. (2015). *Hala Kouri's Trauma-Informed Yoga Teaching Path.* Retrieved from https://www.yogajournal.com/teach/hala-khouris-trauma-informed-yoga-teaching-path

Kouzes, J., & Posner, B. (2003a). The five practices of exemplary leadership. In J. Gallos (Ed.), *Business leadership* (pp. 72–84). San Francisco, CA: John Wiley and Sons.

Kraft, N. (2000). The role of service-learning in critical thinking. In D. Well & H. Anderson (Eds.), Perspectives in Critical Thinking: Essays by Teachers in Theory and Practice (pp. 75-94). New York, NY: Peter Lang Publishing.

Kreitler, H., & Kreitler, S. (1972). *The psychology of the arts.* Durham, NC: Duke University Press.

Krensky, B., & Steffen, S. (2008). Arts-based service-learning: A state of the field. *Art Education, 61*(4), 13–18.

Ladson-Billings, G. (2001). *Crossing over to Canaan: the journey of new teachers in diverse classrooms.* San Francisco: Jossey-Bass.

Lamott, A. (1994). *Bird by bird.* New York, NY: Anchor Books.

Lanius, R. A., Williamson, P. C., Densmore, M., Boksman, K., Neufeld, R. W., Gati, J. S., & Menon, R. S. (2004). The nature of traumatic memories: A T-T FMRI functional connectivity analysis. *The American Journal of Psychiatry, 161*(1), 36–44. doi:10.1176/appi.ajp.161.1.36 PMID:14702248

LaPorte, A. (2002). Intergenerational art education; Building community in Harlem. *The Journal of Social Theory in Art Education., 22*, 51–71.

LaRocca-Pitts, M. (2009). In FACT, chaplains have a spiritual assessment tool. *Australian Journal of Pastoral Care and Health, 3*(2), 8–15. Retrieved from http://www.pastoraljournal.findaus.com/pdfs/ar2.pdf

Larson, R. (2006). Building intergenerational bonds through the arts. *Generations (San Francisco, Calif.), 30*(1), 38–41.

Lauderdale, P. (2008). Indigenous peoples in the face of globalization. *The American Behavioral Scientist, 51*(12), 1836–1843. doi:10.1177/0002764208318934

Lawson-Te Aho, K. (2014). The healing is in the pain: Revisiting and re-narrative trauma histories as a starting point for healing. *Psychology and Developing Societies, 26*(2), 181–212. doi:10.1177/0971333614549139

Lederach, J. P. (1997). *Building peace.* Washington, DC: United Institute of Peace.

Lederach, J. P. (2014). *The little book of conflict transformation.* New York, NY: Good Books.

Leedy, P. D., & Ormrod, J. E. (2005). *Practical research: Planning and design* (9th ed.). Upper Saddle River, NJ: Prentice Hall.

Levick, M. (1998). *See what I'm saying: what children tell us through their art.* Dubuque, IA: Islewest Publishing.

Levine, E. (2015). *Play and art in child psychotherapy: An expressive arts therapy approach*. London: Jessica Kingsley Publishers.

Levine, E. G. (1998). *On the play ground: Foundations of Expressive Arts Therapy: Theoretical and Clinical Perspectives*. London: Jessica Kingsley Publishers.

Lin, N. (2001). *Social capital a theory of social structure and action*. Cambridge, UK: Cambridge University Press. doi:10.1017/CBO9780511815447

Lippman, L. H., Moore, K. A., & McIntosh, H. (2009). *Positive indicators of child well-being: A conceptual framework, measures, and methodological issues*. Innocenti Working Paper No. 2009-21. Florence, Italy: Innocenti Research Centre (UNICEF). Retrieved from http://www.unicef-irc.org/publications/pdf/iwp_2009_21.pdf

Lokon, E., Kinney, J., & Kunkel, S. (2012). Building bridges across age and cognitive barriers through art: College students' reflections on an intergenerational program with elders who have dementia. *Journal of Intergenerational Relationships, 10*(4), 337–354. doi:10.1080/15350770.2012.724318

Loman, S. T. (2005). Dance/movement therapy. In Expressive therapies (pp. 68-89). The Guildford Press.

Lowenfeld, V., & Brittain, W. L. (1987). *Creative and mental growth*. Upper Saddle River, NJ: Prentice Hall. (Original work published 1949)

Lowenstein, L. F. (2010). Attachment Theory and Parental Alienation. *Journal of Divorce & Remarriage, 51*(3), 157–168. doi:10.1080/10502551003597808

Lucchesi, M. (2016). *Voices, Inc*. Retrieved from www.connectwithvoices.org

Lucchesi, M., & Soffer, G. (2015). *Trauma-Informed Lens Yoga*. Retrieved from http://www.traumainformedlensyoga.com/

Lucchesi, M., Matteuchi, A., & Soffer, G. (2018). *Breaking Tradition in Favor of Consent: Results of Trauma-Informed Lens Yoga Survey II*. Retrieved from http://ybicoalition.com/breaking-tradition-favor-consent-results-trauma-informed-lens-yoga-survey-ii/

Lusebrink, V. B. (2004). Art therapy and the brain: An attempt to understand the underlying processes of art expression in therapy. *Art Therapy: Journal of the American Art Therapy Association, 21*(3), 125–135. doi:10.1080/07421656.2004.10129496

Ma, Y.-Y. (2016). *A new way of thinking is possible, a new consciousness – perhaps a new enlightenment – that brings the arts and science back together*. Retrieved from https://www.silkroadproject.org/about-us

Mackenzie, J., & Hamlett, K. (2005). The Music Together program: Addressing the needs of. *Australian Journal of Music Therapy, 16*, 43.

Macpherson, H., Hart, A., & Heaver, B. (2015). Building resilience through group visual art activities: Findings from a scoping study with young people who experience mental health complexities and/or learning difficulties. *Journal of Social Work, 0*(0), 1–20. doi:10.1177/1468017315581772

Makin, S. R. (2000). *Therapeutic Art Directives & Resources: Activities & Initiatives for Individuals & Groups*. London: Jessica Kingsley Publishers.

Malchiodi, C. (2009, February 19). *Be here now: Mindfulness and the creative spirit*. Retrieved from https://www.psychologytoday.com/blog/arts-and-health/200902/be-here-now-mindfulness-and-the-creative-spirit

Malchiodi, C. A. (2003). Art therapy and the brain. Handbook of Art Therapy, 16-24.

Malchiodi, C. (2014). *Creative arts and play therapy for attachment problems*. New York: Guilford Publications.

Malin, H. (2013). Making meaningful: Intention in children's art making. *International Journal of Art & Design Education, 32*(1), 6–17. doi:10.1111/j.1476-8070.2013.01719.x

Marche, T. (2002). Discipline before discipline-based art education: Federal support, curricular models, and the 1965 Penn State seminar in art education. *Arts Education Policy Review, 103*(6), 25–33. doi:10.1080/10632910209600743

Mariano, J. M., & Damon, W. (2008). The role of spirituality and religious faith in supporting purpose in adolescence. In R. M. Lerner, R. W. Roeser, & E. Phelps (Eds.), *Positive youth development & spirituality: From theory to research* (pp. 210–230). West Consohocken, PA: Templeton Foundation Press.

Maslow, A. H. (2011). *Hierarchy of needs: A theory of human motivation* [Kindle Edition]. Retrieved from Amazon.com.

Maslow, A. H. (2013). *A theory of human motivation. origin 1943*. Martino Fine Books.

Masten, A. S. (2009, June). Ordinary magic: Lessons from research on resilience in human development. *Education Canada*, 28–32.

Matousek, M. (2017). *Writing to awaken*. Oakland, CA: Reveal Press.

Mayo Clinic. (n.d.). *Mental Illness*. Retrieved from https://www.mayoclinic.org/diseases-conditions/mental-illness/symptoms-causes/syc-20374968

McCann, I. L., & Pearlman, L. A. (1990). *Psychological trauma and the adult survivor: Theory, therapy, and transformation*. New York, NY: Brunner/Mazel.

McCann, I. L., & Pearlman, L. A. (1990). Vicarious traumatization: A framework for understanding the psychological effects of working with victims. *Journal of Traumatic Stress, 3*(1), 131–149. doi:10.1007/BF00975140

McCann, I. L., & Pearlman, L. A. (1992). Constructivist self-development theory: A theoretical framework for assessing and treating traumatized college students. *Journal of American College Health, 40*(4), 189–196. doi:10.1080/07448481.1992.9936281 PMID:1583241

McCartney, C., Harris, S., & Farrow, V. (2012). Experiences of secondary Hispanic immigrant students: Their stories of challenge and triumph. *Journal of School Leadership, 22*(1), 26–54.

McLaren, B. (2004). Learn to give the gift of a story. *The News*. Retrieved from https://search.proquest.com/docview/374985926

McLean, D. (2011). *Relationship agility and its impact on leader success – a case study*. Unpublished manuscript, Leadership and Change Program, Antioch University, Yellow Springs, OH.

McLean, D. (2014). *Understanding relational agility exploring constructs of relational leadership through story* (Doctoral Dissertation). Culver City, CA: Antioch University.

McLean, L., & Truong-White, H. (2015). Digital storytelling for transformative global citizenship education. *Canadian Journal of Education, 38*(2).

McNiff, S. (1998). *Art-based research*. London: Jessica Kingsley.

McNiff, S. (2011). Artistic expressions as primary modes of inquiry. *British Journal of Guidance & Counselling, 39*(5), 385–396. doi:10.1080/03069885.2011.621526

Medina, Y. (n.d.). *Critical Aesthetic Pedagogy: Toward a Theory of Self and Social Understanding*. Retrieved October 6, 2011, from http://qcpages.qc.cuny.edu/Education/AE%20Conference%20Proceedings/articles/Critical%20A esthetic%20 Pedagogy.pdf

Mehlomakulu, C. (2012, November 2). *Creativity in therapy: Mandalas*. Retrieved from http://creativityintherapy.blogspot.com/2012/11/mandalas.html

Mendez-McLeish, S. (2017). *The art of arriving* (Video File) Magnolia Moon Healing Arts. Retrieved at https://youtu.be/RnlZSsVIZ_Q

Metzl, E., & Morrell, M. (2008). The role of creativity in models of resilience: Theoretical exploration and practical applications. *Journal of Creativity in Mental Health, 3*(3), 303–318. doi:10.1080/15401380802385228

Militello, M., & Guarjardo, F. (2013). Virtually speaking: How digital storytelling can facilitate organizational learning. *Journal of Community Positive Practice., 13*(2), 80–91.

Mindfulness-based cognitive therapy. (2018). *Psychology Today*. Retrieved from https://www.psychologytoday.com/us/therapy-types/mindfulness-based-cognitive-therapy

Miraglia, K. (2017). Creating authentic preservice art teacher experiences through service-learning. In L. N. Hersey & B. Bobick (Eds.), Handbook of Research on the Facilitation of Civic Engagement through Community Art (pp. 116-151). Hershey, PA: IGI Global.

Mistry, A. (2017). The art of storytelling: Cognition and action through stories. *The International Journal of the Arts in Society, 09*(04), 301–324.

Moon, B. L. (2010). *Art-based group therapy: Theory and practice*. Springfield, IL: Charles C. Thomas Publisher, Ltd.

Moore, C. L., & Yamamoto, K. (2012). *Beyond words: Movement observation and analysis*. New York, NY: Routledge.

Moore, D. G., Burland, K., & Davidson, J. W. (2003). The social context of musical success: A developmental account. *British Journal of Psychology, 94*(4), 529–549. doi:10.1348/000712603322503088 PMID:14687460

Mother Goose on the Loose. (2015). Retrieved from http://www.mgol.net/home/why-mgol/

Moyers, B. (Producer), & Grubin, D. (Director). (1997). *The Moyers Collection - Bill T. Jones: Still Here with Bill Moyers* [Motion Picture]. United States: Films for the Humanities and Sciences.

National Art Education Association. (n.d.). Retrieved from arteducators.org

National Institute of Mental Health. (2017). *Major depression*. Retrieved from URL https://www.nimh.nih.gov/health/statistics/major-depression.shtml

National Institute of Mental Illness (NIMH). (2016a). *Bipolar Disorder*. Retrieved from https://www.nimh.nih.gov/health/topics/bipolar-disorder/index.shtml

National Institute of Mental Illness (NIMH). (2016b). *Schizophrenia*. Retrieved from https://www.nimh.nih.gov/health/topics/schizophrenia/index.shtml

National Research Council and Institute of Medicine. (2002). *Community programs to promote youth development*. Washington, DC: National Academy Press.

National Storytelling Network. (2018, Spring). *Healing Story Alliance Member's Newsletter*.

Nebraska Department of Veterans Affairs. (2016). *Post traumatic stress disorder*. Retrieved from http://www.ptsd.ne.gov/what-is-ptsd.html

Neff, K. (2011). *Self compassion: the proven power of being kind to yourself.* New York, NY: HarperCollins.

Nelson, T. S. (1996). *Vicarious trauma: bearing witness to another's trauma* (Doctoral dissertation). University of Illinois. Retrieved from http://www.uic.edu/orgs/convening/vicariou.htm

Nevin, A., Bradshaw, L., Cardelle-Elawar, M., & Diaz-Greenburg, M. (2009). *Becoming a Teacher: A Cross-Cultural Analysis of Motivation and Teacher Identity Formation.* Retrieved October 6, 2011, from the ERIC database.

New Indian Express. (2015). *Healing through storytelling.* Retrieved from https://search.proquest.com/docview/1655891942

Ng, R., Ang, R. P., & Ringo Ho, M. H. (2012). Coping with anxiety, depression, anger, and aggression: The meditational role of resilience in adolescents. *Child and Youth Care Forum, 41*(6), 529–546. doi:10.100710566-012-9182-x

Nicholson, H. (2005). *Applied drama: the gift of theater.* New York: Palgrave. doi:10.1007/978-0-230-20469-0

Nicholson, J. M., Berthelsen, D., Abad, V., Williams, K., & Bradley, J. (2008). Impact of music therapy to promote positive parenting and child development. *Journal of Health Psychology, 13*(2), 226–238. doi:10.1177/1359105307086705 PMID:18375628

Niequist, S. (2016). *Present over perfect.* Grand Rapids, MI: Zondervan.

Nurrie-Stearns, M., & Nurrie-Stearns, R. (2013). *Yoga for emotional trauma. Meditations and practices for healing pain and suffering.* Oakland, CA: New Harbinger Publishing, Inc.

O'Grady, L., & McFerran, K. (2007). Community music therapy and its relationship to community music: Where does it end? *Nordic Journal of Music Therapy, 16*(1), 14–26. doi:10.1080/08098130709478170

Oliveros, P. (2005). *Deep listening: A composer's sound practice.* Lincoln NE: iUniverse.

Ottey, S. D. (1996). Critical Pedagogical Theory and the Dance Educator. *Arts Education Policy Review, 98*(2), 31–39. doi:10.1080/10632913.1996.9935096

Pals, J. L., & McAdams, D. P. (2004). The transformed self: A narrative understanding of post-traumatic growth. *Psychological Inquiry, 15*(1), 65–69.

Parker-Pope, T. (2011. February). Healing through storytelling. *New York Times.*

Pavlicevic, M., & Impey, A. (2013). Deep listening: Towards an imaginative reframing of health and well-being practices in international development. *Arts & Health: An International Journal for Research. Policy & Practice, 5*(3), 238–252. doi:10.1080/17533015.2013.827227 PMID:25729413

Pearlman, L. A., & Saakvitne, K. A. (1995). *Trauma and the therapist.* New York, NY: W.W. Norton & Company.

Pena, D. C. (1998). *Three Teachers' Histories.* Retrieved October 11, 2011, from the ERIC database.

Pendzik, S., Emunah, R., & Johnson, D. R. (2017). The self in performance: Context, definitions, directions. In S. Penkzik, R. Emunah, & R. J. David (Eds.), *The Self In Performance: Autobiographical, Self-Revelatory, and Autoethnographic Forms of Therapeutic Theatre* (pp. 1–18). Palgrave Macmillian.

Pennebaker, J. W., & Smyth, J. M. (2016). *Opening up by writing it down.* New York, NY: The Guilford Press.

Pennsylvania Office of Mental Health and Substance Abuse Services. (2005). *A Call to Change: Towards A Recovery-Oriented Mental Health Service System For Adults.* Retrieved from http://www.dhs.pa.gov/cs/groups/webcontent/documents/document/s_002537.pdf

Phillips, A. (2012, March 7). *Art and trauma: Creativity as a resiliency factor*. Retrieved from https://www.goodtherapy.org/blog/art-and-trauma-creativity-as-a-resiliency-factor-0307124

Pizarro, J. (2004). The efficacy of Art and writing therapy: Increasing positive mental health outcomes and participant retention after exposure to traumatic experience. *Art Therapy: Journal of the American Art Therapy Association*, *21*(1), 5–12. doi:10.1080/07421656.2004.10129327

Plante, P., & Bernèche, R. (2008). A phenomenological study addressing the reinforcement of emotional ties between parent and child through the elaboration and evaluation of dyadic art therapy groups. *Canadian Art Therapy Association Journal*, *21*(1), 18–34. doi:10.1080/08322473.2008.11432297

Ponteri, A. K. (2001). The effect of group art therapy on depressed mothers and their children. *Art Therapy: Journal of the American Art Therapy Association*, *18*(3), 148–157. doi:10.1080/07421656.2001.10129729

Potash, J., & Ho, R. T. (2011). Drawing involves caring: Fostering relationship building through art therapy for social change. *Art Therapy: Journal of the American Art Therapy Association*, *28*(2), 74–81. doi:10.1080/07421656.2011.578040

Powell, H. (2004). A dream wedding: from community music to music therapy with a community. In M. Pavlicevic & G. Ansdell (Eds.), Community Music Therapy (pp. 167–185). Philadelphia, PA: Jessica Kingsley Publishers.

Powell, K. (2010). Making sense of place: Mapping as a multisensory research method. *Qualitative Inquiry*, *16*(7), 639–555. doi:10.1177/1077800410372600

Procter, S. (2011). Reparative musicing: Thinking on the usefulness of social capital theory within music therapy. *Nordic Journal of Music Therapy*, *20*(3), 242–262. doi:10.1080/08098131.2010.489998

Proctor, S. (2004). Playing politics: Community music therapy and the therapeutic redistribution of music capital for mental health. In M. Pavlicevic & G. Ansdell (Eds.), Community Music Therapy (pp. 214–230). Philadelphia, PA: Jessica Kingsley Publishers.

Proulx, L. (2002). Strengthening ties, parent-child-dyad: Group art therapy with toddlers and their parents. *American Journal of Art Therapy*, *40*(4), 238.

Proulx, L. (2003). *Strengthening emotional ties through parent-child-dyad art therapy: Interventions with infants and preschoolers*. London: Jessica Kingsley Publishers.

Pryce, J., Shackelford, K., & Price, D. (2007). Educating child welfare workers about secondary trauma stress. In *Secondary trauma stress and the child welfare professional* (pp. 51-71). Retrieved from http://lyceumbooks.com/pdf/stsch3.pdf

Psychiatric Rehabilitation Association (PRA) and Psychiatric Rehabilitation Foundation (PRF). (n.d.). Retrieved from https://www.psychrehabassociation.org/who-we-are/core-principles-and-values

PTSD United. (2013). *PTSD statistics*. Retrieved from http://www.ptsdunited.org/ptsd-statistics-2/

Pugh McCutchen, B. (2006). *Teaching dance as art in education*. Champaign, IL: Human Kinetics.

Putnam, R. D. (2000). *Bowling alone: The collapse and revival of American community*. New York: Simon & Schuster. doi:10.1145/358916.361990

Rankin, L. (2013). *Mind over medicine*. Carlsbad, CA: Hay House.

Rankin, L. (2015). *The fear cure*. Carlsbad, CA: Hay House.

Rappaport, L. (1998). Focusing and art therapy: Tools for working through post-traumatic stress disorder. *Focusing Folio, 17*(1), 1-6. Retrieved from https://www.focusing.org/pdf/rappaport_focusing_and_art_therapy_tools_for_working_through_trauma.pdf

Rausch, S. L., van der Kolk, B. A., Fisler, R. E., & Alpert, N. M. (1996). A symptom provocation study of posttraumatic stress disorder using positron emission tomography and script-driven imagery. *Archives of General Psychiatry, 53*(5), 380–387. doi:10.1001/archpsyc.1996.01830050014003 PMID:8624181

Regehr, C. (2001). Crisis debriefing groups for emergency responders: Reviewing the evidence. *Brief Treatment and Crisis Intervention, 1*(2), 87–100. doi:10.1093/brief-treatment/1.2.87

Reynolds, F., & Prior, S. (2006). Creative adventures and flow in art-making: A qualitative study of women living with cancer. *British Journal of Occupational Therapy, 69*(6), 255–262. doi:10.1177/030802260606900603

Rhodes, A. M., & Schecter, R. (2012). Fostering resilience among youth in inner city community arts centers: The case of the artists collective. *Education and Urban Society, 46*(7), 826–848. doi:10.1177/0013124512469816

Riaño-Alcalá, P. (2015). Emplaced witnessing: Commemorative practices among the Wayuu in the Upper Guajira. *Memory Studies, 8*(3), 282–297. doi:10.1177/1750698014563970

Roberts, L. M. (2007). From proving to becoming: How positive relationships create a context for self-discovery and self-actualization. In J. Dutton & B. Rose (Eds.), *Exploring positive relationships at work: Building a theoretical and research foundation* (pp. 29–45). New York, NY: Psychology Press.

Robitschek, C. (1998). Personal growth initiative: The construct and its measure. *Measurement & Evaluation in Counseling & Development, 30*, 183–198.

Robles, D. A. (2008). *Beyond assimilation vs. cultural resistance: Wayuu market appropriation in Riohacha, La Guajira, Colombia* (Master's thesis). Retrieved from www.kuscholarworks.ku.edu

Rodriguez, C. (2015). *The Journey of a digital story: A Healing performance of mino-bimaadiziwin: The Good life* (Doctoral Dissertation). Retrieved from https://search.proquest.com/3731363

Rodseth, D. (2011). Dealing with bipolar disorder in general practice. *South African Family Practice, 53*(6), 549–553. doi:10.1080/20786204.2011.10874150

Romano, T. (2013). *Fearless writing*. Portsmouth, NH: Heinemann.

Romano, T. (2015). *Write what matters*. Lexington, KY: Zigzag.

Rosenberg, R. (2002). Ceremonial healing and the multiple narrative tradition in Louise Erdrich's Tales of Burning Love. *Melus, 27*(3), 113. doi:10.2307/3250658

Rossetto, E. (2012). A hermeneutic phenomenological study of community mural making and social action art therapy. *Art Therapy: Journal of the American Art Therapy Association, 29*(1), 19–26. doi:10.1080/07421656.2012.648105

Rothschild, B. (2000). *The body remembers: The psychophysiology of trauma and trauma treatment*. New York, NY: W.W. Norton.

Rothschild, B. (2010). *8 keys to safe trauma recovery: Take-charge strategies to empower your healing*. New York, NY: W. W. Norton.

Rubin, S. (2017). Embodied life stories: Transforming shame through self-revelatory performance. In S. Penkzik, R. Emunah, & R. J. David (Eds.), *The Self In Performance: Autobiographical, Self-Revelatory, and Autoethnographic Forms of Therapeutic Theatre* (pp. 129–139). Palgrave Macmillian.

Rushnell, S., & DuArt, L. (2017). *The Godwink effect.* New York, NY: Howard Books.

Russell, R., & Hutzel, K. (2007). Promoting social and emotional learning through service-learning art projects. *Art Education, 60*(3), 6–11.

Sager, G. (2012, May). The art of storytelling. *Natural Life Magazine*, 21-23. Retrieved from https://search.proquest.com/2048

Sajnani, N. (2017). Relational aesthetics in performance of personal story. In S. Penkzik, R. Emunah, & R. J. David (Eds.), *The Self In Performance: Autobiographical, Self-Revelatory, and Autoethnographic Forms of Therapeutic Theatre* (pp. 85–95). Palgrave Macmillian.

Sandberg, S., & Grant, A. (2017). *Option B.* New York, NY: Knopf.

Sandel, S. L., Judge, J. O., Landry, N., Faria, L., Ouellette, R., & Majczak, M. (2005). Dance and movement program improves quality-of-life measures in breast cancer survivors. *Cancer Nursing, 28*(4), 301–309. doi:10.1097/00002820-200507000-00011 PMID:16046894

Savin-Baden, M., & Howell Major, C. (2013). *Qualitative research: The essential guide to theory and practice.* New York, NY: Routledge.

Saxberg, L. (1996). Storytelling comes alive as an art form. *The Ottawa Citizen.* Retrieved from https://search.proquest.com/docview/239974028

Scarlett, W. G. (2008). Spirituality and positive youth development: The problem of transcendence. In R. M. Lerner, R. W. Roeser, & E. Phelps (Eds.), *Positive youth development & spirituality: From theory to research* (pp. 42–54). West Consohocken, PA: Templeton Foundation Press.

Schütz, A. (1951). Making music together: A study in social relationship. *Social Research*, 76–97.

Seigel, D. (2015). *Brainstorm: the power and purpose of the teenage brain.* New York: Penguin Random House.

Servan-Schreiber, D. (2003). *The instinct to heal: Curing depression, anxiety, and stress without drugs and without talk therapy.* Paris, France: Rodale.

Setti, I., & Argentero, P. (2014). The role of mindfulness in protecting firefighters from psychosomatic malaise. *Traumatology, 20*(2), 134–141. doi:10.1037/h0099398

Shakespeare-Finch, J. (2011). Primary and secondary trauma in emergency personnel. *Traumatology, 17*(4), 1–2. doi:10.1177/1534765611431834

Shank, M., & Schirch, L. (2008). Strategic arts-based peacebuilding. *Peace and Change, 33*(2), 217–242. doi:10.1111/j.1468-0130.2008.00490.x

Shapiro, S. B. (1998). *Toward Transformative Teachers: Critical and Feminist Perspectives in Dance Education. Dance, Power, and Difference.* Champaign, IL: Human Kinetics.

Shapiro, S. B. (1999). *Pedagogy and the politics of the body: A critical praxis.* New York: Garland Pub.

Sharp, C. (2000). *A writer's workbook.* New York, NY: St. Martin's Press.

Showalter, S. E. (2010). Compassion fatigue: What is it? Why does it matter? Recognizing the symptoms, acknowledging the impact, developing the tools to prevent compassion fatigue, and strengthen the professional already suffering the effects. *American Journal for Hospice and Palliative Medicine, 27*(4), 239–242. doi:10.1177/1049909109354096 PMID:20075423

Shue, L. L., & Beck, C. S. (2001). Stepping Out of Bounds: Performing Feminist Pedagogy within a Dance Education Community. *Communication Education*, *50*(2), 125–143. doi:10.1080/03634520109379239

Silva, E. (2008). *Conociendo a mis hermanos Wayuu*. Author.

Small, C. (1999). *Musicking: The meanings of performing and listening*. New York, NY: Music Library Association.

Smith, K. (2018, February 13). *Anxiety vs depression: Tips to help understand the difference.* Retrieved from https://www.psycom.net/anxiety-depression-difference

Smith, C. (1998). *On Authoritarianism in the Dance Classroom. Dance, Power, and Difference*. Champaign, IL: Human Kinetics.

Snow, S. (2017). Influences of experimental theatre on the emergence of self-revelatory performance. In S. Penkzik, R. Emunah, & R. J. David (Eds.), *The Self In Performance: Autobiographical, Self-Revelatory, and Autoethnographic Forms of Therapeutic Theatre* (pp. 21–35). Palgrave Macmillian.

Spouse, J. (2000). Talking pictures: Investigating personal knowledge through illuminative art-work. *Nursing Times Research*, *5*(4), 253–261. doi:10.1177/136140960000500404

Stams, G. J. J., Juffer, F., & van IJzendoorn, M. H. (2002). Maternal sensitivity, infant attachment, and temperament in early childhood predict adjustment in middle childhood: The case of adopted children and their biologically unrelated parents. *Developmental Psychology*, *38*(5), 806–821. doi:10.1037/0012-1649.38.5.806 PMID:12220057

Steiner-Adair, C., & Barker, T. H. (2013). *The big disconnect: Protecting childhood and family relationships in the digital age*. Harper Business.

Stets, J. E., & Burke, P. J. (2000). Identity Theory and Social Identity Theory. *Social Psychology Quarterly*, *63*(3), 224–237. doi:10.2307/2695870

Stewart, M. (2005). *Rethinking Curriculum in Art*. Worcester, MA: Davis Publications.

Stige, B. (2002, November). The relentless roots of community music therapy. *Voices: A World Forum for Music Therapy*, *2*(3). Retrieved from https://www.voices.no/index.php/voices/article/view/98/75

Stige, B. (2003). *Elaborations toward a notion of community music therapy*. Oslo: Unipub AS.

Stige, B. (2006). On a notion of participation in music therapy. *Nordic Journal of Music Therapy*, *15*(2), 121–138. doi:10.1080/08098130609478159

Stige, B., & Aaro, L. E. (2012). *Invitation to community music therapy*. New York, NY: Routledge Taylor and Francis Group.

Stige, B., Ansdell, G., & Elefant, C. (2010). *Where music helps: community music therapy in action and reflection.* Burlington, VT: Ashgate Publishing Company.

Stinson, S. W. (2004). *My Body/Myself: Lessons From Dance Education. In Knowing bodies, moving minds: towards embodied teaching and learning* (pp. 153–167). New York: Kluwer Academic Publishers.

Strickler, J. (1990). Tell me a story: Storytellers hope ancient art can survive in modern society. *Star Tribune*. Retrieved from https://search.proquest.com/docview/418103779

Stroebe, M. S., & Schut, H. (1999). The dual process model of coping with bereavement: Rationale and description. *Death Studies*, *23*(3), 197–224. doi:10.1080/074811899201046 PMID:10848151

Stuckey, H. L., & Nobel, J. (2010). The Connection Between Art, Healing, and Public Health: A Review of Current Literature. *Am J. Public Health, 100*(2), 254-263. Retrieved from https://www.ncbi.nlm.nih.gov/pmc/articles/PMC2804629/

Stuckey, H. L., & Nobel, J. (2010). The connection between art, healing, and public health: A review of current literature. *American Journal of Public Health, 100*(2), 254–263. doi:10.2105/AJPH.2008.156497 PMID:20019311

Substance Abuse and Mental Health Services Administration (SAMHSA). (2015). *Trauma-Informed Approach and Trauma-Specific Interventions.* Retrieved from https://www.samhsa.gov/nctic/trauma-interventions

Substance Abuse and Mental Health Services Administration. (2014). *SAMHSA's concept of trauma and guidance for a trauma-informed approach. HHS Publication No. (SMA) 14-4884.* Rockville, MD: Substance Abuse and Mental Health Services Administration.

Substance Abuse and Mental Health Services Administration. (2014). *SAMHSA's Concept of Trauma and Guidance for a Trauma-Informed Approach. HHS Publication No. (SMA) 14-4884.* Rockville, MD: Substance Abuse and Mental Health Services Administration.

Substance Abuse and Mental Health Services Administration. (2015, November). *A guide to GPRA data collection using trauma-informed interviewing skills.* Retrieved from https://www.integration.samhsa.gov/about-us/Trauma-InformedInterviewingManual-508.pdf

Sutton, J. P. (2002). *Music, music therapy and trauma: International perspectives.* London: J. Kingsley Publishers.

Szabo, R., & Hall, M. (2007). *Behind happy faces.* Beverly Hills, CA: Alegra.

Tajfel, H., & Turner, J. C. (1986). *The Social Identity Theory of Inter-group Behavior. Psychology of intergroup relations* (2nd ed.). Chicago: Nelson-Hall Publishers.

Tan, C. (2008). Manifestations of Hope Chart. In *Manifestations of Hope in Music Therapy with Hospitalized Pediatric Patients.* Philadelphia, PA: Drexel University.

Tapley, E. (2004). Seniors with cognitive disabilities: Assisting visual memory. In A. M. LaPorte (Ed.), *Community connections: Intergenerational links in art education* (pp. 45–56). Reston, VA: National Art Education Association.

Taylor, P. (2002). Service-Learning as postmodern art and pedagogy. *Studies in Art Education, 43*(2), 124–140. doi:10.2307/1321000

Taylor, P. (2005). The children's peace project: Service-learning in art education. *International Education Journal, 6*(5), 581–586.

Tayor, P., & Ballengee-Morris, C. (2004). Service-Learning a Language of "we.". *Art Education, 57*(5), 6–12.

Tedeschi, R., & Calhoun, L. (1996). The post-traumatic growth inventory: Measuring the positive the positive legacy of trauma. *Journal of Traumatic Stress, 9*(3), 455–471. doi:10.1002/jts.2490090305 PMID:8827649

Tedeschi, R., & Calhoun, L. (2004a). Post-traumatic growth: Conceptual Foundations and Empirical Evidence. *Psychological Inquiry, 15*(1), 1–18. doi:10.120715327965pli1501_01

Tedeschi, R., & Calhoun, L. (2004b). The foundations of post-traumatic growth: New considerations. *Psychological Inquiry, 15*(1), 93–102. doi:10.120715327965pli1501_03

Thayer, R. E., Newman, J. R., & McClain, T. M. (1994). Self-regulation of mood: Strategies for changing a bad mood, raising energy, and reducing tension. *Journal of Personality and Social Psychology, 67*(5), 910–925. doi:10.1037/0022-3514.67.5.910 PMID:7983582

The Center for Somatic Studies. (2014). *Developmental somatic psychotherapy*. Retrieved from somaticstudies.com/

The Merriam-Webster Dictionary. (2015, April 13). *Trauma*. Retrieved from: http://www.merriam-webster.com/dictionary/

The Straits Times. (2016, Feb 22). *Figure at 25-year low; social workers say teens now more savvy about using contraceptives*. Retrieved from http://www.straitstimes.com/singapore/big-drop-in-number-of-teen-pregnancies

Theron, L. C. (2013). Black students' recollections of pathways to resilience: Lessons for school psychologists. *School Psychology International*, *34*(5), 527–539. doi:10.1177/0143034312472762

Theron, L., Cameron, C. A., Didkowsky, N., Lau, C., Liebenger, L., & Ungar, M. (2011). A 'day in the lives' of four resilient youths: Cultural roots of resilience. *Youth & Society*, *43*(3), 799–818. doi:10.1177/0044118X11402853

Thobaben, A. M. (2013). The role of art and literacy activities in Children's healing process. *Home Health Care Management & Practice*, *25*(3), 123–125. doi:10.1177/1084822313476299

Tindle, H. (2013). *Up: How positive outlook can transform our health and aging*. New York, NY: Hudson Street Press.

Tortora, S. (2006). *The dancing dialogue: Using the communicative power of movement with young children*. Baltimore, MD: Paul H. Brookes Publishing Co.

Tovar-Restrepo, M., & Irazábal, C. (2013). Indigenous women and violence in Colombia. *Latin American Perspectives*, *41*(1), 39–58. doi:10.1177/0094582X13492134

Trauma and PTSD in the WHO World Mental Health Surveys. (2017). Retrieved from https://www.tandfonline.com/doi/full/10.1080/20008198.2017.1353383

Trent, T. (2017). *The Awakened Woman: Remembering and reigniting our sacred dreams*. New York: Simon & Schuster.

Trieschman, A., Whittaker, J., & Brendtro, L. (1969). *The other 23 hours: Child-care work with emotionally disturbed children in a therapeutic milieu*. Piscataway, NJ: Transaction.

Tulinius, C., & Holge-Hazelton, B. (2011). When the spiral of action research collapses: Using the arts to interpret and continue the process in collective research dialogues. *Action Research*, *9*(1), 42–64. doi:10.1177/1476750311398307

U.S. Department of Health and Human Services, Administration for Children & Families. (2015). *Child Maltreatment 2013*. Retrieved from http://www.acf.hhs.gov/programs/cb/resource/child-maltreatment-2013

U.S. Department of Health and Human Services. (2017). *What is Mental Health*. Retrieved from https://www.mentalhealth.gov/basics/what-is-mental-health

United Nations International Children's Emergency Fund. (2013). *UNICEF annual report 2013 - Colombia*. Retrieved from www.unicef.org

University of Phoenix. (2017, April 17). *Majority of first responders face mental health challenges in the workplace*. Retrieved from http://www.phoenix.edu/about_us/media-center/news/uopx-releases-first-responder-mental-health-survey-results.html

Updegraff, J. A., & Marshall, G. N. (2005). Predictors of perceived growth following direct exposure to community violence. *Journal of Social and Clinical Psychology*, *24*(4), 538–560. doi:10.1521/jscp.2005.24.4.538

Urcuyo, K. R., Boyers, A. E., Carver, C. S., & Antoni, M. H. (2005). Finding benefit in breast cancer: Relations with personality, coping, and concurrent well-being. *Psychology & Health*, *20*(2), 175–192. doi:10.1080/08870440512331317634

Uriana, G. M. (2008). Impactos ambientales de la extraccion de recursos naturales y el rol de la mujer wayuu frente a los cambios climáticos en el departamento de la Guajira, Colombia. *Mujeres Indígenas y Cambio Climático: Perspectivas latinoamericanas*, 120-131. Retrieved from www.bivipas.unal.edu.co

US Department of Health and Human Services. (2005). *A guide to managing stress in crisis response professions* (SMA 4113). Retrieved from http://store.samhsa.gov/shin/content//SMA05-4113/SMA05-4113.pdf

Vaillancourt, G. (2012). Music therapy: A community approach to social justice. *The Arts in Psychotherapy*, *39*(3), 173–178. doi:10.1016/j.aip.2011.12.011

Van den Dries, L., Juffer, F., van IJzendoorn, M. H., & Bakermans-Kranenburg, M. J. (2009). Fostering security? A meta-analysis of attachment in adopted children. *Children and Youth Services Review*, *31*(3), 410–421. doi:10.1016/j.childyouth.2008.09.008

Van der Kolk, B. (2006). Clinical Implications of Neuroscience Research in PTSD. *Annuals of the New York Academy of Sciences,* 1-17.

Van der Kolk, B. (2014). *The body keeps score: Brain, mind and body in the healing of trauma*. New York, NY: Penguin Group.

Van der Kolk, B. A. (1994). The body keeps the score: Memory and the evolving psychobiology of post-traumatic stress. *Harvard Review of Psychiatry*, *1*(5), 253–265. doi:10.3109/10673229409017088 PMID:9384857

Van der Kolk, B. A., Stone, L., West, J., Rhodes, A., Emerson, D., Suvak, M., & Spinazzola, J. (2014). Yoga as an Adjunctive Treatment for Posttraumatic Stress Disorder: A Randomized Controlled Trial. *The Journal of Clinical Psychiatry*, *75*(6), e559–e565. doi:10.4088/JCP.13m08561 PMID:25004196

Van Lith, T. (2014). Painting to find my spirit: Art making as the vehicle to find meaning and connection in the mental health recovery process. *Journal of Spirituality in Mental Health*, *16*(1), 13–36. doi:10.1080/19349637.2013.864542

Veblen, K. K. (2008). The many ways of community music. *International Journal of Community Music*, *1*(1), 5–21. doi:10.1386/ijcm.1.1.5_1

Vennet, R. V., & Serice, S. (2012). Can coloring mandalas reduce anxiety? A replication study. *Art Therapy: Journal of the American Art Therapy Association*, *29*(2), 87–92. doi:10.1080/07421656.2012.680047

Virginia Department of Education Standards of Learning (SOL) & Testing. (n.d.). Retrieved from www.doe.virginia.gov/testing/sol/standards_docs/

Virginia Mennonite Retirement Community. (n.d.). Retrieved from www.vmrc.org

Volkas, A. (2017). Autobiographical therapeutic performance as individual therapy. In S. Penkzik, R. Emunah, & R. J. David (Eds.), *The Self In Performance: Autobiographical, Self-Revelatory, and Autoethnographic Forms of Therapeutic Theatre* (pp. 113–127). Palgrave Macmillian.

Walker, S. (2001). *Teaching Meaning in Artmaking*. Worcester, MA: Davis Publications.

Wanner, E. T., & Bird, J. L. (2017). Incorporating a new technology for patient education. In Information Resources Management Association (Ed.), Healthcare ethics and training (pp. 662-675). Hershey, PA: Information Science Reference. doi:10.4018/978-1-5225-2237-9.ch030

Wanner, E. T., & Bird, J. L. (2015). Strength from spirituality. In J. L. Bird (Ed.), *Innovative collaborative practice and reflection in patient education* (pp. 218–232). Hershey, PA: Information Science Reference. doi:10.4018/978-1-4666-7524-7.ch014

Watkins, M., & Shulman, H. (2008). *Toward psychologies of liberation*. New York, NY: Palgrave Macmillan. doi:10.1057/9780230227736

Watson, D., Clark, L. A., & Tellegen, A. (1988). Development and validation of brief measures of positive and negative affect: The PANAS scales. *Journal of Personality and Social Psychology*, *54*(6), 1063–1070. doi:10.1037/0022-3514.54.6.1063 PMID:3397865

Weir, K. N., Lee, S., Canosa, P., Rodrigues, N., McWilliams, M., & Parker, L. (2013). Whole Family Theraplay: Integrating Family Systems Theory and Theraplay to Treat Adoptive Families. *Adoption Quarterly*, *16*(3-4), 175–200. doi:10.1080/10926755.2013.844216

Wellman, A. (2018). *Long beach community theater.* Retrieved from http://longbeachcommunitytheater.com

Welton, M. R. (n.d.). *Echoes of those now silent: Canadian women's associations as learning sites*. Retrieved from www.populareducation.co.za/sites/default/files

Wengrower, H. (2009). The creative-artistic process in dance/movement therapy. In S. Chaiklin & H. Wengrower (Eds.), *The art and science of dance/movement therapy: Life is dance* (pp. 13–32). New York, NY: Routledge.

Wentling, B., & Behrens, G. A. (2018). Case study of early childhood trauma using a neurobiological approach to music therapy. *Music Therapy Perspectives*, *36*(1), 131. doi:10.1093/mtp/miy003

Wexler, A. (2004). The art of necessity: Pictures of lives reclaimed from trauma. *Art Education*, *57*(1), 21–34.

Whiteland, S. (2012). *Examining visual art experiences for relationship building in shared-site locations*. Retrieved October 28, 2015, from http://digital.library.unt.edu/ark:/67531/metadc115180/m2/1/high_res_d/dissertation.pdf

Whiteland, S. (2013). Intergenerational visual arts programs at shared sites: A step toward sustainability. *Journal of Intergenerational Relationships*, *11*(4), 396–409. doi:10.1080/15350770.2013.839324

Whitman, W. (1993). O Me! O Life! In *Leaves of Grass* (p. 341). New York, NY: Random House. (Original work published 1855).

Wielenga, C. (2013). Shattered stories: Healing and reconciliation in the south African context. *Verbum Et Ecclesia*, *34*(1), 1-8. Retrieved from https://search.proquest.com/docview/1635231523

Willson, R. B. (2009). The parallax worlds of the West-Eastern Divan Orchestra. *Journal of the Royal Musical Association*, *134*(2), 319–347. doi:10.1080/02690400903109109

Wright, A. (2017, May 17). *What are the signs of 'high functioning' depression and could you have it?* Retrieved from https://themighty.com/2017/05/signs-of-high-functioning-depression-or-dysthymia/

Yashinsky, D. (2004). *Suddenly they heard footsteps*. Jackson, MS: University Press of Mississippi.

Yassen, J. (1995). Preventing Secondary Traumatic Stress Disorder. In *Compassion fatigue: Coping with secondary traumatic stress disorder in those who treat the traumatized*. New York, NY: Brunner/Mazel.

Yeh, C. J., Pituc, S. T., Kim, A. B., & Atkins, M. (2008). Poverty loss, and resilience: The story of Chinese immigrant youth. *American Psychologist Association*, *55*(1), 34–48. doi:10.1037/0022-0167.55.1.34

Yılmaz, D., Kisa, S., & Zeyneloğlu, S. (2012). University students' views and practices of ageism. *Ageing International*, *37*(2), 143–154. doi:10.100712126-010-9097-5

Young, R. (2005). *EMS stress and paramedic students*. Canadian Emergency News.

Zapach, M. D. (1997). *The sociocultural impact of El Cerrejon Coal Mine on the Wayuu of the Southern Guajira, Colombia* (Master's thesis). Retrieved from www.era.library.ualberta.ca

Zelkowitz, M. (2004). Bringing the outdoors in: An intergenerational community service mural art project. In A. M. La Porte (Ed.), *Community connections: Intergenerational links in art education* (pp. 57–68). Reston, VA: National Art Education Association.

Zimmermann, S. (2002). *Writing to heal the soul.* New York, NY: Three Rivers Press.

Zimna, K. (2010). *Play in the theory and practice of art.* Academic Press.

Znoj, H. (2006). Bereavement and post-traumatic growth. In L. G. Calhoun & R. G. Tedeschi (Eds.), *Handbook of Posttraumatic Growth: Research and Practice* (pp. 176–196). Mahwah, NJ: Lawrence Erlbaum Associates.

Zohar, D., & Marshall, I. (2004). *Spiritual capital: Wealth we can live by. Kindle Edition.* San Francisco, CA: Berrett-Koehler Publishers.

About the Contributors

Jenny Bopp received a B.A. in Political Science from Hillsdale College in 2008, and in 2014 she graduated with an M.A. in Urban Studies and Community Arts from Eastern University where she focused on trauma-informed, arts-based practices for effecting positive change in communities both locally and globally. Jenny has been working and teaching at Westtown School in Pennsylvania since 2012 as the school's Dance Program Coordinator. Prior to Westtown, Jenny taught ballet and modern dance techniques in various studios, and she has recently opened her own dance studio in West Chester, Pennsylvania. Jenny performed and choreographed for four years with the Hillsdale Tower Dancers dance company, and has performed as a guest artist with Go! Contemporary Dance Works and with Circle Modern Dance in Knoxville, Tennessee. In addition to teaching dance, Jenny has worked as a teaching artist at a local drug and alcohol rehabilitation facility, and she serves as a leader for the dance ministry program at her church.

Amy M Grebe holds an MA in Urban Studies with a concentration in Community Arts from Eastern University. She has been a practicing community artist for over a decade after accidentally stumbling upon this path. Over the years, Ms. Grebe has danced with contemporary dance companies in Pittsburgh and D. C., designed and constructed costuming for dance and theater companies, illustrated children's books, and painted numerous murals. The birth of her daughter prompted her to explore the intersection of creativity, art-making, and positive youth development. This exploration then led to her founding of ACPPA Community Art Center, a celebrated, multidisciplinary arts organization just outside Philadelphia. Currently, Ms. Grebe serves as a consultant, guiding organizations to become safe places where youth can envision a positive future for themselves and gain the tools necessary to attain that future.

***

Sarah Baker is a practicing community artist who holds her M.A. in Urban Studies and Community Arts. She currently lives in intentional community in Bogotá, Colombia and works with the Wájaro Foundation, a non-profit organization working for the holistic wellbeing of the indigenous church in Colombia. Sarah seeks to use her creativity and the arts to engage marginalized communities around the world, inspiring grassroots community action and mutual transformation.

Jennifer Lynne Bird teaches literature and writing classes at Oxbridge Academy in West Palm Beach, Florida. She previously taught current and future teachers at Florida Atlantic University. She received her Bachelor of Science in Education in Secondary English Education, Master of Education in Secondary English Education, and Doctor of Philosophy degrees from Miami University in Oxford, Ohio and her health coach certification from Duke University Integrative Medicine in Durham, North Carolina. Her research in writing and healing led to the publication of her book Innovative Collaborative Practice and Reflection in Patient Education (2015).

Julia A. Crawford is a dance artist and educator originally from Philadelphia, PA. She started JCrawfordDance in 2016, leading women's movement groups, youth dance classes, and using art-making to build community and tell stories for healing and wholeness. She is adjunct faculty at Eastern University in the Dance and Urban Studies programs. She has worked with BuildaBridge International as a teaching artist, Institute Faculty, and trainer. Also with BuildaBridge, she has had the opportunity to dance with resilient people in Bukavu, Democratic Republic of Congo, Kitale, Kenya, and Bangkok and Chiang Mai, Thailand. She also directed the upper and middle school dance programs at a boarding school for eight years along with teaching in several other contexts. She earned her Master of Arts from Eastern University in Urban Studies: Community Arts where she received an Outstanding Thesis award in 2012. She graduated cum laude from Temple University with a BFA in dance where she received the BFA outstanding dance performance award in 2005.

Callie Dean is an adjunct instructor in the Urban Studies program at Eastern University. Her research and professional interests include qualitative and arts-based research methods, arts-integrated curriculum development, program evaluation, and positive youth development. She currently serves as the Education and Community Engagement Manager for the Shreveport Symphony Orchestra, where she develops and directs programming for children, youth, and adults. She lives in Shreveport, LA, with her husband and two sons.

Linda Marie Ellington is a Professor of Business, (2014-current) Director of Graduate Studies (2004-2014) IBM Corporation (1981-2003) Associate Editor, Journal of Adult Vocational Education and Technology (IJAVET) Published Writer Academic Research Peer Reviewer Children's Book Author Volunteer Florida Literacy Doctoral Dissertation Committee Member.

Sue Gauthier-Pin is a Marriage and Family Therapist Associate in California who specializes in integrative expressive arts therapy. She received her Master's Degree in Counseling Psychology with a concentration in Expressive Arts Therapy from the California Institute of Integral Studies in 2015. For the past 10 years, Sue has worked with children, teens, adults and families in community mental health, addiction recovery, and educational settings. She specializes in helping those who are struggling with grief and loss, codependency, addiction, relational and spiritual trauma, creative blocks, life transitions, depression and anxiety. Sue works in Southern California with children and teens in schools with Freedom 4 U, women in recovery from addiction and trauma at Rising Roads Recovery, and sees individuals and families at a group private practice, Peninsula Center for Children and Families.

Tessa Hitz resides in south-central Pennsylvania. As a K-12th grade art educator, she has spent the last ten years sharing her love of making and creating with adults and children alike. She holds her Bachelors in Art Education from Messiah College and her Masters in Urban Studies and Collaborative Arts from Eastern University. Tessa has a passion for making collaboratively alongside adults, building creative confidence in her students and fostering the "aha" moments that bring the joy of discovery into the classroom.

Janelle Junkin, PhD, MT-BC, is a board-certified music therapist and an independent researcher currently conducting a Program Impact Evaluation for the Armed Services Arts Partnership, Washington DC. She has taught at various universities in the Philadelphia region and is currently an adjunct professor at Harrisburg University, Philadelphia campus. Dr. Junkin works with BuildaBridge International providing support and coordination for community artists and creative arts therapists working with refugees, survivors of torture and vulnerable populations and is the founder of Orchestral Dialogues: Accepting Self, Accepting Others. She is the co-founder of unlock Ngenuity, LLC which focuses on consulting, creativity, and community through therapy, coaching and research; she and her business partner serve as anti-oppression and anti-racism consultants. Dr. Junkin has worked in 15 countries on five continents. She is published in the Journal of Applied Arts & Health and the International Journal of Education & the Arts. Her areas of research include child and youth identity development, the role of the arts in conflict transformation, and understanding the community arts and creative arts therapies as vehicles that provide hope and healing to people and communities in crisis.

Melissa Lucchesi is the founder and director of the nonprofit Voices, Inc. She is a fierce survivor of sexual violence who works hard to break the silence and create trauma-informed spaces and communities everywhere. She is a public speaker who shares her story with the wish that survivors will feel hopeful and less alone. She lives in Media with her son, a bright little light named Greyson Liam.

Suet Ferng Tan holds a MA from Eastern University in Urban Studies specializing in Community Arts. She is also trained in education and urban planning, and is certified by Buildabridge International as a trainer to facilitate arts-based programmes in trauma intervention. She has worked alongside artists, therapists and volunteers in Japan, Singapore and the United States, serving a spectrum of population from diverse background. Suet Ferng is based in Singapore and is currently serving in Yellowren Productions as a Community Arts Director. She takes lead in the design of art programmes and has been the Festival Director of Yellowren Arts Festival from 2015 to 2018. Beyond community arts, Suet Ferng has an interest in film, theatre and youth development.

Karin Tollefson-Hall is Associate Professor, Art Education Area Coordinator, and Director of Summer Art, at James Madison University with previous teaching experience in grades 7-12 art and Spanish. Dr. Tollefson-Hall was awarded Higher Education Art Educator of the Year by the Virginia Art Education Association in 2012. Her research interests include, alternative educational settings, non-traditional pedagogy, scholarship of teaching and learning, and qualitative methodologies. She is also a book artist.

Kristine Vuocolo attended Lock Haven University where she earned her Bachelors of Science in Education degree. She has worked in the Mental Health Field for over 14 years working with both adults and children alike. She is a Certified Psychiatric Rehabilitation Specialist and has earned the name of Recovery Champion due to her dedication to the people she serves. Kristine has been the Supervisor of the Transitions Psych. Rehab. Program, Certified Peer Specialist Program, Resource Coordination Program, and helped establish two Decision Support Centers. She currently is the Director of Stepping Stones Clubhouse in Coatesville, PA. In her free time Kristine volunteers for Justice Rain, Inc. for the purpose of helping to educate on acts of injustice.

Rodney Luther Whittenberg is an Emmy Award winning modern "renaissance man". Rodney is founder of Melodyvision where he works as a Creative Consultant by using his skills as a composer / song writer/ multi instrumentalist, producer / engineer / filmmaker and educator. He has received a regional Emmy for his score for the TV Documentary Mother Dot's Philadelphia and Best Sound Design at the Terror Film Festival for Toll Taker. Rodney's work as a filmmaker centers around his passion for telling a story from start to finish in a creative way. Rodney began his career in teaching in 1989 at Project Learn.He also designed and developed many after school programs and intergenerational programs

Index

I

J

L

M

N

O

P

R

S

T

U

V

W

Y

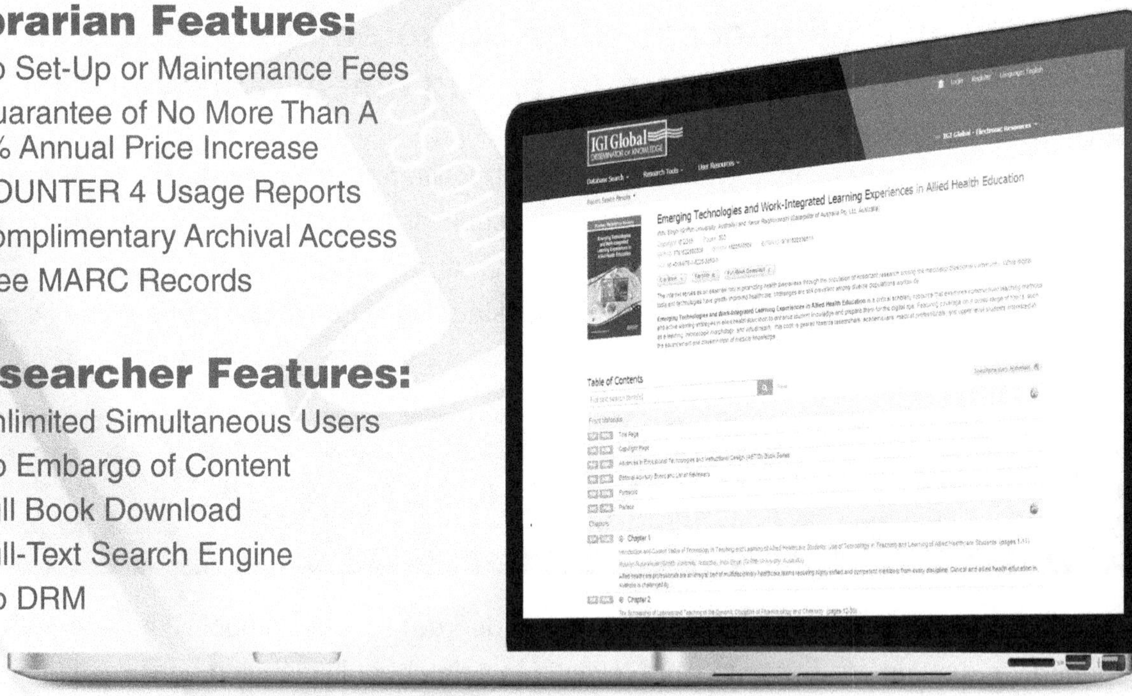
IGI Global
Emerging Technologies and Work-Integrated Learning Experiences in Allied Health Education
Table of Contents

www.ingramcontent.com/pod-product-compliance
Lightning Source LLC
LaVergne TN
LVHW060422300926
849162LV00006B/1502